Spinal Cord Injuries
Anaesthetic and Associated Care

Spinal Cord Injuries
Anaesthetic and Associated Care

J.D. Alderson MB, ChB, FFARCS(I)
Consultant Anaesthetist to Sheffield Health Authority; Honorary Clinical Lecturer, University of Sheffield, Sheffield, UK

Elizabeth A.M. Frost MD
Professor, Department of Anesthesia, Albert Einstein College of Medicine/ Montefiore Medical Center, New York, USA

Butterworths
London   Boston   Singapore   Sydney   Toronto   Wellington

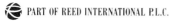
First published 1990

© **Butterworth & Co. (Publishers) Ltd, 1990**

British Library Cataloguing in Publication Data

Alderson, J. D.
  Spinal cord injuries: anaesthetic and associated care.
  1. Man. Spinal cord. Injuries
  I. Title   II. Frost, Elizabeth A. M.
  617.482044

  ISBN 0-407-01148-X

Library of Congress Cataloging in Publication Data

Spinal cord injuries: anaesthetic and associated care/
  [edited by] J.D. Alderson. Elizabeth A.M. Frost.
      p.   cm.
  Includes bibliographical references.
  Includes index.
  ISBN 0-407-01148-X
  1. Spinal cord—Wounds and injuries.
  2. Anesthesia in neurology.
  3. Spinal cord—Wounds and injuries—Treatment.
  [DNLM: 1. Anesthesia. 2. Spinal Cord
  Injuries—therapy. WL 400 S7569]
  RD594.3.S666 1990
  617.4'82044—dc20
  DLC
  for Library of Congress   90-1973
                                              CIP

Typeset by EJS Chemical Composition, Midsomer Norton, Bath
Printed and bound in Great Britain by Courier International Ltd, Tiptree, Essex

Preface

Prior to World War I, the prevailing view on spinal cord injuries was that this was a condition that should be left alone for nature to take its course. Medical management had changed little from about 2500 BC when an Egyptian physician wrote on papyrus 'an ailment not to be treated'. In World War II, 90% of patients with spinal cord injury died within a year of injury, and only about 1% survived 20 years (Swain, Grundy and Russell, 1985).

Following pioneering work by Sir Ludwig Guttman and colleagues in the UK, and Munro and Bors in the USA, on the aggressive treatment of complications there began a gradual reduction in mortality from spinal cord injuries, falling to 35% by the 1960s and 2% by the end of the 1970s. Mortality rates have continued to decrease, the highest incidence occurring within the first 1–2 years. The mortality curve then runs parallel to that for neurologically normal individuals (Carter, 1987). Multi-disciplinary approaches to rehabilitation, including family support, have led to great improvements in the patients' quality of life.

This changing attitude, and resultant success in the management of spinal cord injuries, has come about with the development of specialist teams and centres for spinal cord injury patients. Ideal management now demands immediate evacuation from the scene of the accident to a centre where intensive care of the patients can be supervised by a specialist in spinal cord injuries (Swain, Grundy and Russell, 1985).

Complementing the improved management of spinal injuries is the increasing awareness of the need for education to reduce the incidence of new spinal cord injuries. In the USA, for example, the American Association of Neurological Surgeons sponsor the National Head and Spinal Cord Injury Prevention Program. This programme has been in operation since 1986 and teaches safety and prevention to approximately 300 000 students annually in the USA and Canada. It has received much praise including a Presidential Citation, and continues to grow – it is currently in 41 states. The film 'Harm's Way', which is the main focus of the programme, has alone won five film festival awards. Safety and traffic laws have mandated the use of seat belts in many countries both for front seat and back seat passengers. Indeed in the USA, a driver may be held legally responsible if his passenger does not use a seat belt. Also, in the USA, children under the age of 3 may only be transported in cars in a specially designed, and government-approved, chair in the back seat. In the very near future, air bags will be installed in all new cars, hopefully further reducing accidents involving the chest and spinal column.

The tremendous development seen since World War II in the medical speciality of anaesthesia has seen it become involved and have closer cooperation with many other medical disciplines. Anaesthetists now not only have their traditional role in the operating theatre, but also have become vital members of the medical teams in accident and emergency and trauma units, in the intensive care environment and in the relief of pain. In the preparation of this book it was felt that it was time the expertise gained by anaesthetists in all these fields in the management of patients with spinal cord injuries should be presented in one anaesthetic textbook. Naturally there are overlaps into other disciplines, and we are delighted to include chapters from our colleagues in accident and emergency medicine (traumatology), in neurosurgery and in spinal injury medicine, where it was felt these would be appropriate. Nursing for spinal cord injury patients also requires specialized knowledge, and any book on spinal cord injuries would be incomplete without such a chapter.

While the expertise in the management of spinal cord injuries has been built up in specialized units, these patients may now present, either in the acute phase after the injury or during the chronic rehabilitation phase, to any doctor in any hospital. What we have tried to do in this book is to give information as to the problems these patients will present, and give guidance from specialists in the field as to the appropriate methods of treatment.

Many spinal cord injury patients are young, with excellent survival prospects now available to them if correctly managed. It is important that they are given this optimal care. We hope this book goes some way to giving anaesthetists, wherever they may work, the ability to help achieve this goal.

J.D. ALDERSON
ELIZABETH A.M. FROST

References

Carter, R.E. (1987) Respiratory aspects of spinal cord injury management. *Paraplegia*, **25**, 262–266
Swain, A., Grundy, D. and Russell, J. (1985) A.B.C. of spinal cord injury. *British Medical Journal*, **291**, 1558–1560

Foreword

Great advantages have come to medicine by way of the specialist's concentration on his knowledge and skills. Hippocrates taught us, many years ago, to treat the man and not the part alone. It is thus that the best specialist opens his mind to all other disciplines and none more so than those involved in the management of the sequelae of spinal cord injury.

The late Dr George Riddoch, Consultant Neurologist to the London Hospital and the National Hospital for Nervous Diseases, saw the need for the establishment in England of centres for the treatment of casualties with spinal cord injuries arising from World War II. These centres brought together the expertise of all the disciplines involved in and associated with the management of spinal paraplegia and tetraplegia. In the initial instance this expertise revolved round the neurologist and surgical neurologist, the orthopaedist, the urologist, the plastic surgeon, the rehabilitationist and all the paramedical services, with nursing care of paramount importance at all times. Always there had to be a holistic approach to the patient.

With the passage of the years the ever increasing sophistications of the technologies associated with investigations and treatment have added countless benefits for both specialist and patient. The present book highlights the role of the anaesthetist throughout all stages of the investigative and therapeutic processes. The application of his knowledge and expertise in all phases of management from acute care to long-term follow-up is now set out in chapters written by specialists on both sides of the Atlantic. I pay tribute to the work they do and particularly acknowledge the excellent cooperation that I have always had with my former colleagues at the Spinal Injuries Unit at Lodge Moor Hospital, Sheffield.

A.G. HARDY FRCS
Emeritus Consultant in Spinal Cord Injuries

Contributors

J.D. Alderson MB, ChB, FFARCS(I)
Consultant Anaesthetist to Sheffield Health Authority and Honorary Clinical Lecturer, University of Sheffield, Sheffield, UK

Jeffrey Askanazi MD
Associate Professor, Department of Anesthesiology and Critical Care, Albert Einstein College of Medicine/Montefiore Medical Center, New York, USA

Mary Carlisle RGN
Theatre Nurse, Lodge Moor Hospital, Sheffield, UK

D. Couldwell RGN
Senior Nurse, Spinal Unit Sheffield (retired), Sheffield, UK

Kathleen Marie Dixon PhD
Assistant Professor, Philosophy Department, Bowling Green State University, Bowling Green, Ohio, USA

Elizabeth A.M. Frost MD
Professor, Department of Anesthesia, Albert Einstein College of Medicine/ Montefiore Medical Center, New York, USA

Chris Glynn MB, BS, DCH, FFARCS, MSc
Consultant, Oxford Regional Pain Relief Unit, and Lecturer, Nuffield Department of Anaesthetics, University of Oxford, Oxford, UK

Alan Hirschfeld MD
Assistant Professor, Department of Neurosurgery, Albert Einstein College of Medicine/Montefiore Medical Center, New York, USA

Olli Kirvelä MD, PhD
Senior Staff Anesthesiologist, Department of Anesthesiology, Turku University Central Hospital, Turku, Finland

Patrick A. LaSala MD
Assistant Professor, Department of Neurological Surgery, Albert Einstein College of Medicine/Montefiore Medical Center, New York, USA

G. Ravichandran BSc, MB, BS, FRCS(Ed)
Consultant in Spinal Injuries and Honorary Clinical Lecturer, University of Sheffield, Sheffield, UK

T.C. Shaw FFARCS
Consultant Anaesthetist to Sheffield Health Authority and Honorary Clinical Lecturer to the University of Sheffield, Sheffield, UK

Peter Teddy MA, BM, BCh, DPhil, FRCS
Consultant Neurosurgeon, Department of Neurological Surgery and Senior Research Fellow, St Peter's College, University of Oxford, Oxford, UK

Somasundaram Thiagarajah MD, FFARCS
Associate Clinical Professor of Anesthesiology, Beth Israel Medical Center, New York, USA

J. Wardrope FRCS
Consultant in Accident and Emergency Medicine and Honorary Clinical Lecturer, University of Sheffield, Sheffield, UK

Peter J. Wright FFARCS
Consultant Neuroanaesthetist, Royal Hallamshire Hospital and Honorary Clinical Lecturer, Sheffield University Medical School, Sheffield, UK

Wise Young MD, PhD
Associate Professor, Department of Neurosurgery, New York University Medical Center, New York, USA

Contents

Chapter 1

Pathophysiology of acute spinal cord injury

G. Ravichandran

Introduction

Spinal cord trauma leading to temporary or total paralysis continues to cause major hardship to society to an inordinate degree, especially as it has not been possible to find the means to reverse its effect so far. The organization and anatomical complexities of the neural and osseous tissues surrounding the neuraxis have made it impossible to mend surgically the initial effects of acute traumatic spinal cord injury (SCI). Various systemic effects of SCI are observed by physicians specializing in different branches of medicine. Failure to appreciate the overall effect of SCI on individual systems has led to disastrous consequences in these patients, while under medical management.

In this chapter, an attempt will be made not merely to outline the biochemical and histological changes that happen to the spinal cord as a result of trauma, but also to highlight the various factors that contribute to an informed handling of the patient with SCI.

Historical aspects

Traumatic lesions to the vertebral columns have been uncovered in palaeopathological studies (Schlosser, 1982). Bearsted (1930), in his translation of the famous Edwin Smith papyrus which is dated to have been written between 3000 and 2500 BC, states that the ancient Egyptian surgeons classified the injury to the spinal cord as 'an ailment not to be treated'. The Greek philosopher Hippocrates (460–377 BC) gave details of the paralysis affecting extremities and its association with the dislocation of the vertebrae. It was known to Celsius (30 BC) that paralysis following an injury to the spinal cord in the neck usually led to the rapid onset of death. Ambroise Paré (Bennett, 1964) advocated the cure of spinal dislocation by traction, but this made no difference to the neurological recovery. Prior to the advent of antiseptic agents, most surgical procedures led to death as a result of secondary infection. During World War I, 95% of war casualties with SCI died. Harvey Cushing, a surgeon with the American army during World War I, gave a good description of the neglect and ignorance in the handling of traumatic SCI that led to death. The mortality rate of traumatic paraplegics in the British army was very similar. The survival following SCI improved dramatically towards the end of World War II, largely as a result of improved understanding of the multisystem effect of SCI on the patient. The dedicated and pioneering work done by Sir Ludwig Guttman has formed a basis for the modern care of SCI (Guttman, 1973).

Most SCIs are caused by trauma. Certain local factors influence the incidence of such injuries. Thus, coconuts falling on the heads of labourers are a relatively common cause of SCI in Malaysia and Singapore. Deliberate damage to the spinal cord, using sharpened bicycle spokes is not an uncommon cause of paraplegia in South Africa. Accidents at building sites tend to be a major cause of paraplegia in developing countries, whereas gunshot injuries are the leading cause of paraplegia in California, USA. By and large, in the western world, road traffic accidents contribute to more than 50% of all SCIs. Various forms of sport, such as diving, rugby and horse-riding, are responsible for a further 10–20% of injuries. Domestic accidents and industrial accidents are again a significant contributor in the causation of SCI.

Spinal cord injury has resulted from non-traumatic causes, such as a period of hypoxia following a major myocardial infarction or following surgery for aneurysm of the aorta. Spinal cord lesions have been seen after normally uneventful medical procedures such as renal angiography and epidural injections for pain control. Below is an illustrative example of one such iatrogenic spinal cord lesion following a normally uneventful therapeutic medical procedure:

> A 40-year-old ex-nurse contacted an anaesthetist specializing in pain control through her general practitioner. She complained of severe localized inframammary chest pain that followed an attack of angina that her husband had suffered. The general practitioner had previously performed the relevant cardiac investigations to exclude angina in this lady. In his referral letter he had also mentioned that he had been treating her for anxiety for over 3 years. The letter also mentioned that the husband had since died as a result of coronary artery disease. A senior anaesthetist performed an intercostal block to the left thoracic T4, 5 and 6 intercostal nerves. This produced satisfactory pain control and the lady returned for further injections. On her second visit, an epidural injection of bupivacaine was performed in the dorsal spine, which produced satisfactory pain control for about 8 h. A repeat epidural was performed the following day with similar success. Eight hours after the second injection the patient reported to the nurses that she was unable to move her toes, but the nurses noticed that she was unconcerned about the loss of movements in her lower limbs. The following morning it was noted that she had been incontinent and that she had developed a complete paraplegia below D3. On admission to the spinal injuries unit 3 days later, it was noted that her anxiety state had completely cured itself and that she remained flaccid paraplegic below D3.

Applied neuroanatomy

The spinal cord

Neuraxis develops early in the life of an embryo. A human embryo measuring no more than 1 mm already shows the development of a neural groove as a result of condensation of paraxial mesoderm. At 19 days the neural crest begins to appear and eventually closes to form the neural tube (Figure 1.1). The cranial end of the neural tube develops to produce the brain. When the embryo measures about 2.1 mm (at 3 weeks), the condensation of the paraxial mesoderms and the intermediate cell layers

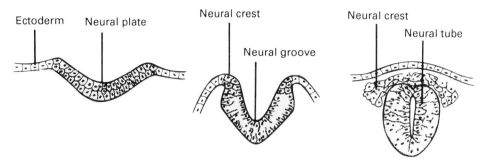

Figure 1.1 Neural plate develops from primitive ectoderm. Condensation of paraxial ectoderm produces neural crest. Lateral migration of crest cells becomes sympathetic ganglia

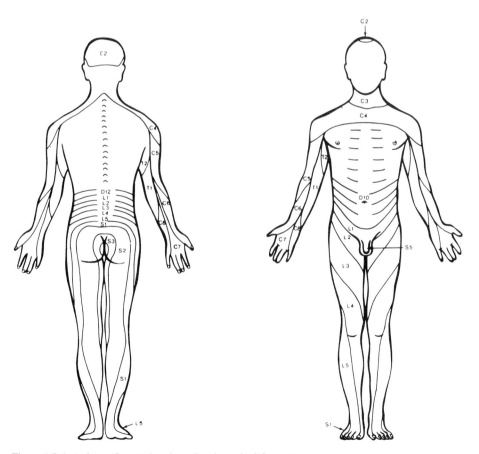

Figure 1.2 Anterior and posterior views showing spinal dermatomes

leads to the development of somites and the primitive notochord. Lateral migration of the neural crest cells eventually leads to the development of the sympathetic chain. The cells of the neural tube, initially of the columnar type, multiply rapidly with accumulation of glial cells dorsally and ventrally. The processes from the ventrally situated nerve cells extend outward along the somites, eventually reaching their end-organs. The bodies of the cells of the dorsal nerves are situated in the spinal ganglia and the dentritic processes extend along the somites and axially towards the brain. By the time the fetus is of 2 months gestation, the spinal cord extends from the base of the skull to the coccyx. However, by 6 months there is a very substantial reduction in the length of the spinal cord in relation to the developing vertebrae. While the neurones and the nerve cells of the spinal cord continue to grow and elongate during adult existence, they lose their ability to multiply and divide. Thus neuroectodermal defects and cysts that develop during the first 2 months of intrauterine life remain patent through life. Figure 1.2 shows the segmental innervation in the adult, and Table 1.1 gives an outline of the various key muscles that are innervated by spinal nerves.

In the adult, the blood supply to the spinal cord comes chiefly from the anterior median sulcal artery and the two posterior spinal arteries. The anterior median sulcal artery is formed by the fusion of branches from the vertebral artery, whereas the posterior spinal arteries originate from the posterior inferior cerebellar arteries or the vertebral arteries themselves. These three longitudinal arterial columns are segmentally reinforced from the radicular branches of the vertebral, subclavian, intercostal and lumbar arteries. By and large, the anterior median sulcal artery

Table 1.1 Segmental innervation of muscles

Muscle	Segmental innervation
Sternomastoid	C1–C4
Trapezius	C2–C4
Diaphragm	C3–C5
Deltoid	C4–C6
Biceps	C5–C6
Brachioradialis	C5–C6
Pectoralis	C5–T1
Triceps	C7–C8
Extensor carpi radialis longus	C6–C7
Flexor carpi radialis	C7–C8
Extensor digitorum	C7–C8
Flexor digitorum	C7–C8
Opponens pollicis	C8–T1
Interossei	C8–T1
Iliopsoas	L1–L4
Sartorius	L1–L2
Adductors	L2–L4
Quadratus femoris	L2–L4
Extensor digitorum longus	L4–S1
Flexor digitorum	L5–S2
Peronei	L5–S2
Tibialis posterior	L5–S2
Gastrocnemius	S1–S2
Biceps femoris	L5–S2
Gluteus maximus	L5–S2

supplies at least two-thirds of the spinal cord at any given level. The posterior third of the spinal cord is usually supplied with blood by the two posterior spinal arteries.

Two areas of reduced vascular perfusion have been recognized in the spinal cord – one in the upper dorsal spine and the other in the lower dorsal spine. This is due to poor collateral circulation in these areas. A major communicating branch to the anterior spinal artery, usually referred to as the artery of Adamkiewicz, often arises in one of the lower thoracic or upper lumbar arteries, most often on the left side.

The vertebral column

The vertebral column develops from bilaterally situated, serially arranged pairs of mesodermal somites alongside the embryonic notochord. By the 4th week, each somite differentiates into sclerotomes which migrate and surround the notochord. The notochord eventually becomes part of the nucleus pulposus, while the sclerotomes form the ribs and the vertebrae. Intersegmental arteries develop which separate the sclerotomes. The caudal half of the sclerotome thickens and combines with the cranial half of the sclerotome just caudal to it. Thus the adult vertebrae do not correspond to the primitive somite or scleroderm, but rather to combinations of two halves of the same. By the 6th week, centres of chondrification appear and by 3 months centres of ossification appear. Several secondary centres of ossification do not fuse with other parts of the vertebrae until several years after birth.

A typical vertebra consists of a body, an arch and at least three processes, the spinal cord lying within the spinal canal. The arch is formed by two lateral masses from which arise articular processes, transverse processes and spinous processes. The meeting of the two laminae which form the spinous process completes the neural arch. The angle of articulation of the adjacent apophyseal joint gradually alters from the neck downward. In the neck, the articulations between the skull and the first cervical vertebra are almost horizontal. The articulation between axis and atlas is directed obliquely downwards. The articulations between the other cervical vertebrae gradually increase in obliquity, providing the greatest degree of rotational movement in the cervical spine. The thoracic vertebrae increase in size gradually. The inferior apophyseal joints are directed anteriorly, caudally and medially to articulate with the superior apophyseal joints of the vertebra below, which are directed posteriorly, and a little laterally and cranially. The movements of the vertebral column are limited by the fibrous ring of the intervertebral disc and by the shape and position of the intervertebral joints. In the thoracic spine, rotation and ventral bending are virtually free, whereas lateral flexion and extension are restricted (Figure 1.3). The lumbar spine is characterized by the freedom of dorsal and ventral flexion, restricted lateral flexion and minimal rotational movements. Lateral flexion occurs, essentially in the thoracolumbar and lumbosacral junction. Lumbar vertebrae are the largest and have square spinous processes, in contrast to the pointed spinous processes in the thoracic and cervical areas.

The sacrum usually is composed of five fused vertebrae. The lumbosacral junction essentially acts as a shock absorber, absorbing the undue loads caused by the erect human torso. The size of the spinal canal at the point of injury has great significance in determining the severity of neurological damage.

The integrity of the various ligaments – anterior longitudinal, posterior longitudinal, ligamentum flavum and interspinous ligaments – is essential for maintaining a normal range of spinal movement. When these ligaments are diseased or damaged, then even minor changes in posture can lead to neurological consequences.

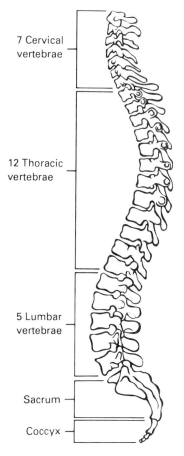

7 Cervical
vertebrae

12 Thoracic
vertebrae

5 Lumbar
vertebrae

Sacrum

Coccyx

Figure 1.3 Adult vertebral column, lateral view

Applied physiology

It is not intended to give details of neurological assessment of the patient in this
chapter, but this should be performed. The examination should, in all cases, include
assessment of higher function, cranial nerves and spinal nerves, including assessment
of sensory and motor function. The various motor and sensory innervations from the
spinal nerves have already been shown in Table 1.1 and Figure 1.2. Injury to the
spinal column leads to either partial or total paralysis of sensory and motor function
below that level. Table 1.2 gives the innervation of commonly used reflexes. Their
presence or absence will be of great value in establishing the level of lesion in both the
conscious and the unconscious patient. In addition, in patients with mid-dorsal
paraplegia an attempt to lift the head usually draws the umbilicus towards the head,
this being due to the unopposed actions of the proximal part of rectus abdominis.
This is often referred to as the Beevor sign.

Table 1.2 Motor innervation of common reflexes

Reflex	Segmental innervation
Biceps	C5–C6
Supinator	C6
Triceps	C7
Abdominal	D7–D12
Cremasteric	L2
Knee	L3–L4
Ankle	L5–S1
Plantar	S1
Bulbocavernosus	S3–S4
Anal	S5

Autonomic nerves

Major autonomic disturbances occur as a result of SCI. The effect of autonomic disturbance is more clearly seen in patients with cervical lesions than in those with dorsal or lumbar lesions. Patients with complete spinal cord lesions above C6 are essentially sympathectomized. During the phase of spinal shock, the heart rate is influenced by the uninhibited activity of the vagus which has cranial innervation. Thus, severe bradycardia with a pulse of 50 or less is not uncommonly seen in patients with tetraplegia. Soon after SCI there is profound sympathetic vasodilatation. This manifests with warm extremities and a low systolic blood pressure. Arterial saturations, as measured with a pulse oximeter, do not show a dramatic fall even in tetraplegic patients with a C4 lesion. In male patients with high cervical lesions, it is not uncommon to see pseudopriapism. Such ill-sustained but frequent erections of the penis may also be seen in patients with minimal neurological deficit, and are often the only sign of impending neurological compromise as a result of vertebral injury.

Reflexes

'Spinal shock' is a term coined by Marshall Hall in 1850, and is still used in spite of its vagaries. Spinal shock represents the state of the patient in whom there is an absence of tendon reflexes following SCI. Cremasteric and bulbocavernosus reflexes may return soon after injury. An abnormal plantar response, in the form of a withdrawal of the lower limb, also develops soon after SCI. The knee and ankle reflexes in paraplegics and the upper extremity reflexes in tetraplegics often take several weeks to return.

During this state of spinal shock paralytic ileus may ensue, a few hours after SCI. The recovery from paralytic ileus, however, is comparatively rapid and in patients appropriately treated, normal bowel sounds can be heard within 48–72 h. The reflex bladder function, on the other hand, may take several weeks, even though reflex defaecation could be achieved with suppositories in 3–4 days. Thus the rate of return of various reflexes varies. Return of tendon reflexes is also delayed in patients with multiple injuries and patients who require prolonged ventilatory support.

The peripheral autonomic nervous system is an efferent system and is made up of neurones which lie outside the central nervous system and are concerned with the visceral innervation. Both sympathetic and parasympathetic neurones have central connections. The hypothalamus is still considered as the highest centre for autonomic activity which in turn is under the control of the cortex via the limbic system. The preganglionic fibres release acetylcholine whose effect is not abolished by atropine. The postganglionic cholinergic fibres release acetylcholine whose effect is abolished by atropine. The postganglionic sympathetic fibres, except for the pseudomotor nerves, release noradrenaline (norepinephrine).

A variety of neuropeptides have now been identified which seem to influence the relative activity of sympathetic, parasympathetic and somatic innervation inside the spinal cord. Recent observations imply that several peptides, in particular neuropeptide Y, encephalins, substance P, angiotensin II, along with other monoamines and amino acid transmitters, play a very vital role in the autoregulation of the spinal cord perfusion (Bannister, 1988).

Neurologic syndromes

Paraplegia

'Paraplegia' is a term used to describe a state where there is either sensory or motor weakness affecting the two lower extremities. Strictly speaking, anyone with a lesion below T2 will be called paraplegic. Tetraplegia, on the other hand, implies sensory motor deficit affecting four extremities.

Anterior spinal cord syndrome

An anterior spinal cord syndrome is said to exist when, as a result of trauma, most of the damage to the cord is confined to the anterior part of the spinal cord. These patients have varying degrees of motor deficit, but will have intact light touch and joint position sense. Pain and temperature sense are compromised. Injuries, where there is a severe flexion force to the vertebral column, often lead to retropulsion of disc material and/or bony fragments leading to this type of lesion. Angiomatous lesions of the head may also cause anterior SCI (Figure 1.4).

Posterior cord syndrome

Posterior cord syndrome is more common following neurosurgical procedures where a cyst or intraspinal tumour is removed. These patients have profound loss of joint position sense and light touch, with a relatively intact motor function below the lesion. They may also have a reasonably well-preserved pinprick and temperature sense (Figure 1.4).

Central cord syndrome

Central cord syndrome is relatively common in elderly patients with spondylitic spine. Often the trauma involved is trivial and the lesion incomplete. The cord appears to have been temporarily compressed in the anteroposterior direction between the thickened ligamentum flavum and the osteophytes over the disc space. This results in a central haemorrhagic necrosis gradually spreading outwards. Because of the laminated orientation of the various sensory motor tracts inside the spinal cord (Figure 1.4), the tracts of the upper extremities are more severely compromised from these lesions than the lower extremities. These patients have varying degrees of sensory motor preservation in the lower extremities and are often

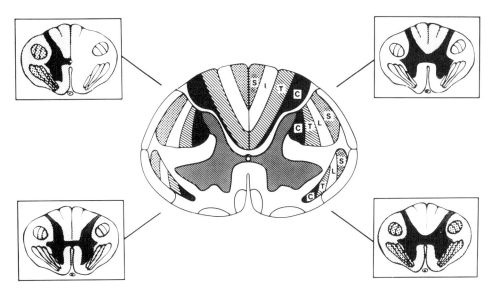

Figure 1.4 Section showing major sensory and motor tracts (S, sacral; L, lumbar; T, thoracic; C, cervical). Light grey area in the smaller pictures shows damage to the cord. Top left: Brown-Séquard syndrome; top right, posterior cord syndrome; bottom left, central cord syndrome; bottom right, anterior cord syndrome

able to walk eventually. Pre-existing cardiovascular and muscular skeletal problems of these elderly patients, however, pose a major challenge to the rehabilitation team.

Brown-Séquard syndrome

A Brown-Séquard syndrome often results from a stab injury to the spinal cord, leading to paralysis of the motor tract on the side of the lesion together with preservation of spinothalamic function (pain, temperature), whereas there is motor preservation and loss of spinothalamic function on the contralateral side of the injury. Where the lesion is produced due to an accident leading to disc herniation in the thoracic spine, the Brown-Séquard lesion is often incomplete (Figure 1.4).

Vertebral fractures and their management

Cervical spine fractures

Several types of classification of cervical and thoracolumbar fractures exist. Essentially the injuries are produced either by a violent flexion force or an extension force. Invariably there is an associated axial force involved in most cervical spine injuries. A person falling on his head from a height might suffer disruption of the ring of atlas resulting in a Jefferson fracture. There usually is no neurological compromise associated with such injuries and these fractures are treated conservatively. If, during such a fall, the neck is extended, resulting in axial loading–extension injury, a distinct traumatic lesion characterized by bilateral fractures through the neural arch of the second cervical vertebra results. This is referred to as the hangman fracture.

The separation of the neural arch initially may be insignificant. However, during mobilization of these patients further axial loading leads to separation of the neural element with forward drifting of the body of C2. Conservative treatment with traction in extension often results in satisfactory union of such fractures. Occasionally there is an indication for surgical stabilization, usually from behind. These fractures are stable in extension, and as long as the neck is not flexed during intubation, there is seldom any danger of neurological compromise resulting from endotracheal intubation.

Fractures of the odontoid process have traditionally been divided into three types. A type 1 fracture is often an avulsion fracture to the upper part of the dens. This is relatively uncommon. There may be associated injury to the transverse ligaments of the atlas. The gap between the posterior edge of the anterior arch of the atlas and the anterior edge of the odontoid peg should not exceed 4 mm in health. If in lateral cervical spine x-rays this gap measures 7 mm or more, a complete rupture of the transverse ligament of atlas should be assumed. Such injuries are unstable, with a potential to lead to neurological loss during endotracheal intubation. These patients need to be nursed in extension. In general, however, when there is no associated injury to the transverse ligament of the atlas, conservative management is the rule. Type 2 fractures, which are the commonest fractures of C2, occur when there is a separation between the dens and the body of C2. Immobilization initially by skull traction and subsequently with appropriate halo-vest jacket, often leads to satisfactory union. Type 3 fractures involve the body of C2. These fractures generally unite.

Fractures of C3–7 often occur as a result of violent injury. Diving in shallow water may result in fracture and dislocation of one or more vertebrae when the head hits the bottom of the pool and the force of the body produces a severe flexion injury to the neck. The flexion force can not only dislocate the vertebrae, but might produce a teardrop fracture of the vertebral body. The spinal cord is severely compressed during the injury. If there is no flexion force during the accident, as might happen when the head hits the windscreen during a car accident, the forces may be such as to cause a burst fracture of a cervical vertebra. The fragments of the vertebral body during the injury explode towards the spinal cord, crushing and severely damaging the spinal cord. Dislocations of cervical vertebrae with or without a fracture of the vertebral body are generally considered unstable.

Initially they are stabilized with sandbags and skull traction. Unsupervised increase in traction force and changes in the line of traction could lead to further neurological compromise. Fractures and dislocations of C4/5 carry an additional risk of producing respiratory compromise as a result of ascending neurological lesions. Prolonged traction with large weights will lead to a gradual deterioration of respiratory function needing, in some instances, ventilatory support. Any attempt at reducing cervical fractures should be done with appropriate skill and under ideal conditions (Figure 1.5). It is equally important to apply skull tongs in the right place with the least amount of patient discomfort. In contemporary medical practice, Gardner-Wells calipers are by far superior to other forms of skull traction.

Dislocations of cervical spine without associated fractures can be reduced either by gradual increase in traction or by manipulation under anaesthesia with x-ray control. No major cardiorespiratory complications are encountered if manipulations are carried out soon after injury in a previously fit individual. The traction force require to reduce unilateral facet dislocation with locked facets is often higher than when the dislocation is bifacetal. Relief of pain and reduction of spasm of the cervical muscles

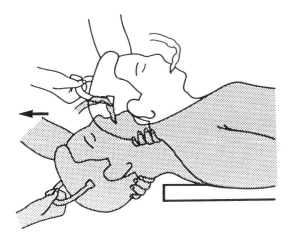

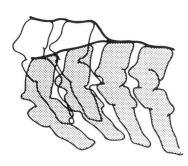

Figure 1.5 Closed reduction of bilateral facet dislocation of cervical spine. Under general anaesthesia, and with patient relaxed, the neck is flexed to about 45°, maintaining manual traction. This will disengage the dislocation. Maintaining the traction the neck is gradually extended to reduce the dislocation. Traction pull is then reduced. It is preferable to manipulate the neck under x-ray control

often encourages reduction with lower weights. Most spinal centres believe that reduction should be achieved as soon as possible, and when closed manipulation does not achieve satisfactory realignment of the fracture in the neck, an open reduction should be performed. Patients may require a degree of ventilatory support in the postoperative phase following such surgery.

Dorsal (thoracic) and dorsolumbar fractures

Fractures of the dorsal (thoracic) spine often occur as a result of major violence. Car and motorcycle accidents usually lead to upper dorsal fractures and often there are associated rib and chest injuries. The spinal canal in the thoracic spine is narrow and any violence producing a fracture of the thoracic vertebrae normally results in complete paraplegia. Fractures of the upper dorsal spine are difficult to visualize and plain x-rays of the dorsal spine taken a few hours after injury may show a localized paravertebral haematoma. In many of these patients the haematoma disappears with the production of haemothorax after a few days. It is worth remembering that fractures of T3/4/5 may be associated with a fractured sternum and possibly injury to the intima of the aorta. Plain radiographic and ultrasound examinations of the arch of the aorta are often inconclusive in excluding aortic injury, and on occasions patients have required arch aortogram to be performed to exclude associated aortic injury.

Fractures of the thoracolumbar junction (T11–L2) occur with regular frequency, often following road traffic accidents. Radiological demonstration of these injuries is relatively easy and, because of the large diameter of the spinal canal, some of the lesions tend to be incomplete. Pain is a major factor in the management of these patients. When bony structures are considered unstable or neurological evaluation implies a slow progressive neurological deterioration, then surgical intervention is indicated. Several orthopaedic and/or neurosurgical exposures and methods of stabilization are available. Most patients suffer a prolonged paralytic ileus following surgery to their thoracolumbar spine.

Metrizamide myelography to delineate cord compression is not hazard free during the acute phase, and cord oedema occurring during the first 24–48 h after SCI restricts the value of myelography. Computed tomography (CT) and magnetic resonance imaging (MRI) techniques give valuable information to understand the bony architecture following trauma (Figure 1.6). Decompressive procedures, particularly in the cervical spine, need to be carried out only if there is residual compression of the neural elements after reduction of the cervical spine. There are no large-scale studies that show unequivocal evidence of neurological recovery due to primary surgical decompression either to the thoracic or the lumbar spine. The role of surgical stabilization of the vertebral fractures associated with neuraxis trauma remains controversial. In general, if there is a progression of the neurological lesion under observation, then surgery is indicated. In the neck, if manipulation does not achieve successful realignment of the dislocated cervical vertebrae, reduction by surgery is indicated. Occasionally, when there is gross malalignment of the vertebrae with severe pain, surgical stabilization will be indicated. Septic wounds, the presence of a foreign body in the spine and locked facets of the cervical spine are other indications for surgical intervention. The choice of surgical procedure is often determined by the available expertise, but in general decompression of the spinal cord from the front is preferable to laminectomies.

Pathophysiology

The spinal cord

Immediately after injury, in most instances there is no externally visible change in the appearance of the spinal cord. Petechial haemorrhages usually begin at the centre of the spinal cord, releasing catecholamines. There may be a gradual loss in potassium from the injured cord tissue (Lewin, Hansebout and Pappius, 1974); it is possible that this potassium gathers in excess concentrations in the extracellular fluid to cause spinal shock. There is, however, no true increase in serum potassium level following acute SCI.

About 4 h after SCI there is usually a central haemorrhagic necrosis occurring in the cord. At 7 h there is chromatolysis and acute swelling of the nerve cells. Intracellular neurofibrils undergo fragmentation subsequently. It appears that the process of neural disintegration in the spinal cord is slower to occur than in the human cerebral cortex. Ducker, Kindt and Kempe (1971) and Ducker and Perot

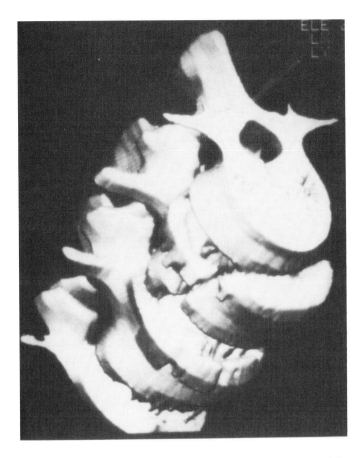

Figure 1.6 Lumbar spine fracture, CT scan. Computer-generated image allows three-dimensional imaging. This patient had *no* neurological deficit

(1971) showed that initially the evolution of SCI does not parallel the clinical neurological conditions. Although clinical signs may improve, pathological changes may progress for a further 7 days. The severity of the trauma seems to influence the extent of central grey matter damage. With a force sufficient to produce only temporary paralysis, in experimental animals it has been shown that chromatolysis, vacuolation and alteration in the cytoplasmic density and stainability occur. Oedema of the white matter is relatively minimal when the trauma produces transient lesion only.

In the later stages of SCI there is resolution of the haemorrhage with phagocytosis. There is cavitation and eventual replacement of the destroyed neural tissue with glial scar. If the haemorrhage during the original lesion extended cranially and caudally, a condition often referred to as haematomyelia, then during the process of resolution several years after SCI a large cavity may result. These cavities may communicate with the subarachnoid space and therefore remain collapsed. Sometimes the cavities continue to distend, producing further neurological change due to syringomyelia.

Damage to the spinal cord can occur as a result of extradural haematoma from vertebral fracture, causing progressive compression. Ischaemia may also result from severe systemic hypoxia, as might happen following a myocardial infarction.

In most instances following a primary spinal cord trauma, the internal spinal cord blood flow is altered. Several chemicals are released at the site of injury whose role in the control of spinal cord blood flow is still being evaluated. It has been shown that immediately after SCI no blood flow occurs in the haemorrhagic areas and about an hour later the entire grey matter is in a state of haemorrhagic non-perfusion. It has also been noticed that there is focal dilatation and constriction of intrinsic arteries. Changes in spinal cord perfusion are partly influenced by P_{CO_2}. Ducker, Saleman and Lucas (1978) and Ducker *et al.* (1978), using an argon washout technique, showed that the blood flow was significantly decreased in paraplegic animals, and this has led to the concept of 'self-destruct' of the spinal cord. There is confusing and contradictory evidence on the role of ischaemia in the production of further neurological damage. Experimental evidence does suggest that the leaking of tissue fluid into the surrounding tissue leads to oedema, which further reduces tissue oxygen levels.

There is controversy over the role of catecholamines in the genesis of secondary damage to the spinal cord. Osterholm (1974) claimed that the release of noradrenaline (norepinephrine) following traumatic SCI led to an autodestruction of the cord. These observations have never been confirmed by other workers and subsequent blood flow measurements after experimental SCI tend to cast further doubt on the catecholamine theory. It has been shown that there is a fall in the level of other biogenic amines, including dopamine, some 7 days after the cord injury. More recently, an impressive array of neuropeptides such as NPY, vasopressin, oxytocin, vasoactive intestinal peptides, substance P and metencephalins has been seen in the lateral horn of the spinal cord. The evidence to date suggests that a complex series of biochemical reactions takes place following SCI. These are influenced by the P_{O_2}, the P_{CO_2} and the arterial blood pressure (Bannister, 1988).

Role of drugs and surgery

There is no convincing evidence to suggest that pharmacological or surgical manipulation of the pathological process will influence the outcome following traumatic SCI. Figure 1.7 shows details of the various observed responses in the spinal cord to trauma. Surgical decompression, oxygenation, administration of steroids or dimethyl sulphoxide (DMSO) and local cooling have all been advocated as a means of improving neural tissue function following SCI. None of them, however, produces unequivocal neurological improvement (Janssen and Hansebout, 1989). There is an association of upper gastrointestinal bleeding and the administration of steroid. Surgical decompression, particularly of the upper dorsal and dorsolumbar spine, has been known to lead to more dense paralysis.

Blood pressure

Following SCI, the mean arterial blood pressure often falls. When the paralysis is incomplete and there is associated pain, the systolic blood pressure may transiently rise. Generally there is peripheral vasodilatation and the central venous pressure remains low. Challenging these patients with large quantities of fluid seldom produces an appropriate increase in the central venous pressure, and inappropriate infusion of crystalloids eventually leads to pulmonary oedema. Once pulmonary

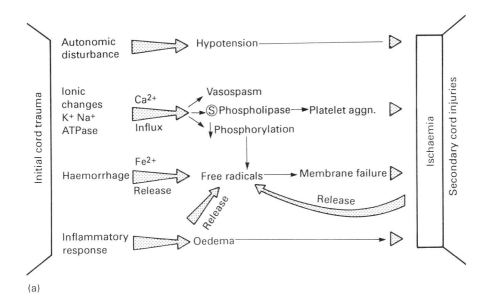

(a)

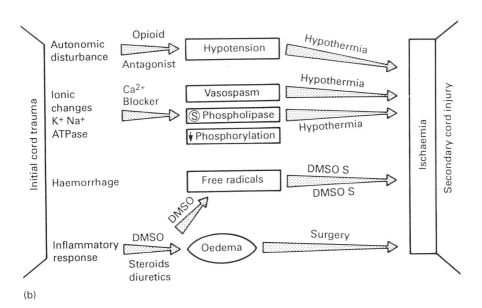

(b)

Figure 1.7 (a) Primary spinal cord trauma leads to several pathological changes as shown. Activation of phospholipase leads to platelet aggregation. Release of free radicals causes nerve membrane failure with loss of conductions. (b) Pharmacological and surgical manipulation currently practised, to reduce cord trauma (DMSO, dimethyl sulphoxide; S, steroid)

oedema has been established in these patients, it is often very difficult to reverse the situation.

Thermoregulation

Largely as a result of peripheral vasodilatation and partly because of loss of temperature sensation, most patients with SCI lower their body temperature. Measurements of temperature made with oral thermometers often give erroneous readings. It is therefore essential to estimate the core temperature on arrival at the accident and emergency department. Patients should be warmed gradually. One of the effects of hypothermia is a degree of confusion which becomes difficult to interpret when there is associated hypoxia from paralysis of respiratory muscles.

Respiratory system

Young adult tetraplegic patients with uncomplicated C4 complete lesions often do not have any respiratory embarrassment purely as a result of the paralysis. The vital capacity may be of the order of 1–1.5 litres (about 30–40% normal). Oxygen saturations, as measured with a pulse oximeter and arterial gas estimations, do not show a significant fall in the early stages. However, within 24 and 48 h there is a gradual, but steady, fall in the oxygen saturation. This is partly due to a fatigue of the diaphragm and partly due to an increased pulmonary shunting (Morgan, Silver and Williams, 1986). Patients with traumatic tetraplegia are unable to cough or sigh, and this leads to progressive, patchy atelectasis. The role of appropriate chest physiotherapy during the acute phase following traumatic SCI cannot be over-emphasized.

   Patients with tetraplegia exhibit paradoxical respiration because of loss of intercostal muscle tone. These patients can also develop acute lung collapse due to a mucus plug which will suddenly and dramatically reduce the respiratory reserve. Prolonged supine recumbent nursing of these patients further increases the chance of lung collapse due to sputum retention. Frequent turning of the patient to allow gravity drainage will be a great advantage in improving physiological respiration in high tetraplegic patients.

Pressure areas

Loss of sympathetic tone soon after SCI, together with loss of muscle tone, predisposes the patient with acute SCI to the development of a pressure sore from a relatively trivial trauma. Thus patients who lie on the roadside after a car accident for about 30 min often have prolonged red marks on those parts of the body that were in contact with the hard, uneven surface. These marks do not disappear for several days following the trauma. If pressure is not relieved from those areas, the 'pre-sore' changes will progress to the formation of a deep and troublesome pressure sore. Pressure sores that develop soon after SCI are often difficult to treat and tend to do badly even after surgical intervention. It is believed that loss of vasomotor control following SCI in some way influences the recovery from superficial skin damage produced by the application of pressure. The prolonged recumbency that follows during the pressure sore management leads to major systemic and psychological effects on the patient. They may develop contractures of the shoulders and elbows.

They also suffer from protracted orthostatic hypotension when mobilized. The eventual outcome after rehabilitation in these patients tends to be very poor indeed.

Gastrointestinal tract

Patients with acute traumatic SCI develop paralytic ileus. This may not be evident soon after the injury, but if they are given inappropriate quantities of fluid by mouth, a protracted paralytic ileus ensues. Patients are normally denied oral fluid for the first 24 h and then clear fluids are given for a further 24 h before gradually introducing flavoured fluids and food. They also run the risk of developing gastrointestinal bleeds, and routine antacid therapy has been a well-accepted practice. Unless the patient has ingested large quantities of fluid or food prior to the accident and there is a risk of vomiting, there is no indication for routine nasogastric aspiration.

Paralytic ileus tends to develop several hours after injury, particularly in patients with thoracolumbar spinal injuries. Patients with lumbar spinal injuries develop late onset of paralytic ileus and, if unrecognized, develop major complications. Patients with dorsolumbar spinal injuries are often nursed with a transverse lumbar pillow in the hope of achieving some postural reduction. Thin patients who rapidly lose weight following SCI develop recurrent upper intestinal obstruction as a result of partial or total occlusion of the third part of the duodenum by the superior mensenteric artery. The condition is caused by the transverse lumbar pillow which exaggerates the lumbar lordosis. This is referred to as the superior mensenteric artery syndrome and can easily be relieved by nursing such patients on their sides rather than supine.

Immediately after SCI some patients have faecal incontinence. Subsequently they develop constipation and bowels do not move for about 3–7 days. Appropriate aperients and suppositories are given to these patients from the third day following SCI. If the patient has an anal reflex or bulbocavernosus reflex, a rectal stimulant in the form of a suppository will lead to bowel evacuation. Any faecal soiling must be cleaned scrupulously in order to avoid natal cleft pressure sores. The diet should be rich in fibre, and bulk-forming laxatives should be instituted as soon as patients are able to take food by mouth.

Bladder

Spinal cord injury generally leads to retention of urine and if the bladder is not catheterized there will eventually be an overflow incontinence. Retention happens both in patients with suprasacral and infrasacral spinal cord lesions. The best method of management of acute SCI, as far as the bladder is concerned, is to use an indwelling catheter initially. Once the patient has been transferred to the appropriate spinal injuries unit, his bladder may be managed by other means such as intermittent catheterization. Acute traumatic SCI patients in Jamaica are routinely treated by suprapubic compression without resorting to catheterization and this has not led to upper tract dilatation or major renal parenchymal damage. Such management is inadvisable without adequate supervision by a specialist team.

Autonomic dysreflexia (hyperreflexia)

Retention of urine as a result of a blocked catheter in patients with SCI leads to a condition referred to as autonomic dysreflexia (or hyperreflexia). This is a clinical syndrome consisting of severe hypertension, headaches, sweating and in some instances bradycardia. Any noxious stimulus below the lesion could produce this syndrome. In patients who have had repeated episodes of autonomic dysreflexia, even a minor degree of bladder distension or constipation could lead to major symptoms of autonomic dysreflexia. Blood pressure changes could be dramatic and systolic blood pressure may easily exceed 200 mmHg (26.6 kPa). It is vital that immediate attempts are made to reduce the blood pressure with the use of appropriate medication such as sublingual glyceryl trinitrate, etc. If the cause of autonomic dysreflexia is retention, this should be relieved forthwith. Autonomic dysreflexia can be produced by many unrelated conditions, such as toenail infection, pressure sores, pathological fracture of the lower extremities and infected piles. Uterine contractions during delivery in the paraplegic female can at times produce hypertension.

Reflex changes

Soon after SCI there is a total abolition of all the tendon reflexes below the lesion. However, sympathetic vasodilatation leading to pseudopriapism can often be seen in male patients immediately after injury. It is often possible to elicit the anal reflex and bulbocavernosus reflex within an hour or so after SCI. In incomplete lesions, a pathological withdrawal response to plantar stimulation is seen. Tendon reflexes do not usually return for 4–6 weeks after SCI. Return of tendon reflexes may be delayed by several weeks in patients with major soft-tissue and bony injuries. Patients who remain on long-term ventilation do not have return of their tendon reflexes for several months. When the SCI is incomplete, the tendon reflexes begin to appear very soon after injury.

Venous thrombosis

Recumbency and loss of movements in the lower extremities predispose a spinal cord injured patient to the development of deep venous thrombosis. Routine anticoagulation therapy is necessary and accurate monitoring of the state of coagulation is important. Certain spinal injury centres use subcutaneous heparin as the sole method of anticoagulant therapy, whereas others combine it with warfarin after a few days. Application of anti-embolism stockings in the lower extremity is an advantage and is preferable in the early days after cord injury. Anticoagulation therapy is continued for a minimum of 6 weeks and often until the patient is mobilized.

Emotional support

Every conscious patient is fully aware of the extent of his neurological deficit before a physician confirms his doubts. It is important that any information divulged to the patient is accurate and appropriate. Often patients do not solicit information soon after the injury and it is unwise to force them to face the possibility of a wheelchair existence when they are not psychologically prepared to do so. Casual inconsiderate remarks made in the accident and emergency department are often remembered by patients, who then feel very hostile towards the receiving hospital. Because it is difficult to make a realistic prognosis soon after SCI, it is useful to let the patient have some hope of possible recovery. In specialized spinal injuries units, patients are handled by experienced staff through whom they eventually ascertain the full implications of a paraplegic existence.

In some instances, informed counselling from an experienced clinical psychologist is an advantage. Pre-morbid psychiatric states, such as might be seen in patients who have attempted suicide, will need to be handled with appropriate medication.

References

Bannister, R. (1988) *Autonomic Failure*, Oxford Medical Publications, Oxford, pp. 511–521

Bearsted, J.H.I. (1930) *The Edwin Smith Papyrus*, Vol. 1, University of Chicago Press, Chicago, pp. 316–342, 425–428

Bennett, G. (1964) Chapter 1. In *Injuries of the Spine* (eds M.B. Howarth and J.G. Petrie), Williams and Wilkins, Baltimore, pp. 1–59

Ducker, T.B., Kindt, G.N. and Kempe, L.G. (1971) Pathological findings in acute experimental spinal cord trauma. *Journal of Neurosurgery*, **35**, 700–708

Ducker, T.B. and Perot, P.L., Jr (1971) Local tissue oxygenation and blood flow in the acutely injured spinal cord. In Proceedings of the 18th Veterans Administration Spinal Cord Injury Conference, Harvard Medical School, Boston, pp. 29–32

Ducker, T.B., Saleman, M. and Lucas, J.T. (1978) Experimental spinal cord trauma II. Blood flow tissue oxygen, evoked potentials in both paretic and plegic monkeys. *Surgical Neurology*, **10**, 64–70

Ducker, T.M., Saleman, M., Perot, P.L., Jr and Ballantine, D. (1978) Experimental spinal cord trauma I. Correlation of blood flow, tissue oxygen and neurologic status in the dog. *Surgical Neurology*, **10**, 60–63

Guttman, L. (1973) *Spinal Cord Injuries, Comprehensive Management and Research*, Blackwell Scientific Publications, Oxford, pp. 9–21

Janssen, L. and Hansebout, R.R. (1989) Pathogenesis of spinal cord injury and newer treatments – a review. *Spine*, **14**(1), 23–33

Lewin, M.G., Hansebout, R.R. and Pappius, H.M. (1974) Chemical characteristics of traumatic spinal cord oedema. *Journal of Neurosurgery*, **40**, 65–75

Morgan, M.D., Silver, J.R. and Williams, J. (1986) The respiratory system of the spinal cord patient. In *Management of Spinal Cord Injuries* (eds R.F. Bloch and M. Basbaum), Williams and Wilkins, Baltimore, pp. 78–116

Osterholm, J.L. (1974) Noradrenergic mediation of traumatic spinal cord injury — autodestruction. *Life Science*, **14**, 1363–1384

Schlosser, A. (1982) Wirebe sa Ulenverletzungen in der Urzeit. *Zeitschrift für Orthopädie*, **116**, 902–904

Chapter 2

Initial care of spinal cord injury

T. C. Shaw, J. Wardrope and Elizabeth A. M. Frost

Introduction

Spinal injuries are a common finding in accident victims; 10% of fatal road traffic accident victims are found to have severe spinal injuries (Tolonen *et al.*, 1986). Falls and sports injuries are an increasing source of such problems, while in the USA penetrating trauma accounts for 14% of spinal cord injury (SCI) (Stover and Fine, 1987).

Emergency medical personnel at the scene of an accident are not presented with a patient bearing a label saying 'I have a spinal injury', but are often faced with a confused and sometimes dangerous situation where the *ideal* care of the spine conflicts with other priorities. On rare occasions there may be dangers to other patients or to the rescuers themselves.

However, it is in these difficult circumstances that it is vital to think of the possibility of spinal injury. Unskilled handling of the patient in these situations might lead to further irreparable damage of the spinal cord. The scope of this chapter is to review the initial care of the injured patient as a whole and to discuss the major difficulties that might sometimes arise in the extrication, early assessment and transport of these patients.

In most areas of medicine there is often more than one method of treatment which is acceptable. There are quite marked differences in the routine management of the injured patient between different countries. An attempt will be made to look at the methods of management currently used in the UK and the USA. Readers should be familiar with the protocols, methods and equipment used in their own local situation.

The priorities in the care of these patients are:

1. *Maintenance of adequate oxygenation to the spinal cord*, which implies the management of an adequate airway, breathing and circulation in order to prevent secondary hypoxic neural damage.
2. *Stabilization of the spine* to prevent further *mechanical* damage to the spinal cord.

Out-of-hospital organization

United Kingdom

Before 1974 the emergency care of accident victims was the responsibility of local government, and a number of different services were used to provide this emergency service. The Ambulance Service was then made part of the National Health Service and is now funded through the Regional Health Authorities.

Until 1986 (Vincent, 1986) most ambulance crews had basic skills in resuscitation and the care of the accident victim. Most regions are now implementing advanced training of ambulance personnel. Experienced ambulance crews with basic training wishing to undertake advanced training are subject to a rigorous selection procedure. If successful, they undertake the recently introduced course from the National Health Service Training Authority consisting of three parts:

1. One week (40 hours) of anatomy, physiology and patient assessment.
2. Three weeks (120 hours) of applied anatomy and physiology. During this time the ambulanceman is taught about all the commonly used emergency skills including the care of the airway, oral endotracheal intubation, advanced cardiac life support and the management of the injured patient including spinal injury.
3. Four weeks' clinical work in hospital. This time is spent practising the skills of intravenous cannulation, airway care and the care of the unconscious patient.

Candidates who successfully complete the course are subjected to annual re-certification. These ambulancemen carry the equipment necessary to use their skills: defibrillators, intravenous cannulae, intravenous fluids and a few drugs, and equipment for endotracheal intubation. All emergency ambulances carry the equipment needed for basic life support such as suction apparatus, oxygen and self-inflating bags and mask.

In the UK the spinal care equipment which is routinely carried by the emergency ambulance service has recently been modernized and consists of:

(a) Cervical collars. The rigid cervical collar (Ambu Stifneck; Figure 2.1) is now used in preference to soft collars. There is little doubt that soft collars *do not provide adequate immobilization of the cervical spine*. It is estimated that a soft collar only restricts neck rotation by 11%, but the range of flexion, extension and lateral flexion remains completely unrestricted (Podolsky *et al.*, 1983). A rigid collar gives a 50% reduction in movement (Graziano *et al.*, 1987). The application of a collar may give a false sense of security to the rescuer.
(b) Extrication devices such as the Kendrick (Figures 2.2 and 2.3). These are used in the removal of victims from a vehicle and are designed to immobilize the head, neck and the whole of the trunk.
(c) Scoop stretcher. This is used to transfer patients with suspected spinal injuries from the accident scene to the ambulance.
(d) Transport stretcher (York). This firm stretcher is the usual method of transport in the ambulance.

United States

In the USA the Emergency Medical Services were completely reorganized during the latter part of the 1960s. All states now have a comprehensive service. There are three levels of training: the Basic EMT and EMT-A (Emergency Medical Technician Ambulance), the EMT-I (Emergency Medical Technician Intermediate) and the EMT Paramedic grade. The course to become an EMT takes approximately 110 hours of classroom training, plus field work in hospital emergency departments, fire departments and ambulance service. Also, every 3 years, a refresher course lasting 40 hours must be completed to maintain certification.

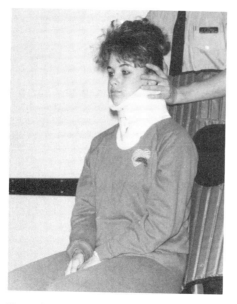

Figure 2.1 Rigid neck collar applied and in-line stabilization maintained. Extrication device positioned behind patient

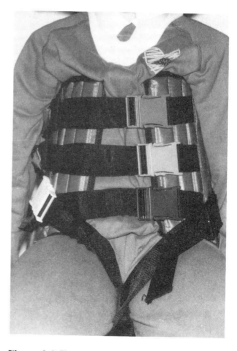

Figure 2.2 Torso secured to extrication device by straps

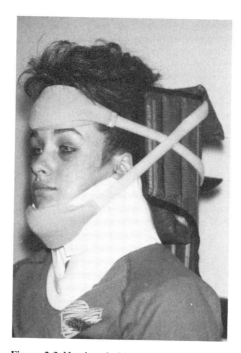

Figure 2.3 Head and chin straps complete the manoeuvre

The EMT-I graduate is an EMT-A who has passed specific training courses to provide specialist skills, and may be designated by these skills, e.g. EMT – Defibrillator Technician.

The EMT – Paramedic will have completed rigorous paramedic training up to the standards specified by the Department of Transport Standard Paramedic Curriculum.

The EMT will therefore have a comprehensive training in the use of a wide range of emergency equipment as well as experience with safety and security procedures that are used in hostile conditions.

It is worth noting that the medicolegal system in the USA has had an impact on EMT practice. There are problems of alleged negligence, i.e. not providing proper care to a standard expected of a trained EMT. The EMT must also be aware of patients' rights not to be touched or to refuse treatment.

West Germany and France

Other countries have their own systems of emergency care of the injured. For instance, the Federal Republic of Germany has an integrated system using helicopters which are staffed by doctors. Similarly the SAMU (Emergency Medical Assistance Services) in France is led by trained physicians specializing in immediate care.

Epidemiology of spinal injury

The estimated incidence of SCI in the UK is 20 new cases per annum per million population. This results in over 1000 new cases of SCI per year (Swain, Grundy and Russel, 1985).

The incidence in the USA is estimated to be 30 new cases of SCI per annum per million population. Since the life expectancy of patients with SCI has greatly increased over the past 40 years, the estimated prevalence of patients suffering from SCI is 906 cases per million (Stover and Fine, 1987).

Injury to the spinal cord results in almost equal numbers of quadriplegics and paraplegics (Stover and Fine, 1987). It is of interest to note that there is some evidence from the USA that the proportion of complete neurological lesions has fallen since the introduction of well-organized Emergency Medical Services, thus emphasizing the great importance of the pre-hospital phase in the care of the accident victim (Green, Eismont and O'Heir, 1987).

It is important to be aware of the types of accident which commonly cause spinal trauma. The exact figures will vary from country to country, but overall about 50% of SCI will be due to road traffic accidents, 25% to falls and 25% to other causes, predominantly sport and assault (Swain, Grundy and Russel, 1985; Green, Eismont and O'Heir, 1987).

In a road traffic accident the large changes in velocity involved subject the whole body to tremendous forces. In the UK many SCIs occur in motorcyclists. These accidents are often front collisions where the rider falls over the handlebars, taking most of the impact on the head and receiving cervical and thoracolumbar fractures.

Recent seat belt legislation for cars has reduced the severity of injuries to other organs, but there is evidence that there are more neck injuries occurring (Rutherford, 1986). There is a risk that if the seat belt is not properly worn, serious thoracolumbar fractures such as the Chance fracture will occur, with or without associated abdominal injury (Hope and Houghton, 1986).

The commonest type of collision is when two cars meet head on. The car decelerates and the driver, wearing his seat belt, continues forward due to his momentum until his trunk is restrained by the belt. The head flexes forward with its 7 lb (3 kg) of weight, often striking the steering wheel. The body and head then recoil back into the seat. The backward motion of the body is stopped by the seat, but if there is no adequate headrest then the head may be hyperextended over the back of the seat.

Falls from a height cause a fifth of SCI (Stover and Fine, 1987). Lumbar fractures are extremely common in falls onto the heels. Diving accidents are a common source of high cervical spinal injuries. The mechanism of injury is often a forced flexion.

Accident site management

The priorities of the emergency services in the initial care of the injured are as follows:

1. Prevention of further injury to patient, bystanders and the emergency service personnel and a rapid assessment of the accident scene and the patient.
2. Extrication from the place of injury to a place of relative safety.
3. Assessment of the injuries with basic lifesaving measures to ensure adequate airway, ventilation and the control of external haemorrhage.
4. Stabilization of the spine and the splintage of fractures or potential fractures.
5. Transport to an appropriate hospital with the facilities to deal with the level of injury.

Scene assessment and primary examination

A swift but careful examination is needed by those arriving at the scene of an accident. The rescuer must take into account the overall setting of the accident to secure the safety of the patient, other civilians and the emergency personnel themselves. The first crucial question to answer is: 'How much time do I have?' In the majority of situations there will be *no* reason to rush.

Examination of the scene and the mechanism of the accident will give important clues to the pattern of injury which might be expected. The injuries sustained by a driver in a head-on collision are different from those in a side-to-side collision or a rear impact.

There should then follow a rapid appraisal of the patient. Obviously, full examination at this stage is not possible, but in the first few seconds the conscious level of the patient can be assessed. If the patient is alert, not in obvious shock and with a normal respiratory rate, then it is likely that the airway, breathing and circulation are adequate to allow time for a careful extrication from the accident scene. At this stage it is simple to ask the patient if he can move his fingers and toes and if he can feel normally. The rescuer should ask the patient if he has neck or back pain. *Even if the patient appears neurologically intact and has no neck or back pain, it should not be assumed that there is no spinal injury.* The pain of other injuries or the effects of the accident may obscure the symptoms of a spinal injury. Similarly there may be difficulties in diagnosis if the patient has been drinking or taking drugs.

A major problem arises if the patient is unconscious following an accident. It is easy to attribute the unconsciousness to head injury, but it is essential to establish that the unconsciousness is not due to hypoxia or hypovolaemia. In the unconscious patient following trauma, hypoxia and hypovolaemia are the major problems in over 40% of cases (Gentleman and Jennet, 1981). The best time to detect these problems is in this vital first examination, because if they are missed the patient may die.

Therefore, ascertain first that the patient is *breathing* and, secondly, that there is a *palpable pulse*.

Extrication

Standard extrication from vehicle

In most accidents there will be enough time to perform a careful controlled removal of the victim. One person should take control of the head and keep the neck in a neutral position in line with the trunk. Avoiding any flexion, extension or rotation, a rigid collar of the correct size is applied. Manual in-line support of the neck is maintained and the extrication device is placed behind the patient's back (see Figure 2.1). The patient's trunk is then secured to the device (see Figure 2.2) and finally the head is secured using straps (see Figure 2.3). The patient can then be lifted clear. At this point it is advisable to check the movement and sensation in the limbs.

Emergency extrication from vehicle

On rare occasions the accident scene may be dangerous and there may not be time to apply an extrication device. Furthermore, if the patient's condition is critical then the need for rapid management of the airway, breathing and circulation may dictate emergency extrication. A rigid cervical collar is applied. At least four personnel are needed to remove the victim. One person takes control of the head to maintain stability and the patient is lifted clear, taking as much care as possible to prevent spinal movement.

Motorcycle helmet removal

This may be necessary to gain access to the airway and should be carried out in a controlled manner. Two people are needed for helmet removal. The helmet is held by the first rescuer, who maintains the neck in neutral position to the rest of the body. The second rescuer places one hand behind the neck and, with the other hand, undoes the chin strap. He then supports the head with one hand under the neck and the other hand placed around the jaw. The first rescuer then uses lateral force to spread the helmet and removes it (Figure 2.4). If a full-face helmet is used, then some rotation of the *helmet* is required to allow removal. The first rescuer may then regain control of the head (McSwain, 1987).

Trapped accident victim

In some road traffic accidents and in other accident situations such as fallen buildings, the patient may be trapped for a prolonged period. In these circumstances it is essential to secure the airway and try to obtain intravenous access. The spine should be immobilized using the methods described above.

Victim found on ground

If a patient with a suspected spinal injury is found on the ground, then a rigid cervical collar is applied. If the application of the collar or attempts to place the neck in a

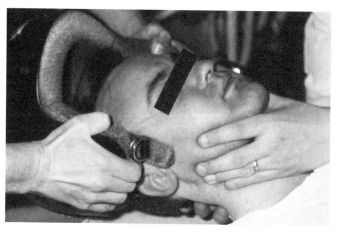

Figure 2.4 Motorcycle helmet removal. One rescuer is maintaining in-line stabilization with one hand placed behind the neck and the other around the jaw. The second applies lateral force to spread the helmet and removes it

neutral position cause pain or increase muscle spasm, then these attempts should be abandoned. The neck is then immobilized in the most comfortable position for the patient. The patient is placed supine and lifted using a scoop stretcher. Alternatively the patient may be 'log-rolled' onto a long spinal board, as discussed later. The neck is immobilized with tape or straps. A roll of material may be placed under the normal curve of the neck.

Victim found in water
Diving into shallow water is a common source of cervical spine injury. With any drowning situation the maintenance of respiration is the first priority. It may be difficult to extricate the victim from a pool and as many helpers as possible should be used. If a board is available, the patient should be placed on it while still in the water.

If it is apparent during the extrication of a conscious and rational patient that there is no motor or sensory function whatsoever in an area consistent with SCI (paraplegia or quadriplegia), then it is unlikely that time spent on careful extrication and stabilization of the vertebral column will be of any benefit. The priority then becomes to secure the airway as expeditiously as possible, re-establish cardiovascular stability and treat other emergent injuries.

Secondary assessment

Once the patient has been removed to a safe area and the spine has been stabilized, then a more formal clinical assessment is performed. The mouth, face and jaw are examined to ensure there are no immediate upper airway problems. The depth and rate of breathing are recorded. The pulse is then felt and the rate recorded. Other signs of shock such as pallor, sweating, restlessness and poor capillary return to the nail bed are noted.

A formal assessment of the Glasgow Coma Scale is made using the level of eye opening, verbal response and motor response. A patient with SCI may not be able to move the limbs, in which case facial responses are noted.

This will lead to a brief examination of spinal cord function. *The patient should not be undressed nor should a long time be spent on detailed neurological examination at this stage.* The patient is asked to gently abduct the shoulder (C5), move the fingers on each hand (C7–8) and spread the fingers (T1). Sensation on the thumb side of the forearm/hand (C6) and little finger side (C8) may be tested. The patient is then asked to move his ankle up (L5) and down (S1). Sensation over the knee cap is tested (L3) and if possible over the Achilles tendon (S1).

Again it must be emphasized that a normal neurological examination at this point does not rule out a potentially unstable spinal injury.

Resuscitation

If a patient with suspected SCI sustains a cardiac arrest, then resuscitation in the field should proceed according to conventional protocols. In high cervical lesions it is likely that the arrest is secondary to hypoventilation resulting in hypoxic arrest. This makes care of the airway the first priority. In these circumstances, intubation is justified in the field. There is some evidence that nasal intubation is the safest technique in unstable cervical injuries, but with a cardiac arrest this approach is not appropriate. Nasal intubation also carries an increased risk of producing intracranial infection if there is concomitant head injury, and may also cause nasal bleeding leading to difficulty in securing the airway.

Most advanced ambulance personnel and many doctors in the UK are only trained in oral endotracheal intubation. In this technique, movement of the head and neck should be restricted as far as possible by an assistant holding the head in a neutral position (Majernick *et al.*, 1986).

Hypovolaemia from massive haemorrhage is another common cause of cardiac arrest in the patient with multiple injuries. The outlook for such patients is very poor unless they have suffered penetrating chest trauma when rapid transport and emergency thoracotomy may save the patient's life.

The other causes of cardiac arrest in the injured victim include tension pneumothorax and cardiac tamponade.

Intravenous infusion

Hypotension in a patient with SCI may be due to that injury, blood loss from other injuries or a combination of both.

Hypotension caused by SCI is due to the loss of normal sympathetic activity (blood loss even from fractures of lumbar vertebrae would not cause significant hypovolaemic hypotension). The severity of any hypotension associated with SCI will depend on the level and the severity of the lesion. The higher the level and the more complete the lesion, the greater the degree of sympathetic paralysis and hypotension. In this situation the vasodilatation causing the hypotension will mean that the skin is pink and warm, at least initially. In a complete cervical cord lesion, the hypotension may be associated with a bradycardia due to the lack of cardiac sympathetic nerve activity. In lower lesions, a tachycardia may develop. Rapid infusion is *not* required if the hypotension is due to SCI alone. Indeed, vigorous fluid therapy may produce pulmonary oedema. A systolic blood pressure of 80–90 mmHg (10.6–12 kPa) is quite satisfactory in these circumstances.

Hypotension due to blood loss classically presents with a tachycardia and pale, cold, clammy skin. These responses may be altered by SCI.

It is controversial whether time should be spent in the field obtaining intravenous access in the trauma patient. If the patient is not trapped and the journey time to hospital is short, it is probably better not to delay transfer. However, if there is going to be a long delay before reaching hospital, then it is reasonable to spend a few minutes establishing intravenous access. Colloid should be given for blood loss. Crystalloid at no more than maintenance levels should be given for the hypotension due to SCI.

Stabilization

The conscious patient
In the UK the conscious patient is transported to hospital in the supine position on a firm stretcher. A rigid cervical collar is used if neck injury is suspected. If an extrication device has been used, then this is left in place. If an extrication device has not been used, then rolls are placed under the natural spinal curves at the back of the neck and in the lumbar region. All hard objects such as keys and coins are removed from the clothing to prevent pressure sores. The arms and legs are immobilized at the sides with straps, and a blanket placed between the legs. The patient is then covered with a blanket in order to conserve heat, since the presence of a spinal cord lesion seriously impairs the normal heat preservation mechanisms.

In the USA much greater use is made of the spinal board, with the trunk firmly strapped to the board and the head also taped or strapped to it.

The unconscious patient
There is much debate over the best way to transport the unconscious, injured patient. An unconscious patient is assumed to have SCI until proven otherwise by radiology. Some authorities maintain that the unconscious victim should be transported in the supine position in the same manner as a conscious patient with SCI. This is the common practice in the USA. However, there are serious disadvantages to this position in the unconscious patient. We believe that the best way to transport the unconscious patient with suspected SCI is the *stable lateral position*. We realize that many authorities will disagree with this advice. In the USA the long spinal board is used extensively and we would not wish to change accepted local practice. However, we believe that the transport of the patient in the stable lateral position avoids serious problems which may occur in other positions.

In the *supine position*, airway maintenance can be a problem. Some airway maintenance manoeuvres, such as extension of the cervical spine, are obviously not recommended in a patient with potential SCI. Normal airway maintenance aids, such as an oropharyngeal airway, may provoke bradycardias and even asystole in a patient with SCI (Grundy, Swain and Russel, 1986). There may be blood or vomit in the mouth which may cause obstruction of the airway. Another problem is that of the patient vomiting or regurgitating during transport. If this occurs in a non-intubated unconscious patient, then he must be turned to prevent aspiration of the vomit into the lungs. Even with a patient firmly secured to a long spinal board this manoeuvre is very difficult to perform quickly and with any degree of spinal control by one person in the back of a moving ambulance. Regurgitation of stomach contents is a silent, passive event and thus may go unnoticed. Aspiration of gastric contents is recognized as an important cause of preventable death in trauma victims, and therefore the risks of this occurring must be weighed against the possibility of damage to the spinal cord.

The obvious answer to the airway problem is to safeguard the airway with an endotracheal tube. However, the risks of intubation in the field in a patient with a possible spinal injury are too great to recommend routine use of this technique. As well as the technical difficulty that may be encountered, there is a danger that stimulation of the vagus during intubation or suction might lead to profound bradycardia or even cardiac arrest in patients with cervical cord lesions (Grundy, Swain and Russel, 1986). The *semi-prone 'recovery'* position is not recommended in this situation, since there is rotation in the cervical and lumbar spine.

The ideal method is to log-roll the patient into a *stable lateral position*, keeping the neck and trunk in a straight line. The patient may then be secured and padded to allow safe transport.

Moving the patient to this position requires considerable care. Three or four people are required. One person, who should be the most experienced available, takes control of the head and coordinates the manoeuvre. The head is held in the neutral position with very slight 'in-line' longitudinal traction. The other rescuers then gently place their arms under the shoulders, trunk and pelvis. On the command of the person controlling the head the patient is log-rolled as one into a lateral position. Pillows or rolls of material are placed to support the head and trunk and straps are placed over the forehead, shoulders and pelvis.

Another method of achieving the stable lateral position is to place the patient on a spinal board in the supine position, with rolls to support the natural curves of the cervical and lumbar spine. The trunk and head are then securely strapped to the board. The patient and board may then be turned to the lateral position, taking care that all the straps are secure.

Problems may arise when a patient needs to be moved into a lateral posture but there are insufficient rescuers to perform a log-roll. Baker has described a manoeuvre (J.H.E. Baker, personal communication) which allows the safe positioning of the patient with possible SCI when there are not enough helpers to effect a proper log-roll.

From the supine position, the arm nearest the rescuer is placed at 90° of abduction at the shoulder, with the far arm placed across the trunk. The leg farthest away from the rescuer is bent into a dog-leg (Figure 2.5). The rescuer's hand nearest the head will support the head while the other hand is placed on the hips and turns the trunk in a non-violent controlled manner (Figure 2.6). Keeping the head under control, the uppermost leg is bent at right angles at the hip and knee. The arms may then be

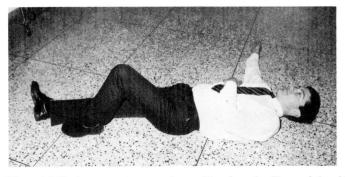

Figure 2.5 Single rescuer turn – supine position (see also Figures 2.6 and 2.7). Arm nearest rescuer is placed at 90°. Far leg bent to dog-leg

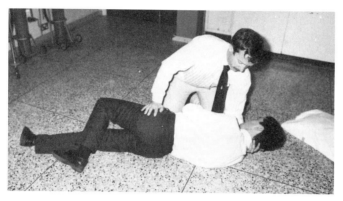

Figure 2.6 Single rescuer turn – controlled turn. One hand controls head and neck, while the other holds the belt area and can easily effect a controlled turn onto side

positioned under the head to add stability to the position and to supplement head support (Figure 2.7). If sufficient rescuers are present, of course, the log-roll technique should be used.

Transport

Once the patient is secure in the appropriate position, he is carefully loaded onto the ambulance. In most countries the transfer to hospital will be made by road, but in

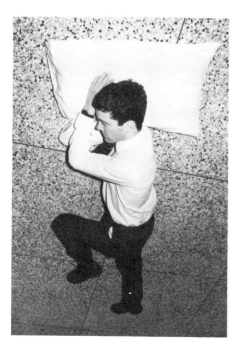

Figure 2.7 Single rescuer turn – end position.
Note the straight thoracolumbar spine

some parts of the USA, Canada and West Germany the transfer may be made by helicopter. During the journey the patient's airway and breathing should be observed. The drive to hospital should be at a *slow* pace and avoiding any major pot-holes in the road.

There is some debate over which type of hospital these patients should go for initial evaluation. Some countries have highly organized trauma centres with on-site spinal injury teams. In the UK such patients are taken to the nearest accident and emergency unit, where there will be surgical, anaesthetic and orthopaedic cover but there may not be specialists in spinal injury. In the UK the care of spinal injuries is concentrated in a dozen or so centres, often in relatively small hospitals. However, it is of vital importance that these centres are informed of spinal injury patients in order that they may advise on the care of the patient as quickly as possible, to help prevent any avoidable complications.

Acknowledgement

We would like to thank Dr J.H.E. Baker, MB, ChB, MRCP, Consultant in Rehabilitation Medicine, Rookwood Hospital, Cardiff, Wales, for the detailed description of the single rescuer turn into the lateral position.

References

Gentleman, D. and Jennet, B. (1981) Hazards of interhospital transfer of comatose head injured patients. *Lancet*, **2**(8251), 853–854

Graziano, A.F., Scheidel, E.A., Cline, J.R. and Baer, L.J. (1987) A radiographic comparison of prehospital cervical immobilisation methods. *Annals of Emergency Medicine*, **16**, 1127–1131

Green, B.A., Eismont, F.J. and O'Heir, J.T. (1987) Pre-hospital management of spinal cord injury. *Paraplegia*, **25**, 229–238

Grundy, D., Swain, A. and Russel, J. (1986) ABC of spinal cord injury. Early management and complications – 1. *British Medical Journal*, **292**, 44–47

Hope, P.G. and Houghton, G. (1986) Spinal and abdominal injury in an infant due to incorrect use of a car seat belt. *Injury*, **17**, 368–369

McSwain, N.E. (1987) Patient assessment and initial management. In *Evaluation and Management of Trauma* (eds N.E. McSwain and M.D. Kerstein), Appleton-Century-Crofts, Connecticut, pp. 77–79

Majernick, T.J., Bieniek, R., Houston, J.B. and Hughes, H.G. (1986) Cervical movement during orotracheal intubation. *Annals of Emergency Medicine*, **15**, 417–420

Podolsky, S., Baraff, L.J., Simon, R.R., Hoffman, J.R., Larmon, B. and Ablow, W. (1983) Efficacy of cervical spine immobilisation methods. *Journal of Trauma*, **23**, 461–465

Rutherford, W.H. (1986) The Maurice Ellis Lecture for 1986: The responsibility of emergency medicine towards the prevention of road accidents. *Archives of Emergency Medicine*, **3**, 163–176

Stover, S.L. and Fine, P.R. (1987) The epidemiology and economics of spinal cord injury. *Paraplegia*, **25**, 225–228

Swain, A., Grundy, D. and Russel, J. (1985) ABC of spinal cord injury: at the accident. *British Medical Journal*, **291**, 1558–1560

Tolonen, J., Santavirta, S., Kiviluotu, O. and Lindqvist, C. (1986) Fatal cervical injuries in road traffic accidents. *Injury*, **17**, 154–158

Vincent, R. (1986) Resuscitation by ambulance crews. *British Medical Journal*, **292**, 1257–1259

Chapter 3

Emergency room care of the patient with spinal cord injury

Alan Hirschfeld

Introduction

As with all forms of major trauma, the care which spinal injured patients receive upon arrival to the hospital's emergency room has an enormous influence on their overall morbidity and mortality. In the past two decades there has been an increasing trend towards the establishment of regionalized systems of trauma centers. Although no scientifically controlled study has ever demonstrated the effectiveness of such systems in the treatment of spinal cord injury (SCI), retrospective reports have indicated a decreased morbidity and mortality rate in hospitals where a high volume, combined with the development of protocols, has led to a routinization of treatment (Green and Eismont, 1984; Sypert, 1984; Tator *et al.*, 1984; Soderstrom and Brumback, 1986). Clinical reviews of the management of trauma patients in general have pointed out that many lives have been lost or compromised because of errors in the management of basic resuscitation problems (Van Wagoner, 1961; Foley, Harris and Pilcher, 1977; Dove, Stahl and Del Guarcia, 1980).

There is some variation in the treatment algorithms proposed by various SCI treatment centers (Green and Eismont, 1984; Cooper, 1986; Soderstrom and Brumback, 1986), but they all emphasize the importance of a multidisciplinary, triaging team approach and the development of treatment protocols. In most cases the team leader is either a trauma surgeon or an emergency room physician. This person, or his designee, can act as the voice contact of the trauma team with the paramedics in the field, and should also initiate the triaging of patients and the implementation of protocols once the patient arrives.

In organizing the approach to the early management of spinal injured patients, it is often helpful to think of it in terms of phases or priorities. Although these phases are generally entered into in a sequential fashion, there may be significant temporal overlap between them. The most commonly utilized phases are: (a) resuscitation; (b) diagnosis; (c) treatment.

Resuscitation

During the first moments of a spinal injured patient's stay in the hospital, he must be considered and treated as a trauma victim primarily and as a spinal injury victim secondarily. The first priority of the trauma team is to insure cardiovascular

32

stability and optimal oxygenation. At this early stage, the neurosurgeon and the anesthesiologist may not be involved. It is important, therefore, for the rest of the team to be well-versed in the exigencies of handling a person who may have had a spinal fracture or SCI.

Over 80% of patients with SCI are under 40 years of age (Green *et al.*, 1981). Significant past medical problems, such as atherosclerotic vascular disease, emphysema, hypertension, and hepatic or renal failure, usually do not further complicate the resuscitation process. Most cervical cord injuries result from motor vehicle accidents, however, and the majority of these have significant associated trauma to the limbs, thorax, brain, abdomen, pelvis or face, in decreasing order of frequency (Ducker and Saul, 1982). Even higher rates of associated injury to the thorax and abdomen are seen in patients with thoracic SCI. Polytrauma may also compromise the cardiovascular and respiratory systems in other causes of spinal injury, such as falls, assault, industrial accidents and sports accidents. A frequent scenario in diving accidents is that the patient may lie at the bottom of a swimming pool for several minutes before his companions realize he is in serious trouble, so the trauma team is faced with a near-drowning victim as well as SCI.

As with all major trauma, the 'ABCs' consist of establishing an Airway and maintaining Breathing, to optimize oxygenation of the blood, and treating shock and cardiac arrhythmias to restore and support Circulation. There is strong evidence that survival rate and morbidity, and possibly even neurological outcome, is adversely affected by systemic insult (i.e. hypoxia or ischemia) at this early stage (Sypert, 1984; Tator *et al.*, 1984; Soderstrom and Brumback, 1986).

Airway and breathing

The causes of compromised airway and breathing may be divided into two groups – non-neurological and neurological. Among the non-neurological causes are secretions, vomitus, blood or foreign bodies such as dentures in the airway, a prolapsed tongue in obtunded patients, tracheal injury, and rib fractures causing splinting, a flail chest, or hemo- or pneumothorax.

Neurological causes include cervical cord injury, especially at mid- or high cervical levels, and severe brain injury with compromised brainstem function. Most cervical cord injuries will result in the loss of thoracic and abdominal muscles normally used in breathing (Luce, 1985). Air exchange will then depend upon the function of the two hemidiaphragms, which are innervated by the phrenic nerves, composed of small branches of the third, fourth and fifth cervical nerve roots. As the hemidiaphragms contract they descend – the increased intra-abdominal pressure forces the abdominal wall outward. This is called abdominal breathing. The higher the level of injury, the more these nerves are themselves detached from supraspinal drives. At levels above C3, the actions of the accessory breathing muscles, the scalenes, sternocleidomastoids, and trapezei, cause minimal inspiratory movements, mostly through increasing the anteroposterior diameter of the chest. The atonic hemidiaphragms ascend due to the negative intrathoracic pressures, causing the abdominal wall in turn to be sucked in. This is called abdominal paradoxical breathing and is a poor prognostic indicator for patient survival, because it implies long-term ventilator dependence. Neurogenic pulmonary edema, a form of adult respiratory distress syndrome, can be seen in spinal cord injured (Poe, Reisman and Rodenhouse, 1978) as well as brain injured patients, but usually manifests itself later.

Assessment of a patient's ventilatory status can be made quickly and easily, by visual inspection, palpation and auscultation. By inspection, the respiratory rate, volume and drive can be estimated. Skin color can be a clue to the efficiency of the patient's inspiratory efforts in oxygenating the blood. There may be a great deal of inspiratory effort in a patient with airway obstruction, abdominal paradoxical breathing, and other causes of air hunger. This may often make the patient appear to be combative. Paradoxical movement of a flail segment may also be detected by visual inspection.

Palpation of the anterior thoracic wall permits an estimation of ventilatory excursions, and the detection of subcutaneous emphysema caused by a fractured rib. A flail chest can also be felt on palpation, but if pain causes respiratory splinting, this movement may be minimal.

Auscultation of the chest will also give useful information on the quality and quantity of the patient's ventilations. Diminished or absent breath sounds indicate the presence of a hemothorax or pneumothorax. In tension pneumothorax, the additional finding of distended jugular veins may be present. Rhonchi may indicate the presence of upper airway obstruction from vomitus, blood or water.

The role of the chest x-ray in this early phase is not very great. It is useful primarily to confirm diagnoses made by inspection, palpation and auscultation. An example is small pneumothoraces in patients who are not in respiratory distress. Of much greater usefulness is the arterial blood gas, which should be drawn immediately upon admission of all seriously injured patients. Ideally this should be obtained while the patient is breathing room air, so that the Pao_2/Fio_2 ratio can be easily determined (Soderstrom and Brumback, 1986). The Pao_2/Fio_2 ratio gives an estimation of the degree of pulmonary shunting. This is often impractical to do, however. In any event, in patients with respiratory compromise, the arterial blood gas is often useful in helping the physician decide whether or not to intubate.

Management of the airway should begin, as soon as the patient enters the emergency room, by removal of any upper airway obstruction. This is usually performed with a suction device, but it may be necessary to don gloves and feel in the patient's oropharynx for solid objects. For the elevation of a prolapsed tongue, the chin lift maneuver has been preferred over the jaw thrust, because the latter is risky in patients with potential cervical spinal instability. Until the cervical spine is cleared, adequate oxygenation is usually attainable using an oropharyngeal or nasopharyngeal airway and oxygen supplied by face mask. If adequate oxygenation cannot be maintained with unassisted breathing, an 'Ambu' bag will often temporize until the patient can be intubated. No rigid rules exist which can be used to determine which patients require intubation. In general, patients with a $Pao_2 < 70$ mmHg (9.3 kPa) or a $Paco_2 > 45$ mmHg (6.0 kPa) on room air will require ventilatory support, as will patients whose Pao_2/Fio_2 ratio indicates a pulmonary shunt of greater than 20% (Soderstrom and Brumback, 1986). This will be true of most patients with a cervical cord injury at the C5 level or above.

Once the decision to intubate a patient has been made, it is necessary to rule out cervical spinal injury. This is true of all patients with blunt trauma, regardless of the neurological findings. This is best performed with a lateral cervical spine x-ray. Occasionally there may not be enough time available to perform this test, in which case one of several methods may be employed which do not involve hyperextending the patient's neck. The most commonly used technique is nasotracheal intubation, which is essentially a blind procedure and requires that the patient be breathing. If the patient is apneic, more rapid oral intubation, using a laryngoscope, with the patient's head in the neutral position, may be tried. Some feel that axial traction applied during intubation reduces the degree of displacement of spinal fracture dislocations when the neck is extended. However, Bivins *et al.* (1988) found that this maneuver caused an unacceptable degree of distraction in the unstable spine and posterior subluxation in their patient with a C6–7 fracture dislocation. They felt that cricothyroidotomy should be the procedure of choice in patients when nasotracheal intubation cannot be performed. Cricothyroidotomy is also recommended when severe facial fractures or bleeding prevent endotracheal intubation.

If time permits, a nasogastric tube should be placed prior to intubation. Many patients with severe blunt trauma or with cervical cord injury will have significant acute gastric dilatation which can compromise respiratory excursions. A nasogastric tube will alleviate this as well as remove stomach contents which could be vomited and aspirated. Placement of a nasogastric tube is contraindicated in patients with head or facial trauma because of the risk of inserting it into the cranial cavity through a basilar skull fracture.

Finally, tension pneumothoraces may be immediately life threatening and, if suspected on the clinical grounds of absent breath sounds, distended jugular veins, and cardiovascular lability, should be decompressed immediately, even without radiographic confirmation. This may be done by inserting a large-bore needle into the second or third intercostal space. For non-tension pneumothoraces and hemothoraces, the chest x-ray may be used to confirm the diagnosis. If they are of sufficient volume to compromise gas exchange, a chest tube should be placed in the standard fashion by the trauma surgeon or emergency room physician.

Pulmonary contusion is an uncommon injury which can compromise respirations. It should be suspected in patients presenting with respiratory distress, bloody secretions, chest injury, hypoxia and non-segmental infiltrates on chest x-ray. The treatment of choice consists of positive pressure ventilatory support. This co-morbidity was found in 1.2% of a recent series of 408 patients with cervical spinal injury (Soderstrom and Brumback, 1986).

Circulation

The cause of circulatory collapse may also be divided into non-neurological and neurological categories. The most common cause of shock in patients with major trauma is blood loss. Paramedics will often place patients in a Military Anti-Shock Trousers (MAST) device at the scene of injury because of hypotension. Once the patient arrives at the hospital, a thorough search must be made for the source of bleeding. This will require completely disrobing the patient. Most external sources are obvious and may readily be stopped by external compression. Occasionally a bleeding artery may have to be ligated or clamped. Bleeding from occipital scalp wounds or from the perineum occasionally goes unnoticed until several liters are lost onto the stretcher. Common areas of internal bleeding in blunt trauma are the thoracic cavity, abdomen, retroperitoneum, pelvis and thighs.

Young trauma victims are usually able to maintain a normal blood pressure with losses of up to 25% of their circulating blood volume. Earlier indicators of significant blood loss include a persistent tachycardia and signs of peripheral vasoconstriction such as skin pallor, coolness and clamminess. Because of decreased renal perfusion, urine output will also be low.

Other, less common causes of shock should always be kept in mind. These include tension pneumothorax, pericardial tamponade and cardiac contusion. Pericardial tamponade is usually caused by penetrating wounds and may be diagnosed by finding high central venous pressures in the face of hypotension. Cardiac contusion is a diagnosis of exclusion in patients with evidence of cardiac failure and arrhythmias, with low central venous pressure and no detectable source of blood loss. An electrocardiogram should be obtained upon admission in all severe trauma patients, and those in whom an abnormality is detected should be placed on a cardiac monitor in the emergency room.

Neurogenic shock may also occur in SCI. It results from the loss of sympathetic tone and leads not only to hypotension and hyperthermia, but to bradycardia as well. This is in marked contradistinction to hemorrhagic shock. In the absence of bradycardia, the diagnosis of 'spinal shock' should still be considered, if there are no other injuries which would account for the patient's hypotension. In the 408 patients reported by Soderstrom and Brumback (1986), a neurogenic etiology was diagnosed in 82.6% of those with incomplete and 81.7% of those with complete cord injuries who presented in shock. Some centers insert Swan-Ganz catheters to monitor the cardiac outputs in all bradycardic patients (Green and Eismont, 1984).

Patients with SCI may have other types of cardiac arrhythmia, even in the absence of cardiac contusion. Atrioventricular block, supraventricular tachycardia and cardiac arrest may all occur in the first week following SCI, but the incidence in the first few hours is unknown (Piepmeier, Lehmann and Lane, 1985; Lehmann *et al.*, 1987). In humans these abnormalities have been related to loss of autonomic control of cardiac rhythm. Studies by Evans, Kobrine and Rizzoli (1980), using a balloon compression model in monkeys, implicated hyperactivity of both sympathetic and parasympathetic systems.

Treatment of circulatory failure requires the placement of at least one large-bore intravenous line to enable rapid fluid replacement. These may be peripheral or central venous lines. Subclavian lines, though often placed reflexively by trauma teams, may not be desirable because of an increased risk of creating pneumothoraces in poorly cooperative patients under emergency conditions compared with more controlled, elective situations. They can be useful if the diagnosis of cardiac tamponade is being considered.

Foley catheters should be placed in all severe trauma victims upon arrival to the hospital. They are more useful than central lines for monitoring the effectiveness of fluid resuscitation, as they permit frequent measurement of urine output, which is directly related to cardiac output. There is little role for arterial lines in the early resuscitative measures.

The initial fluid used to resuscitate patients in shock is usually either a crystalloid or a colloid solution. Considerable controversy exists concerning which type is preferable. There is a growing body of evidence that implies that recovery from a variety of central nervous system injuries is compromised when glucose-containing solutions are used (Ginsberg, Welsh and Budd, 1980; Sieber *et al.*, 1987). Lactated Ringer's solution or normal saline are most commonly administered, though there has been recent interest in hypertonic saline (Todd, Tommasino and Moore, 1985) and in the combination of hypertonic and hyperoncotic fluids (Whittley, Prough and DeWitt, 1988). Once blood is available, transfusions should be considered in patients with continued shock or low hematocrits. In highly unstable patients, O-positive blood should be given, after the initial large volume of fluids, rather than waiting for blood to be cross-matched.

Patients suffering from neurogenic shock will not benefit from large fluid infusions, and may even develop pulmonary edema, which is why it is important to differentiate neurogenic from hemorrhagic shock at the outset. Pressor agents such as dopamine may be necessary to maintain vascular tone, and atropine should be used in patients with bradycardia to maintain cardiac output. Insertion of a Swan-Ganz catheter may eventually be required to assist in this differential, but it is usually not performed in this phase of patient care.

Diagnosis

Initial clinical examination

While the patient is being resuscitated, the initial attempts at diagnosis are made. In the suspected spinal injured patient, the goals are to establish the extent of neural injury and to determine the extent of associated injuries. Spinal instability is assumed unless proven otherwise in this early phase. All manipulations are performed with the patient supine and his head in the neutral position. Sandbags on either side of the head or other forms of immobilization may be required. After immediately life-threatening airway and cardiovascular problems are addressed, a simple neurological evaluation should be performed and the results documented in the chart. This examination, similar to that performed by the paramedics in the field, assesses the patient's mental status, brainstem function and motor response in an objective fashion. The mental status is described in terms of how alert the patient appears and how oriented he is. Brainstem function is tested by observing the pupillary response to bright light and, in deeply obtunded patients, the presence or absence of the corneal and gag reflexes. The doll's eye maneuver to test the occulocephalic reflex should not be performed unless cervical spine stability has been demonstrated. Motor response to noxious stimuli should be tested in all four extremities and pathological responses noted as well as the absence of response. By visual inspection of the patient, one can often detect significant cord injuries. Diaphragmatic and paradoxical breathing, priapism and the complete absence of movement are all ominous signs. The last of these is not strictly diagnostic, as patients with long bone fractures may also keep the involved extremity completely motionless.

Initial investigations

In addition to the arterial blood gases (ABG) on admission, other blood work should be sent as stat samples. These include a complete blood count, platelet count, electrolytes, blood urea nitrogen and creatinine, glucose, prothrombin time and partial thromboplastin time, and a sample for blood typing. Under the appropriate circumstances, blood for toxicology should also be drawn. A urinalysis should be performed to look for blood. If found, an emergency intravenous pyelogram should be included in the radiologic workup.

If persistent volume needs indicate ongoing occult bleeding, peritoneal lavage is usually performed at this point to rule out intra-abdominal hemorrhage. Other studies which may be performed in the latter half of the resuscitation phase include the anteroposterior chest x-ray and pelvic x-rays. The former will not only detect traumatic pathology, but can also be used to check the positions of the endotracheal tube and central line, if these had been inserted. The latter will help in the diagnosis of pelvic fractures, which are often the source of life-threatening internal bleeding.

A lateral cervical spine x-ray is also performed at this point, if it has not already been done as a pre-intubation study. This should be routinely performed in anyone with a neurological deficit, anyone complaining of neck pain or tenderness, and anyone whose level of consciousness is impaired. Some centers also include anyone whose mechanism of injury might involve the cervical spine. To evaluate the spine properly, there must be clear visualization of all bony elements from the occiput to the C7–T1 disc space. This may require applying downward traction on the arms to pull the shoulders out of the way, in obese or muscular individuals. If this does not help, other views which can be obtained in the emergency room include the swimmer's view and oblique x-rays. If the patient is deteriorating neurologically or significant intracranial pathology is suspected, a computed tomography (CT) scan should also be performed.

Further diagnosis

After the patient has been resuscitated, a more detailed diagnostic phase begins. This should include taking a history from the patient or witnesses. Family members may be helpful in giving information about previous medical conditions and medications currently being taken by the patient. A detailed description of the injury, if available, may give some clues as to the mechanism of injury.

Clinical examination

A detailed physical examination should also be performed to check for associated, but not necessarily life-threatening injuries, such as long bone fractures. Until the C-spine has been definitely cleared, this must be done with the patient supine and the neck in the neutral position. A thorough neurological examination should also be performed and the results recorded in the chart for comparison with future examinations. Many SCI centers have developed their own standardized examination sheet and grading systems for spinal cord injury (Lucas and Ducker, 1979; Tator et al., 1984; Bracken and Collins, 1985). The main purposes of the neurological examination are to detect neurological injury, establish the level of cord compromise, and follow the progression or resolution of the neurological findings.

In addition to the mental status examination, the neurological examination should include brief cranial nerve and more detailed motor, sensory and reflex examinations. An important part of the neurological examination is testing of the sacral segments. Certain incomplete cord lesions may not be appreciated as such if this is omitted. Sensation in the perineal region is tested with pinprick and by asking the patient if he can feel the Foley catheter. A rectal examination will determine the tone and voluntary control over the anal sphincter. The presence or absence of the anal wink and, in men, the bulbocavernosus and cremasteric reflexes should be noted.

Motor nerve function

The motor examination should test the strength of several muscle groups in each extremity, and an objective grading method should be used to record the results in the patient's chart. In cervical spinal fractures, the interossei and all lower muscle groups will be affected by spinal cord lesions at the T1 level. Because of the differential growth of the spinal cord and the spinal column, the T1 spinal cord segment will be directly behind the C7–T1 disc space. Lesions at the C8 cord level, behind the C7 body, will cause paralysis below and including the lumbricals. At C7 the triceps is affected, at C6 the biceps and at C5 the deltoids. Above C5 the diaphragm will be affected to varying degrees. In patients with thoracic fractures, portions of the abdominal muscles will be paralysed as well as the lower extremities. Beevor's sign is an upward movement of the umbilicus caused by lack of contraction of the lower abdominal muscles and unopposed action of the upper abdominal muscles when the patient tenses his abdomen in trying to get up. It indicates a lesion at the T10 spinal cord level. In cervical cord lesions, the lower extremities should also be examined by testing the motor strength of the ileopsoas, quadriceps, tibialis anterior, hamstrings and gastrocnemius muscles, which are innervated principally by the L2–3, L3–4, L4, L5–S1, and S2 nerve roots, respectively.

Sensory nerve function

Sensation testing should be performed with the sensory dermatomal distribution in mind. Pinprick sensation should be tested on both sides, and the examiner should proceed from areas of sensory loss and note the exact area at which the patient begins to detect the pin. Since some forms of cord injury selectively spare the dorsal columns, joint position sensation at the toes, ankles, knees, fingers, wrists and elbows, should also be tested when possible.

Reflexes

Deep tendon reflexes at the Achilles tendon, patellar tendon, triceps, brachioradialis and biceps tendons should then be tested. As part of the picture of 'spinal shock', patients with severe SCI will have no tendon reflexes below the level of the lesion for several weeks, at which time they reappear and gradually become hyperactive. There will also be loss of superficial reflexes such as the abdominal reflexes and anal wink.

Signs of autonomic disturbance should also be looked for. These include a distended abdomen from paralytic ileus and a distended, atonic urinary bladder. If a nasogastric tube and Foley catheter have been placed, these signs may not be present. Anhydrosis (lack of sweating) over parts of the body may also be present, but it is difficult to detect unless one is specifically looking for it.

Neurological syndromes

Patients with SCI may present with a variety of neurological pictures, some of which are stereotypical enough to be called syndromes. This depends on the mechanism of injury, i.e. the vectors of force, acting on the cord (Raynor and Koplik, 1985). The most common picture are the 'complete' and 'incomplete' cord injuries, in which all neurological functions are either totally or partially lost below the level of the lesion. In patients suffering from hyperextension injuries, the central portion of the cord may be differentially damaged, giving rise to the central cord syndrome, in which the motor and sensory modalities in the upper extremities are more affected than those in the legs. Less common are the anterior cord syndrome, the Brown-Séquard syndrome, and the rare posterior cord syndrome.

The anterior cord syndrome is felt to be due to compression of the anterior spinal artery by a fragment of disc or vertebral body which has moved posteriorly into the canal. The posterior columns, and therefore proprioception, are relatively spared, while motor function and pain and temperature sensations are lost bilaterally. The Brown-Séquard syndrome is usually seen in penetrating wounds and rotational injuries. One side of the spinal cord is significantly more affected than the other, so motor strength is lost ipsilaterally and pinprick sensation is lost contralaterally. In the posterior cord syndrome, only proprioception is affected. Pain in a dermatomal distribution is indicative of nerve root compression. There may be accompanying numbness and weakness in muscles innervated by the nerve root. Every effort should be made to identify such radiculopathy, because by decompressing the nerve root useful neurological function may be regained, which will help considerably in the patient's rehabilitation.

Diagnostic imaging

After the clinical evaluation has been completed, radiographic studies of the spine are performed. The extent and timing of the radiographic workup depends on the clinical picture and the timing with respect to the injury (Cooper, 1986). Patients who have had complete cord lesions for over 24 h have little or no chance for recovery, so the workup is less aggressive and invasive. Patients with incomplete lesions, who are deteriorating neurologically, who have complete lesions for less than 24 h, or who have evidence of nerve root compression, will have more aggressive workups in the hope that, by finding a surgically correctable source of ongoing cord or nerve root compression, an improved outcome may be achieved. The main goal of the radiographic studies is to identify and define static anatomic abnormalities such as fractures and subluxations. Another important goal is to detect spinal instability, which is an indication for either external or internal fixation.

The first and most important of all radiographic studies is the lateral cervical spine x-ray. This should be performed, as early as possible, on the patient's stretcher, in the emergency room, with portable equipment. In this way, there will be minimal movement of the patient's neck. Emphasis should again be placed on the necessity of visualizing the entire cervical spine from the occiput to the C7–T1 disc space. Traction on the shoulders, a 'swimmer's view', or oblique views, in descending order of preference, may be used to help visualize the lower cervical spine in obese or husky individuals. If a fracture or dislocation is detected on the lateral C-spine x-ray, all subsequent studies can and should be performed with the patient in skeletal traction. If it is necessary to move the patient, one person should be in charge of maintaining spinal alignment and traction.

The lateral C-spine film should be reviewed in a systematic fashion by either a radiologist or a neurosurgeon. The vertebral bodies, facet joints, odontoid process and spinous processes, and their alignment with each other, are the main bony concerns. Next come the disc spaces, the relationship of the spine to the occiput, and the degree of curvature of the spine. The prevertebral soft tissues should also be inspected. Widening of this soft-tissue space, usually due to a hematoma, indicates a dislocation or fracture even in spines where the bony alignment appears to be normal.

Other views which may help to demonstrate or confirm the presence of fractures are the anteroposterior view, to check the alignment of the spinous processes in suspected rotatory injuries, and the open mouth view, to visualize the odontoid process and the atlanto-axial and atlanto-occipital relationships from anteriorly. In patients with neck pain but no neurological deficits and no abnormality seen on the static plain x-rays, a dynamic study, such as flexion–extension films, should be performed to check for spinal instability. Under an experienced physician's supervision these movements may be performed actively by the patient, or, if fluoroscopy is available, passively by the physician. Flexion–extension films may also be desirable in patients with neurological deficits if all potential causes of cord compression (e.g. subluxation, epidural hematoma, extruded disc fragment, and spondylotic spurs) have been excluded by other radiographic studies. Any dynamic study should be terminated instantly if a patient complains of severe pain, weakness or numbness. Flexion–extension films should not be performed on an unresponsive patient.

The criteria for diagnosing spinal instability vary from center to center. Spinal stability may be compromised by purely ligamentous injuries, so the isolated presence or absence of fractures is relatively unimportant. Exceptions are certain odontoid fractures, hangman's fractures, and more severe crush fractures of the vertebral bodies, where the kyphotic deformity may increase over time. Most criteria for instability include subluxation with neurological deficit, facet fractures with dislocation, atlanto-axial and atlanto-occipital dislocation, and displacement of greater than 2 mm, in adults, on flexion–extension studies (White, 1975). The ligamentous elements of the spine can be divided into three 'columns'. The anterior column is comprised of the anterior and posterior longitudinal ligaments and the annulus fibrosis. The middle column consists of the facet joint capsules. The posterior column contains the ligamentum flavum and interspinal ligament. It is generally accepted than any displacement sufficient to disrupt two of the three columns should be considered unstable. Examples from the literature (Gentzbein, 1982) are saggital displacement greater than 3.5 mm, kyphotic angulation of greater than 11%, and distraction greater than 1.7 mm. A new 'stretch test' has also been devised to test spinal stability (White, 1979).

Additional studies which may be performed while the patient is still in the emergency room include CT scanning, myelography and polytomography. The CT scan, which should be performed with thin cuts and saggital reconstruction, can often define the anatomic details of spinal fractures better than plain x-rays. Because of its ability to differentiate soft-tissue densities, CT scanning is also used when a diagnosis of epidural hematoma or extruded disc fragment is being entertained. Its main limitation is in detecting small, axially oriented fractures without displacement.

Since the advent of CT scanning, the use of myelography has diminished considerably. Its indications have also changed as more experience is gained by spinal cord trauma centers. Currently, myelography is performed in patients with progressive neurological deficits despite good spinal alignment, in patients with fixed partial myelopathy or radiculopathy and suspected disc material or blood in the epidural space, and, in some centers, in patients with complete deficits of less than 24 h duration and normal spinal alignment. It is not performed in patients with non-reducible fractures or subluxations, in patients with complete neurological deficits of greater than 24 h duration, or in patients without neurological deficits. Since patients undergoing myelography should be moved as little as possible, a lateral cervical rather than lumbar puncture is performed to introduce the dye. After preparing the skin with iodine and anesthetizing it with 1% lidocaine, a spinal needle is introduced, under x-ray guidance, between the posterior arches of C1 and C2, from a point just inferior and posterior to the mastoid process. The contrast material used is usually a water-soluble one, such as metrizamide. This material will mix well in the cerebrospinal fluid rather than layering in the posterior gutters as is often the case with oil-based contrast agents. If available, a CT scan should be obtained after the myelogram is completed, as this will provide additional information especially in the lower cervical region.

Polytomography, though infrequently performed today, still is an excellent study to visualize the facet joints and odontoid process (Harris, 1986). It may demonstrate small horizontal fractures through the vertebral body, pedicles and lamina, and small teardrop fractures better than plain x-rays or CT scans. Polytomography may also help differentiate between old or chronic pathological displacements and acute traumatic displacements. Finally, it is at least as good as CT scanning for examining lower cervical spinal alignment in those few patients in whom other methods have failed.

A high index of suspicion for cervical spine fracture and instability must be maintained in all blunt trauma patients with neck pain, regardless of their neurological condition, until all of the necessary studies are adequately performed to rule it out. In one recent study, as many as 24% of C-spine fractures remained undetected for the first 24 h post-injury, and 3% are undetected for up to a month (Reid *et al.*, 1987). In children, the elasticity of the vertebral ligaments may allow a momentary subluxation to occur, creating a neurological deficit, but presenting with normal x-rays (Pollack, Pong and Sclabassi, 1988).

The occurrence of multiple spine fractures, either adjacent to or distant from one another, is not uncommon in motor vehicle accidents and in high falls. It is therefore strongly advisable to obtain a plain x-ray survey of the entire spine if a fracture or dislocation has been identified.

The usefulness of magnetic resonance imaging (MRI) in evaluating SCI after the acute phase is now well established (Quencer *et al.*, 1986). A recent study has also indicated that a variety of pathological entities can also be detected in the acute setting (Kalfas *et al.*, 1988). These include anatomic cord transection, focal cord enlargement, hyperintense intramedullary lesions, disc herniation and other causes of epidural cord compression. However, despite the development of spinal traction and stabilization devices constructed of non-ferromagnetic materials, the performance of an MRI scan remains impractical for many patients, particularly those on ventilators or with cardiovascular lability.

Neurological function tests

Another study which is often performed in the acute stage of SCI is the somatosensory evoked potential (SEP), which measures the ability of the dorsal column white matter tracts to conduct electrical impulses. SEPs are particularly useful to detect subclinical spinal cord function and changes in function (Young, 1982; Chabot *et al.*, 1985). In the acutely injured or partially injured patient, they have also been shown to be a useful prognostic tool in estimating the probability and extent of eventual neurological recovery. More occasionally, cystometry is performed to study bladder function. These studies are generally not performed until the patient has reached the intensive care unit.

Treatment

The goals of treatment in the emergency room are: (a) to prevent or reverse neurological dysfunction; (b) to re-establish normal spinal alignment; and (c) to assure spinal stability. Treatment modalities may be either physical/mechanical (further subdivided into non-surgical and surgical) or pharmacological/ physiological. Some of these have already been discussed. Perhaps the most important treatment for preventing further neurological deficit is spinal immobilization. Improper immobilization at the scene of the accident can lead to neurological deterioration (Podolsky *et al.*, 1983). Immobilization is usually attempted with either a hard cervical collar or by using the short board technique, with sandbags on either side of the patient's head and tape across his forehead and under the chin (Podolsky *et al.*, 1983; Graziano *et al.*, 1987). This is continued in the emergency room at least until the lateral cervical spine x-ray is obtained. The other treatment modality of which we have spoken is the administration of oxygen and the correction of any other identifiable causes of potential systemic insult.

If subluxation or facet fracture dislocation is present on x-ray, or if spinal instability is suspected, the next maneuver is to apply axial traction to the skull. The devices used most commonly are the Gardner-Wells tongs and the halo ring, although many other devices exist (Grundy, Swain and Russell, 1986). Both are easy to apply. Gardner-Wells tongs should be placed about 2 cm above the pinnae of the ears, so that the vector of force lies along the main axis of the body. If slight extension is desired, they should be placed slightly anteriorly. In awake patients about 1–2 cc (ml) of local anesthetic, usually 1% lidocaine (lignocaine) or 0.5% bupivacaine, is used to infiltrate the proposed pin sites. The same is true of applying the halo ring, which is fixed to the skull by four pins. The halo ring is preferable to other traction devices if it appears likely that the patient will be placed in a halo-vest for long-term stabilization in the next couple of days.

Traction is usually applied incrementally starting with about 5 lb (2.5 kg) for every cervical vertebra cephalad to the subluxation. If the only purpose is stabilization, no further weight is applied. A lateral x-ray should be obtained to make sure that the spine has not been distracted by the weights. If reduction of a subluxation is being attempted, additional weights, in increments of 5 lb (2.5 kg), may be necessary because of paraspinal muscle spasms. X-rays should be obtained between each weight increment to verify the need for more weight. Up to 80 lb (36 kg) may often be required in lower cervical spine subluxations. Rarely is this exceeded. If traction alone is unsuccessful, additional measures which may be taken, with extreme caution, include the administration of muscle relaxants and general anesthesia, or mild hyperextension in anterior subluxations. Occasional case reports have given reason to hope that the recent and successful use of cervical traction may facilitate neurological recovery even in patients with complete cord injury (Brunette and Rockswald, 1987). Occasionally a subluxation with locked facets may not be reducible, in which case open reduction is necessary. If an emergency laparotomy or the surgical procedure is required, the patient should be kept in traction at all times during the procedure. Axial skeletal traction has little role in the treatment of thoracic and lumbar spine fractures. These are occasionally treated with positional adjustment, such as placing rolled sheets under the back to hyperextend the spine at a kyphotic gibbus.

The decision about whether and when to operate on a spinal injury is often made in the emergency room, on the basis of information obtained during the diagnostic phase. The variety of surgical options is too great to discuss in this chapter, and surgical indications do vary from center to center. The main point of difference between centers is whether or not it is of any use at all to operate on a patient who has had instantaneous and complete loss of cord function for less than 24 h. The halo-vest is often used adjunctively following internal fixation of unstable cervical spines, but the development of new internal fixation systems, such as the Kaspar plate and Halifax clamp, may obviate the need for such bulky and clumsy apparel, while still permitting early patient mobilization.

All forms of mechanical therapy, even when applied by experienced personnel, may result in decline in function of spinal injured patients. In a recent study of 283 SCI patients, 14 deteriorated neurologically during their acute hospital management (Marshall *et al.*, 1987). In 3 of these patients, deterioration was directly associated with skeletal traction application. This represented 5% of all patients in whom this form of therapy had been used. Four of 134 patients undergoing operative intervention also deteriorated, whereas 5 of the remaining 7 patients declined as the result of other forms of mechanical intervention. Only 2 of the 14 were felt to have deteriorated independently of their management.

Specific medical therapies have been developed to treat SCI. These are usually initiated as soon as possible in order to maximize their effectiveness. The theoretical basis for these treatments is the subject of a later chapter and will not be discussed at length here. The most commonly used medical therapy is high-dose steroids, which is felt to decrease spinal cord edema, improve blood flow, and prevent damage to neuronal membranes caused by free radical species (Hall and Braughler, 1982). Other medical therapies that have been tried include the administration of hypertonic solutions such as mannitol, the opiate antagonist naloxone, and calcium channel blockers (Flamm *et al.*, 1985; Benthuysen, 1987; Janssen and Hansebout, 1989). None of the medical therapies has been proven to be of significant benefit in prospective randomized and blinded trials. In most of the clinical trials, all patients with SCI are treated similarly. However, it is possible that a development of more sophisticated, non-invasive ways to investigate spinal cord biochemistry and physiology *in vivo* will permit the selection of subpopulations of patients who may benefit from specific therapies. It may also lead to the development of models which will bring us closer to an understanding of the pathophysiology of SCI, upon which more effective treatment strategies can be formulated.

References

Benthuysen, J.L. (1987) Naloxone therapy in spinal trauma: anesthetic effects. *Anesthesiology*, **66**, 238–240

Bivins, H.G., Ford, S., Bezmalinovic, Z., Price, H.M. and Williams, J.L. (1988) The effect of axial traction during orotracheal intubation of the trauma victim with an unstable spine. *Annals of Emergency Medicine*, **17**, 25–29

Bracken, M.B. and Collins, W.F. (1985) Randomized clinical trials of spinal cord injury treatment. In *Central Nervous System Trauma Status Report* (eds D.P. Becker and J.T. Povlishock), National Institutes of Health, Bethesda, MD, pp. 303–312

Brunette, D.D. and Rockswald, G.L. (1987) Neurologic recovery following rapid spinal realignment for complete cervical spinal cord injury. *Journal of Trauma*, **27**, 445–447

Chabot, R., York, D., Watts, C. and Waugh, W.A. (1985) Somatosensory evoked potentials evaluated in normal subjects and spinal cord-injured patients. *Journal of Neurosurgery*, **63**, 544–551

Cooper, P.R. (1986) Initial clinical evaluation and management. In *Medical Complications of Quadriplegia* (eds P.H. Berzeller and M.H. Bezkor), Yearbook Medical Publishers, Chicago, pp. 1–9

Dove, D.V., Stahl, W.M. and Del Guarcia, L.R.M. (1980) A five-year review of death following urban trauma. *Journal of Trauma*, **20**, 760–766

Ducker, T.B. (1976) Experimental injury of the spinal cord. In *Handbook of Clinical Neurology*, Vol. 25 (eds P.J. Vinker, G.W. Bruyn and R. Braakman), American Elsevier Publishing Co., New York, pp. 9–26

Ducker, T.B. and Saul, T.G. (1982) The poly-trauma and spinal cord injury. In *Early Management of Acute Spinal Cord Injury* (ed. C.H. Tator), Rava Press, New York, pp. 53–58

Evans, D.E., Kobrine, A.L. and Rizzoli, H.V. (1980) Cardiac arrhythmias accompanying acute compression of the spinal cord. *Journal of Neurosurgery*, **52**, 52–59

Flamm, E.S., Young, W., Collins, W.F., Piepmeier, J., Clifton, G.L. and Fischer, B. (1985) A phase I trial of naloxone treatment in acute spinal cord injury. *Journal of Neurosurgery*, **63**, 390–397

Foley, R.W., Harris, L.S. and Pilcher, D.B. (1977) Abdominal injuries in automobile accidents: review of care of fatally injured patients. *Journal of Trauma*, **17**, 611–615

Gentzbein, S.D. (1982) Assessment of cervical spinal instability. In *Early Management of Acute Spinal Cord Injury* (ed. C.H. Tator), Raven Press, New York, pp. 41–52

Ginsberg, M.D., Welsh, F.A. and Budd, W.W. (1980) Deleterious effect of glucose pretreatment of recovery from diffuse cerebral ischemia in the cat. 1. Local cerebral blood flow and utilization. *Stroke*, **11**, 347–354

Graziano, A.F., Scheidel, E.A., Clive, J.R. and Baer, L.J. (1987) A radiographic comparison of prehospital cervical immobilization methods. *Annals of Emergency Medicine*, **16**, 1127–1131

Green, B.A., Callahan, R.A., Klose, K.J. and de la Torre, J. (1981) Acute spinal cord injuries: current concepts. *Clinical Orthopedics and Related Research*, **154**, 125–135

Green, B.A. and Eismont, S.J. (1984) Acute spinal cord injury: a systems approach. *CNS Trauma*, **1**, 173–195

Grundy, D., Swain, A. and Russell, J. (1986) ABC of spinal cord injury. Early management and complications – I. *British Medical Journal*, **292**, 44–47

Hall, E.D. and Braughler, J.M. (1982) Glucocorticoid mechanisms in acute spinal cord injury: a review and therapeutic rationale. *Surgical Neurology*, **18**, 320–327

Harris, H.J. (1986) Radiographic evaluation of spinal trauma. *Orthopedic Clinics of North America*, **17**, 75–86

Janssen, L. and Hansebout, R.R. (1989) Pathogenesis of spinal cord injury and newer treatments. A review. *Spine*, **14**, 23–32

Kalfas, I., Wilberger, J., Goldberg, A. and Prostko, E.R. (1988) Magnetic resonance imaging in acute spinal cord trauma. *Neurosurgery*, **23**, 295–299

Lehmann, K.B., Lane, J.G., Piepmeier, J.M. and Batsford, W.P. (1987) Cardiovascular abnormalities accompanying acute spinal cord injury in humans: incidence, time course and severity. *Journal of the American College of Cardiologists*, **10**, 46–52

Lucas, J.T. and Ducker, T.B. (1979) Motor classification of spinal cord injuries with mobility, morbidity and recovery indices. *American Surgeon*, **45**, 151–158

Luce, J.M. (1985) Medical management of spinal cord injury. *Critical Care Medicine*, **13**, 126–131

Marshall, L.F., Knowlton, S., Garfin, S.R., Klauber, M.R., Eisenberg, H.M., Kopaniky, D., Miner, M.E., Tabbador, K. and Clifton, G.L. (1987) Deterioration following spinal cord injury. A multi-center study. *Journal of Neurosurgery*, **66**, 400–404

Piepmeier, J.M., Lehmann, K.B. and Lane, J.G. (1985) Cardiovascular instability following acute cervical spinal cord trauma. *CNS Trauma*, **2**, 153–160

Podolsky, S., Baroff, L.J. Simon, R.R., Hoffman, J.R., Larmon, B. and Abion, W. (1983) Efficacy of cervical immobilization methods. *Journal of Trauma*, **23**, 461–465

Poe, R.H., Reisman, J.L. and Rodenhouse, T.G. (1978) Pulmonary edema in cervical spinal cord injury. *Journal of Trauma*, **18**, 71–73

Pollack, I.F., Pong, D. and Sclabassi, R. (1988) Recurrent spinal cord injury without radiographic abnormalities in children. *Journal of Neurosurgery*, **69**, 177–187

Quencer, R.M., Sheldon, J.J., Post, M.J.D., Diaz, R.D., Montalvo, B.M., Green, B.A. and Eismont, S.J. (1986) MRI of the chronically injured cervical spinal cord. *American Journal of Roentgenology*, **147**, 125–132

Raynor, R.B. and Koplik, B. (1985) Cervical cord trauma: the relationship between clinical syndromes and force of injury. *Spine*, **10**, 193–197

Reid, D.C., Henderson, R., Saboe, L. and Miller, J.D.R. (1987) Etiology and clinical course of missed spine fractures. *Journal of Trauma*, **27**, 980–986

Sieber, F.E., Smith, D.S., Traystman, R.J. and Wollman, H. (1987) Glucose: a reevaluation of its intraoperative use. *Anesthesiology*, **67**, 72–81

Soderstrom, C.A. and Brumback, R.J. (1986) Early care of the patient with cervical spine injury. *Orthopedic Clinics of North America*, **17**, 3–13

Sypert, G.W. (1984) Early management of spinal injuries. *American Family Physician*, **29**, 113–122

Tator, C.H., Rowed, D.W., Schwartz, M.L., Gertzbein, S.D., Bharatwal, N., Barkin, M. and Edwards, V.E. (1984) Management of acute spinal cord injuries. *Canadian Journal of Surgery*, **27**, 289–293

Todd, M.M., Tommasino, C. and Moore, S. (1985) Cerebral effects of isovolemic hemodilution with a hypertonic saline solution. *Journal of Neurosurgery*, **63**, 944–948

Van Wagoner, F.H. (1961) Died in hospital: a three-year study of deaths following trauma. *Journal of Trauma*, **1**, 401–408

White, A.A., Johnson, R.M., Panjabi, M.D. *et al.* (1975) Biomedical analysis of clinical stability in the cervical spine. *Clin. Orthop.*, **109**, 85–95.

Whittley, J.S., Prough, D.S. and DeWitt, D.S. (1988) Shock plus an intracranial mass lesion in dogs: cerebrosvascular effects of resuscitation fluid choices. *Anesthesia and Analgesia*, **67** (suppl.) S259

Young, W. (1982) Correlation of somatosensory evoked potentials and neurologic findings in spinal cord injury. In *Management of Acute Spinal Cord Injury* (ed. C.H. Tator), Raven Press, New York, pp. 153–165

Chapter 4

Anaesthetic management of acute spinal cord injury

J.D. Alderson and Somasundaram Thiagarajah

Introduction

The anaesthetist may become involved with the management of a spinal cord injury (SCI) patient, first as part of the initial reception and resuscitation team in the accident and emergency department, as described in Chapter 3, or secondly in the operating room where he may be required for surgery necessary to treat the results of the patient's trauma. The specific problem of associated injuries is dealt with in Chapter 5, and this chapter is, therefore, devoted to the anaesthetic management that may be required during treatment within the acute phase of SCI.

The medical management of any trauma to the spine follows three basic principles: (a) protection of the spinal cord; (b) restoration of the integrity of the spinal canal to relieve compression; (c) establishment of spinal stability (Fraser and Edmonds-Seal, 1982). If associated injuries require urgent priority treatment, then temporary methods of achieving these principles of treatment have to be used. The satisfactory stabilization of cervical fracture is temporarily achieved by using a cervical collar, holding the neck in a neutral position (Feur, 1976). Thoracolumbar fractures, on the other hand, are usually more stable, but will require careful positioning of the patient to avoid further damage by keeping the patient supine on a solid flat surface and carefully avoiding rotation or flexion when lifting from bed to operating table. Two main methods are used in the further treatment of the actual spinal injury, either definitive surgery such as open reduction, or conservative management such as traction or posture.

Cervical injuries

Even in the presence of instability it is usual practice to treat the vast majority of cervical fractures and fracture dislocations by conservative means, using a Nickel halo (Perry and Nickel, 1939) or skeletal long traction. The Nickel halo is preferred by many centres as it gives better biplanar control than that achieved by Crutchfield tongs. Either can be applied following local anaesthetic infiltration. With the Nickel halo, screws are inserted into the outer table of the skull, and traction progressively increased in 2.5 kg increments over several days until reduction of the injury is secured – up to 20 kg may be necessary. In injuries with minimal instability and no displacement or neurological loss, this method can be continued satisfactorily for up to 3 months. However, if conservative therapy is used as the sole method of treatment for all cervical injuries, then approximately 42% of cases remain clinically or radiologically unstable at 3 months (Cheshire, 1969).

In the acute phase the major reasons for abandoning conservative treatment are increasing neurological deficit (Tarlov, 1972) and fracture instability. Evidence of ligamentous disruption producing this instability is usually derived from radiographs, with severe wedging, tear-drop fractures, locked facets and multiple spinal fractures all suggesting severe damage to the stabilizing anterior or posterior ligaments (Holdsworth, 1970) and warranting early consideration of surgery. Severe muscle spasm following cervical fractures is common and may prevent early reduction of cervical dislocations by conservative traction. This may require manipulation under muscle relaxation (Evans, 1961), but if this is unsuccessful then open surgical intervention may be required. Anterior or posterior fusion may be required in the acute situation, especially in the presence of disc disruption with pain, spinal compression with an anterior spinal cord syndrome, or instability (Roy-Camille et al., 1979). With all surgical procedures, conservative skull traction must be maintained until surgical stability is assured.

Thoracolumbar spine

The indications for the use of conservative *versus* surgical treatments for thoracolumbar injuries remain controversial. Many centres believe that early surgical intervention to correct and stabilize the spine may improve neurological function and allow rapid mobilization, avoiding the hazards of prolonged bed confinement. Others would argue that a major surgical procedure such as posterior spinal fusion is particularly hazardous in the acute phase of spinal shock, and that conservative therapy of postural realignment should be used at least until the phase of spinal shock has passed.

Dickson, Harrington and Erwin (1978) recommend the use of posterior spinal fusion with Harrington rod instrumentation for urgent reduction and stabilization of a thoracolumbar injury, if there is loss of integrity of the spinal column. This major surgical procedure is associated with considerable blood loss, and with heat loss and poor venous return, and is not well tolerated by patients with the spinal shock syndrome. As part of the operative procedure, intraoperative awakening may be required to ascertain whether too much distraction is produced by the Harrington distraction rods leading to spinal cord stretching and impaired neurological function (Sudhir et al., 1976; Waldman et al., 1977). Abott and Bentley (1980) describe a technique for elective surgery using endotracheal maintenance anaesthesia of morphine and nitrous oxide and oxygen, with a long-acting relaxant. In this technique, the relaxant is allowed to wear off prior to the patient being awakened, by omitting the nitrous oxide and using 95% oxygen with 5% carbon dioxide, allowing verbal communication with the patient.

Alternatively, somatosensory evoked potentials may be used to monitor spinal cord function in patients with compromised cord function during surgery (Grundy, 1984). Permanent neurological deficits can be prevented by recognition of changes and adopting appropriate action. Availability of new computerized monitors makes the interpretation of somatosensory evoked potential less difficult than previously, and diligent and flawless techniques will minimize interference artefacts. However, if the neurological insult is not severe or the dorsal columns are not involved in the injury, then this monitor may fail to detect cord damage. More recently, motor evoked potentials have been used to detect deterioration of motor function. Mobilization of the patient can begin as early as the second day following surgery when Harrington rod distraction is used.

An anterior approach to the thoracolumbar spine may also be used, and is particularly indicated in acute injuries with motor weakness in conjunction with intact touch, pain and proprioception suggesting anterospinal artery syndrome due to trauma compression anteriorly. For access to the thoracic spine, a posterolateral thoracotomy is used, with resection of the vertebral body. Particular care needs to be taken to identify the origin of the spinal arteries of Adamkiewicz by radiography, as this selects the side of the thoracotomy (Paul *et al.*, 1975).

Anaesthetic problems

Following complete transection of the spinal cord, the patient goes through two stages – an acute phase of spinal shock lasting from 3 days up to 6 weeks, and a later reflex phase. It is only the spinal shock phase we are concerned with here, and this poses several problems for anaesthesia.

Respiratory problems

The phrenic nerves receive their roots mainly from C4, with contributions from C3 and C5. Thus with a complete lesion at C5 or below, although intercostal muscle activity is lost, diaphragmatic function is spared, and adequate tissue oxygenation is maintained. Injuries above C3 cause rapid death unless ventilation is controlled immediately.

When the cervical SCI is below C5 there is intercostal paralysis, which on its own decreases alveolar ventilation by the 60% of tidal volume attributable to rib elevation. It also causes a type of paradoxical expiration and prevents effective coughing, for although the diaphragm may work normally, the intercostal and abdominal muscles are flaccid. The unopposed action of the diaphragm contracting pulls the lower ribs together, giving a comparative reduction in lower chest volume in inspiration, and an increase in volume when it relaxes in expiration (Corbett, Kerr and Prys-Roberts, 1969). The average vital capacity for a C5 quadriplegic with accessory respiratory muscles and diaphragm, but without intercostal or abdominal muscles, should be 2200–2500 ml (Carter, 1987). Whatever diaphragmatic activity remains is frequently subjected to mechanical splinting by abdominal distension (Cheshire and Coats, 1975). Respiratory drive may be depressed by high levels of circulating β-endorphin in response to cord trauma (Quimby, Williams and Greifenstein, 1973). Secretions may prove difficult to cough up and are particularly likely to pool, causing atelectasis and pneumonia in the period from 3 to 5 days after injury (Carter, 1987). Hypoxia may lead to further impairment of the conscious level and a further reduction in respiratory drive (Fraser and Edmonds-Seal, 1982).

Aspiration of stomach contents can occur, further decreasing alveolar ventilation (Cheshire and Coats, 1975), and clearly if highly acid may present the anaesthetist with pneumonitis and bronchospasm (Mendelson's syndrome) (Quimby, Williams and Griefenstein, 1973). The latter is not helped by unopposed vagal activity following the total sympathectomy of a cervical transection, causing broncho-constriction.

During the first few days following injury, three pathological events may further reduce respiratory function – extension of the lesion, pulmonary embolism and pulmonary oedema. The latter is covered more fully later in this chapter. Extension of the injury may occur from haemorrhage or from cord oedema which may ascend in two bilateral cones from the level of the injury (Woolman, 1965). If these cones extend to involve the anterolateral portion of the cord in the C2–C4 area, then sleep apnoea (Ondine's curse) can occur without other changes in respiratory function. Respiration is unchanged while the patient is awake, but when he sleeps he becomes apnoeic and can die.

Preoperative assessment should always include simple respiratory function tests (vital capacity), blood gas analyses and chest x-ray examination.

Cardiovascular problems

At the time of the SCI there is a short-lived but explosive autonomic discharge accompanied by bradycardia, hypertension and bizarre dysrhythmias (Greenhoot, Shiel and Mauch, 1972; Evans, Kobrine and Rizzoli, 1980). The higher the level of the injury, the greater the response. The afterload offered to the heart resulting from the intense vasoconstriction can precipitate left ventricular failure and the development of subendocardial infarction (Eidelberg, 1973). This leads to reduced myocardial function over the next few days.

The hypertensive aspect of this sympathetic discharge also may disrupt the pulmonary capillary endothelium giving frank haemorrhage or preparing the stage for pulmonary oedema (Theodore and Robin, 1976).

This sympathetic discharge is very shortlived and succeeded by a longer period of 'shock'. If the SCI is cervical, the spinal shock phase represents the equivalent of a total sympathectomy, and is characterized by hypotension and bradycardia (Troll and Dohrmann, 1975). Sympathectomy increases venous capacitance, thereby increasing the vascular compartment size. The hypotension and bradycardia may further impair cardiac function by reducing coronary blood flow. The lower the level of the injury, the more of the sympathetic outflow remains under the control of the brain, and the less is the effect on the blood pressure. Lesions at T6 and above are likely to give such cardiovascular changes.

It is important to remember that despite the sympathectomy of a high lesion, the parasympathetic vagus nerve is intact, being cranial in origin. Application of this knowledge allows an understanding of several important reflexes that pose problems to the anaesthetist. With unopposed vagus innervation, the response to hypoxia is that of a bradycardia, reversible by giving oxygen, and also by giving atropine. This bradycardia can lead to asystole (Frankel, Mathias and Spalding, 1975). Other important vagal reflexes for the anaesthetist are those in response to endotracheal intubation, and also tracheal suction. Both can produce asystole as above, and such procedures should be pretreated by atropine (Welply, Mathias and Frankel, 1975). With injuries below T5, such effects are unlikely (Figure 4.1).

The normal experience and training of an anaesthetist faced with a hypotensive patient requires him to give intravenous fluid in an attempt to restore the blood pressure. In a tetraplegic this is a hazardous procedure, as there is great risk of pulmonary oedema from overloading the circulation in these patients. Troll and Dohrmann (1975) recommend the use of pulmonary artery wedge pressure to monitor the left atrial pressure, as they believe central venous pressure readings do not adequately warn of left heart failure. In the spinal shock phase, the resting

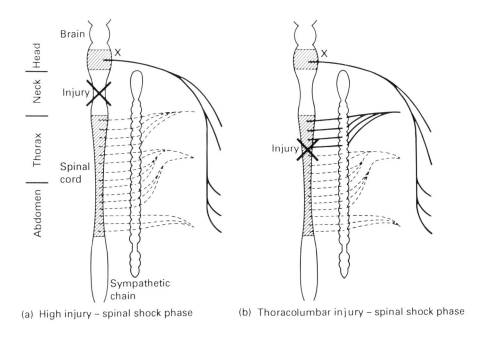

(a) High injury – spinal shock phase

(b) Thoracolumbar injury – spinal shock phase

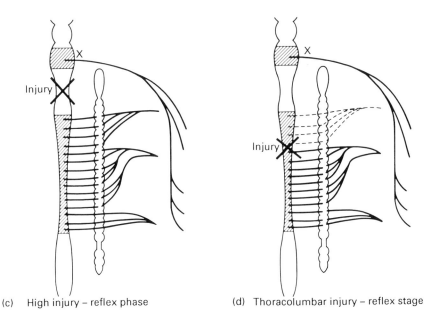

(c)   High injury – reflex phase

(d) Thoracolumbar injury – reflex stage

Figure 4.1 Schematic drawing of effects on the autonomic nervous system of spinal cord injury: (a) unopposed action of the vagus nerve with a cervical injury; (b) lower injuries allow some sympathetic outflow to counteract the vagus nerve; (c, d) in the reflex phase, autonomic hyperreflexia can be provoked by stimuli and produce severe cardiovascular effects in high injuries

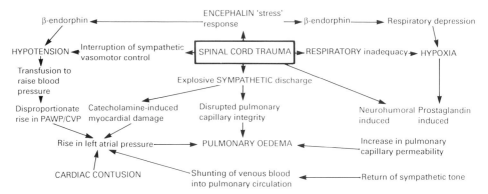

Figure 4.2 Pathophysiological sequelae of spinal cord injury (PAWP, pulmonary arterial wedge pressure; CVP, central venous pressure) (From Fraser and Edmonds-Seal, 1982, by permission)

plasma adrenaline (epinephrine) and noradrenaline (norepinephrine) levels are low (Mathias *et al.*, 1979) and therefore the use of sympathomimetic drugs may be rational (Troll and Dohrmann, 1975), bearing in mind that the return of sympathetic tone a few days after injury may precipitate a rise in left atrial and right atrial pressures (Brisman *et al.*, 1974). Fraser and Edmonds-Seal (1982) have produced an excellent chart of the many factors involved in the production of pulmonary oedema (Figure 4.2).

Artificial ventilation can be regarded as a series of Valsalva manoeuvres, and in tetraplegics this reflex is abnormal, being more likely to cause hypotension because of the absence of compensatory overshoot when the intrathoracic pressure is returned to normal (Welply, Mathias and Frankel, 1975). The quadriplegic is also very susceptible to decreased ventricular filling pressures due to the initial myocardial damage, so positive end expiratory pressure (PEEP) which impedes venous return can also be associated with hypotension (Troll and Dohrmann, 1975). However, PEEP may have a place in the treatment of pulmonary oedema. It is suggested that low inspiratory time/expiratory time ratios may minimize the deleterious cardiovascular effects, a 1:2 ratio being recommended (Quimby, Williams and Greifenstein, 1973).

Because of the effect of the sympathectomy on peripheral capacitance vessels, it is important to prevent venous pooling; therefore, positioning of the patient to prevent this is essential. This loss of control of the capacitance vessels also means that blood loss is not well tolerated, and great care should be taken on fluid replacement.

Deep vein thrombosis can be a major problem in spinal injuries, with limb immobilization and venous pooling as contributory factors. Unless there is an associated head injury, it is, therefore, normal practice to use prophylactic subcutaneous heparin or oral anticoagulants for up to 12 weeks following SCIs. If major surgery is contemplated, subcutaneous heparin should be started 2h preoperatively and continued for at least 2 weeks postoperatively (Fraser and Edmonds-Seal, 1982).

Thermoregulation

With loss of the ability to sweat or vasoconstrict within affected dermatomes the patient becomes poikilothermic and needs careful control of his environmental conditions. In surgery, considerable heat loss can occur, and the means to warm the patient and also warm intravenous fluids are essential. Core temperature should be monitored.

Gastric stasis

Paralytic ileus is relatively common after SCI and may last for 2–3 days. The patient is at considerable risk of aspiration of stomach contents, and a distended stomach can impede respiration, so nasogastric drainage should be instituted immediately and oral fluids withheld until bowel sounds return. Gastric stasis is most troublesome in thoracolumbar injuries, and can lead to a hypokalaemic alkalosis.

Suxamethonium (succinylcholine)

Before discussing anaesthesia management of the acute phase of spinal injuries, mention must be made of the use of suxamethonium in spinal injury patients.

First, the use of suxamethonium in patients with cervical spine injuries may be inappropriate, as the fasciculation of the neck muscles, which are in spasm following the injury, can cause displacement of the fracture.

Secondly, suxamethonium in certain SCIs is associated with a rise in the serum potassium. This potentially lethal condition was highlighted by Commander Tobey of the US navy in 1970, when he reported four cardiac arrests, following suxamethonium, occurring in young marines who had been rendered paraplegic in Vietnam between 44 and 85 days previously (Tobey, 1970). He speculated that suxamethonium had produced hyperkalaemia, and set out to investigate this hypothesis by subjecting 4 more patients to a suxamethonium infusion. The results are shown in Figure 4.3 and clearly substantiate his hypothesis.

Tobey also reported, however, that suxamethonium used within 24 h of trauma was not associated with cardiac effects.

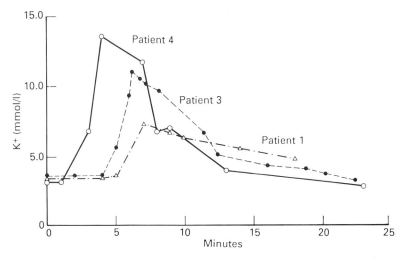

Figure 4.3 Changes in serum potassium with infusion of 0.1% suxamethonium (succinylcholine). Total dose varies between 20 and 80 mg (From Tobey, 1970, by permission)

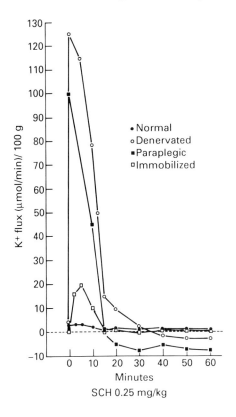

Figure 4.4 Potassium ion fluxes of normal, immobilized, paraplegic and denervated canine skeletal muscle after injection of succinylcholine (SCH) (From Gronert and Theye, 1975, by permission)

Experimental work in baboons by Tobey and co-workers demonstrated that the half-peak increase in serum potassium occurred 8.4 days after injury, with the peak increase (5.5 mmol/litre) occurring 14 days after injury (John *et al.*, 1976). The pathophysiology appears to be a hypersensitivity of the skeletal muscles involved (Gronert and Theye, 1975). There is a spread of acetylcholine receptors from the motor end-plate to include the entire muscle membrane, and the muscle becomes exquisitely sensitive to depolarizing agents. Depolarization, with a rapid increase in ionic permeability, takes place throughout the whole muscle and produces massive ionic fluxes, such that 100 μmol/min potassium can be released from 100 g of denervated muscle. The required dose of acetylcholine to produce depolarization is reduced by a factor of 10^{-4} (Figure 4.4).

This hypersensitivity develops gradually over 8–10 days after injury, and lasts for 8–9 months. The hyperkalaemic response can be attenuated by pretreatment with non-depolarizing relaxants such as gallamine, but full paralysing doses are required to totally prevent it occurring (Figure 4.5). Suxamethonium should certainly be avoided in the period from 3 days to 9 months following the injury (Fraser and Edmonds-Seal, 1982).

Anaesthesia

For the reasons already outlined, anaesthesia in the acute phase of spinal injuries can be particularly hazardous. The indication for anaesthesia should, therefore, be

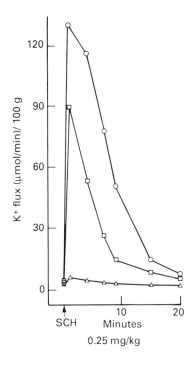

Figure 4.5 Potassium ion fluxes of denervated muscle after succinylcholine (SCH) injection. Gallamine-pretreatment categories are: ○, none; □, gallamine, 0.5 mg/kg, 5 min before SCH; △, total gallamine paralysis (3 mg/kg initial dose plus 4 mg/kg per hour constant infusion begun 15 min before SCH). $N = 5$ in each group   (From Gronert and Theye, 1975, by permission)

carefully discussed with the surgeon so that the hazards are fully understood before a decision to operate is made.

The patient should be assessed for neurological deficit, and note made of the findings. Incomplete lesions in particular should carefully be recorded, in view of potential medicolegal effect should the deficit become worse following anaesthesia. If the injury is complete, and mid-thoracic or above, then thought should be given to the abnormal state of the cardiovascular and respiratory systems as outlined above, with particular reference to reflexes. Simple preoperative tests should include vital capacity, blood gases and chest x-ray. Pulse and blood pressure should be recorded, and if there is evidence of hypotension then further monitoring should be actively considered to assist fluid replacement or inotropic usage.

Workers at Yale suggest that an indwelling arterial cannula be inserted to record arterial pressures and allow blood gases to be repeatedly sampled (Troll and Dohrmann, 1975). They also believe a Swan-Ganz pulmonary artery catheter should be inserted to permit cardiac output measurement, pulmonary artery wedge pressure measurement and pulmonary shunting to be calculated. They believe this allows full assessment of the state of the cardiovascular system, facilitates treatment with either fluid or inotropic agents, and protects against the development of pulmonary oedema. In less complex cases hourly urine output measurements of greater than 0.5 ml/kg per hour may be sufficient indication of adequate cardiovascular function (Fraser and Edmonds-Seal, 1982).

For all but the shortest cases the temperature of the patient should be well controlled, and measured centrally. A warming blanket should be provided, and all parenteral fluids warmed to body temperature. If possible the theatre environment should be kept warm.

As part of the preoperative assessment, other injuries – apart from that requiring surgery – should be excluded. The abdomen will be 'silent', and signs suggestive of possible abdominal injury should be taken seriously. Absent bowel sounds will indicate ileus, and should be treated with nasogastric aspiration and intravenous fluid replacement. For urgent anaesthesia, the prophylactic use of non-particulate antacids should be considered, and metoclopramide may encourage gastric emptying (Fraser and Edmonds-Seal, 1982).

Endotracheal intubation will be required for most surgery. This is a hazardous procedure in a patient with unstable vertebrae (especially cervical) and a possible full stomach, and must be carefully planned. To protect the cervical vertebrae in an unstable cervical injury, the neck must be immobilized.

In an acute situation a cervical collar should be applied, but if time is available then full skull traction implemented with a Nickel halo or Crutchfield calipers as described earlier. This should not be removed, and the traction should remain in place for intubation, as it is important that the head and neck remain in the neutral position. The ward bed and traction should be taken through into the operating theatre.

Intubation may be performed awake or following general anaesthesia. Awake intubation can be used whereby the laryngeal reflexes are not obtunded until the moment of intubation and, therefore, this method is of advantage in a patient with possible full stomach. Awake orotracheal intubation using an ordinary laryngoscope can be performed following topical anaesthesia to the tongue, and gradually advancing the laryngoscope onto the anaesthetized area until the cords are visualized (Sims and Giesecke, 1976). When using a conventional laryngoscope the anaesthetist's assistant, or the surgeon, should fully stabilize the neck, preventing extension by the action of the laryngoscope, although Evans (1961) reported that in cervical injuries following acute flexion, conventional orotracheal intubation may, itself, reduce the cervical fracture (Figure 4.6).

The use of the intubating fibre optic laryngoscope is probably the least traumatic method of intubation, but should be reserved for experienced hands.

Although awake intubation offers advantages in that prevention of aspiration is more likely, intubation under general anaesthesia can be performed, provided that the risk of aspiration is realized. It is difficult to perform cricoid pressure with safety in a cervical injury, and it should probably be abandoned. Inhalational induction allows control of the airway as loss of consciousness is gradual, and is associated with less hypotension than some intravenous induction agents. Intubation can be performed either blind nasally, or by the conventional orotracheal route using a laryngoscope, or by fibre optic means. This technique can be combined with topical local anaesthesia, or non-depolarizing muscle relaxants may be used. Blind nasal intubation has been recommended under light anaesthesia using 5% cocaine solution to shrink the nasal mucosa and reduce the risk of epistaxis (Walts, 1965).

Suxamethonium should be avoided for the reasons mentioned, although some centres believe it has a use in the emergency respiratory failure situation in the accident and emergency department, and can be used safely up to 72 h after the injury (Plunkett, Wilkins and Edwards, 1986).

If respiratory inadequacy is already present, then tracheostomy under local anaesthesia should be considered, to allow postoperative tracheal toileting, and intermittent positive pressure ventilation (IPPV).

The effects of a high lesion, i.e. T5 and above, on vagal reflexes must be considered when intubating or when performing tracheal suction. Preoperative atropine should be given in susceptible patients, and hypoxia avoided.

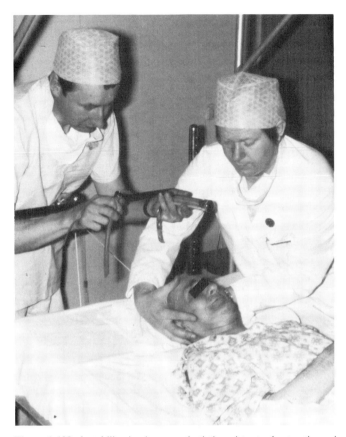

Figure 4.6 Neck stabilization by anaesthetist's assistant, plus traction prior to intubation

Induction of anaesthesia

The use of any anaesthetic agent that causes myocardial depression may be hazardous in a patient who is hypotensive following the sympathectomy of spinal shock, and who has possible myocardial damage following the acute sympathetic discharge at the time of the injury. A preoperative electrocardiogram should be performed to indicate myocardial damage and the electrocardiogram monitored throughout.

The loss of compensatory vasoconstriction leads to greater falls in blood pressure with myocardial depressants, and if there is also associated fluid loss then quite marked falls can occur. Induction agents such as ketamine, which preserve the blood pressure, may be better than barbiturates in these circumstances. Agents which provoke involuntary movements, such as etomidate and propofol, are best avoided. If barbiturates are used, they should be administered cautiously.

Maintenance of anaesthesia

Most operations on the spine will require muscle relaxation to overcome the spasm of the muscles at the site of the injury. Non-depolarizing relaxants, with IPPV, will be required. Atracurium has the advantage of excellent reversal prospects that do not solely rely on neostigmine, but also on temperature and pH. This makes it a valuable drug in neuromuscular disease. Pancuronium has the advantage of maintaining blood pressure and producing a tachycardia, and may be of benefit. Myocardial depressant agents should be used with caution, if at all, and minimal anaesthesia used to prevent awareness.

Intermittent positive pressure ventilation can impede venous return to the heart and the inspiratory/expiratory time ratio should be kept below 1:2, and PEEP avoided unless pulmonary oedema is present.

Some anaesthetists prefer to have a spontaneously breathing patient for neck manipulation – as any further neurological damage performed by the surgeon is then immediately obvious. Others would argue that this method does not relax the spasm of the neck muscles and that full relaxation is preferable.

Summary and checklist for anaesthesia for patients in 'spinal shock'

1. Other injuries?
2. Complete lesion?
3. Lesion T5 and above – affects of sympathectomy – BP ↓ P ↓ CO ↓
   – responses to blood loss, etc.
   – affects of unopposed vagus – hypoxia Rx O_2, atropine
   – tracheal intubation and suction Rx atropine
   – affects respiration – vital capacity
   – blood gases
   – secretions
4. Myocardial damage? – ECG
5. Adequate perfusion? – urine output 0.5 ml/kg per h
   – PAWP and CO; fluids; sympathomimetics
6. Pulmonary oedema? – chest x-ray; pulse oximetry; PAWP
7. Ileus? – nasogastric tube; i.v. fluids
   – antacid; metoclopramide
8. DVT prophylaxis?
9. Temperature? – poikilothermic – warming blanket
   – warm i.v. fluids
   – monitor core temperature
10. Stability of fracture? – cervical collar ⎫
    traction   ⎬ maintain
11. Intubation   – LA ⎭
    (*with traction on for* – GA
    cervical fracture)   – atropine ?required
    – fibre optic
    – blind nasal
    – oral
    – tracheostomy
12. Induction – inhalational ⎫ beware myocardial depressants
    – intravenous ⎭ beware agents → involuntary movements
13. Muscle relaxants – avoid suxamethonium 4 days – 9 months
    – atracurium?
14. IPPV – 1:2 ratio inspiratory to expiratory time
15. Positioning – venous pooling
    – pressure sores
16. Relaxant reversal – ?complete

Figure 4.7

Positioning of the patient on the operating table is very important, as the protective spasm around the fracture will be removed once a relaxant is in operation. Any transfer of the patient from the ward bed to operating table should occur with the anaesthetist and surgeon jointly supervising and supporting the head and fracture site in the neutral position. Besides the stability of the fracture, attention should be turned to avoidance of head-up tilts, or dependent lower limbs, as pooling of blood may occur, worsening the hypotension. Pressure sores are easily provoked below the level of the injury and pressure should, therefore, be avoided on the skin.

Very careful monitoring of cardiovascular parameters is essential throughout surgery, and blood loss must be replaced immediately, as the patient's sympathectomy prevents vasoconstriction in compensation for loss.

Neuromuscular reversal must be fully achieved prior to extubation. Assessment of neuromuscular function above the injury may be useful, and tidal volumes, at least, should be assessed before extubation is performed. Onset of increasing hypoxia during surgery suggests pulmonary oedema formation. Removal of IPPV will worsen this. Pulse oximetry is very useful intraoperatively, and should be continued postoperatively, along with pulse and blood pressure, temperature and hourly urine volume measurements.

Failure to obtain adequate respiratory function following muscle relaxant reversal may require IPPV ± PEEP. Non-irritant endotracheal tubes (PVC or silicone) should be employed, or tracheostomy performed.

Spinal injury patients should always be nursed postoperatively by nurses familiar with their problems. In particular, respiratory problems need careful assessment and appropriate action taken promptly. The management of intravenous fluids in the operative and postoperative period is critical if pulmonary oedema is to be avoided.

This section, dealing with anaesthesia in the acute phase of spinal injuries, is summarized in Figure 4.7.

References

Abott, T.R. and Bentley, G. (1980) Intra-operative awakening during scoliosis surgery. *Anaesthesia*, **35**, 298–302

Brisman, R., Kovach, R.M., Johnson, D.O., Roberts, C.R. and Ward, G.S. (1974) Pulmonary edema in acute transection of the cervical spinal cord. *Surgery, Gynecology and Obstetrics*, **139**, 363–366

Carter, R. (1987) Respiratory aspects of spinal cord injury management. *Paraplegia*, **25**, 262–266

Cheshire, D.J. (1969) The stability of the cervical spine following the conservative treatment of fractures and fracture-dislocations. *Paraplegia*, **7**, 193–203

Cheshire, D.J.E. and Coats, D.A. (1975) Respiratory and metabolic management in acute traumatic tetraplegia. *Paraplegia*, **3**, 178–181

Corbett, J.L., Kerr, J.H. and Prys-Roberts, C. (1969) Cardiovascular responses to aspiration of secretions from the respiratory tract in man. *Journal of Physiology*, **201**, 51P–52P

Dickson, J.H., Harrington, P.H. and Erwin, W.D. (1978) Results of reduction and stabilization of the severely fractured thoracic and lumbar spine. *Journal of Bone and Joint Surgery*, **60-A**, 799–805

Eidelberg, E.E. (1973) Cardiovascular response to experimental spinal cord compression. *Journal of Neurosurgery*, **38**, 326–331

Evans, D.E., Kobrine, A.I. and Rizzoli, H.V. (1980) Cardiac arrythmias accompanying acute compression of the spinal cord. *Journal of Neurosurgery*, **52**, 52–59

Evans, D.K. (1961) Reduction of cervical dislocations *Journal of Bone and Joint Surgery*, **43-B**, 552–555

Feur, H. (1976) Management of acute spine and spinal cord injuries. Old and new concepts. *Archives of Surgery*, **111**, 638–645

Frankel, H.L., Mathias, C.J. and Spalding, J.M.K. (1975) Mechanisms of reflex cardiac arrest in tetraplegic patients. *Lancet*, **2**, 1183–1185

Fraser, A. and Edmonds-Seal, J. (1982) Spinal cord injuries. *Anaesthesia, 37*, 1084–1098

Greenhoot, J.H., Shiel, F.O. and Mauch, H.P., Jr. (1972) Experimental spinal cord injury: electro-cardiographic abnormalities and myocardial degeneration. *Archives of Neurology, 26*, 524–529

Gronert, G.A. and Theye, R.A. (1975) Pathophysiology of hyperkalemia induced by succinylcholine. *Anesthesiology, 43*, 89–99

Grundy, B.L. (1984) Electrophysiologic monitoring. In *Clinical Anaesthesia in Neurosurgery* (ed. E.A.M. Frost), Butterworths, Boston, pp. 83–91

Holdsworth, F. (1970) Review article: fractures, dislocations and fracture-dislocations of the spine. *Journal of Bone and Joint Surgery, 52-A*, 1534–1551

John, D.A., Tobey, R.E., Homer, L.D. and Rice, C.L. (1976) Onset of succinylcholine induced hyperkalaemia following denervation. *Anesthesiology, 45*, 294–299

Mathias, C.J., Christensen, N.J., Frankel, H.L. and Spalding, J.M.K. (1979) Cardiovascular control in recently injured tetraplegics in spinal shock. *Quarterly Journal of Medicine,* New Ser XLVIII, **190**, 273–287

Paul, R.L., Michael, R.H., Dunn, J.E. and Williams, J.P. (1975) Anterior transthoracic surgical decompression of acute spinal cord injuries. *Journal of Neurosurgery, 43*, 299–307

Perry, J. and Nickel, V.L. (1939) Total cervical-spine fusion for neck paralysis. *Journal of Bone and Joint Surgery, 41-A*, 37–60

Plunkett, P.K., Wilkins, R.G. and Edwards, J.D. (1986) Early management of spinal cord injury. *British Medical Journal, 292*, 485

Quimby, C.W., Williams, R.N. and Greifenstein, F.E. (1973) Anesthetic problems of the acute quadriplegic patient. *Anesthesia and Analgesia, 52*, 333–340

Roy-Camille, R., Saillant, G., Berteaux, D. and Marie-Anne, S. (1979) Early management of spinal injuries. In *Recent Advances in Orthopaedics*, Vol. 3 (ed. B. McKibbin), Churchill Livingstone, Edinburgh, pp. 57–87

Sims, J. and Giesecke, A.H., Jr. (1976). Airway management. In *Anesthesia for the Surgery of Trauma* (ed. A.H. Giesecke), F.A. Davis, Philadelphia, pp. 71–77

Sudhir, K.G., Smith, R.M., Hall, J.E. and Hansen, D.D. (1976) Intraoperative awakening for early recognition of possible neurologic sequelae during Harrington rod spinal fusion. *Anesthesia and Analgesia, 55*, 526–528

Tarlov, I.M. (1972) Acute spinal cord compression paralysis. *Journal of Neurosurgery, 36*, 10–20

Theodore, J. and Robin, E.D. (1976) Speculations on neurogenic pulmonary edema. *American Review of Respiratory Diseases, 113*, 405–411

Tobey, R.E. (1970) Paraplegia, succinylcholine and cardiac arrest. *Anesthesiology, 32*, 359–364

Troll, G.F. and Dohrmann, G.J. (1975) Anaesthesia of the spinal cord-injured patient: cardiovascular problems and their management. *Paraplegia, 13*, 162–171

Waldman, J., Kaufer, H., Hensinger, R.N., Callaghan, M.L. and Leiding, K.G. (1977) Wake up technic to avoid neurologic sequelae during Harrington rod procedure. *Anesthesia and Analgesia, 56*, 733–735

Walts, L.F. (1965) Anesthesia of the larynx in the patient with a full stomach. *Journal of the American Medical Association, 192*, 705–706

Welply, N.C., Mathias, C.J. and Frankel, H.L. (1975) Circulatory reflexes in tetraplegics during artificial ventilation and general anaesthesia. *Paraplegia, 13*, 172–182

Woolman, L. (1965) The disturbance of circulation in traumatic paraplegia in acute and late stages: a pathological study. *Paraplegia, 2*, 213–226

Chapter 5

Associated injuries

Elizabeth A.M. Frost

Introduction

In the multiple traumatized patient, spinal cord injury (SCI) may be associated with many other systemic injuries.

The incidence of head injury associated with SCI has been estimated at 15–50% (Shrago, 1973; Davidoff *et al.*, 1988). There is a significantly increased risk for closed head injury for patients involved in traffic accidents (risk ratio = 3.7) (Davidoff *et al.*, 1988). It is, however, important to note that head injuries are infrequently associated with cervical spine injury (58 : 1) (Gbaanador, Fruin and Taylor, 1986; Bayless and Ray, 1989). When head injuries are present they are usually not occult and patients are often comatose. The recommendation has been made that emergency cervical radiography is not efficacious and should not be routine in the management of head trauma (Bachulis *et al.*, 1987).

Thus SCI may be missed. In one study, the diagnosis of cervical spine and thoracolumbar fractures was delayed from 1 to 36 days in 22.9% and 4.9% of cases, respectively (Reid *et al.*, 1987). Causes of delayed diagnosis were failure to obtain x-rays, misinterpretations of radiographs or absence of medical care.

Patients, paraplegic or quadriplegic after SCI, may not appreciate abdominal pain. Sympathetic interruption can mask internal hemorrhage. Chest trauma in the head and spinal cord injured patient may also be hidden (Hart, 1986).

Thus although all patients with head injury should not be assumed to have SCI, in all patients who have SCI other injuries must be excluded.

Head injury

Head injury has remained one of the major causes of mortality in young people (Mendelow, 1988). In fact, head injury remains the commonest cause of coma, raised intracranial pressure and of admission for acute neurological intensive care (Jennett, 1988).

Emergency measures include intubation, ventilation, oxygenation and stabilization of the circulatory system (Singbartl and Cunitz, 1987).

Respiratory status

Respiratory abnormalities occur almost immediately after severe head injury. Blood gas values obtained at the scene of the accident and at admission to hospital following craniocerebral trauma found that hypercapnia correlates with the severity of head injury (Pfenninger *et al.*, 1987). More severe injuries were associated with Pa_{CO_2} levels over 50 mmHg (6.6 kPa). Also, patients who have sustained a pre-hospital hypoxic event have significantly poorer outcomes (Eisenberg *et al.*, 1983).

Transient respiratory arrest at the time of injury is not uncommon and may cause diffuse microatelectasis and hypercarbia. Time to intubation is critical. In a study of almost 2000 patients over a 28-month period, the adjusted mortality rate was 22.5% in those intubated within 1 h of injury and 38.4% in those in whom intubation was delayed for more than 1 h ($p < 0.01$) (Gildenberg and Makela, 1982).

The airway is best secured after oxygenation (hyperventilation, if possible), intravenous thiopental and/or lidocaine and a short-acting muscle relaxant. Cricoid pressure should be used. Diazepam and midazolam have long half-lives and, at the doses required to allow atraumatic intubation, significantly interfere with neurological examination for hours. Nasal intubation is not indicated because of the risk of hemorrhage and contamination if the patient has a basal skull fracture.

Clearly, care must be taken in securing the airway of patients with neck injuries. However, in a review of several thousand patients with multiple trauma, of whom at least 15 had cervical injury, no further complications were sustained following oral intubation (Grande and Barton, 1988). Rather, difficulties with nasointubation are not insignificant. If the practitioner is well skilled in fiberoptic intubation, this technique is a reasonable alternative in safely securing the airway. However, equipment and skill are required that may not always be available in the emergency situation (Grande, 1988).

Cardiovascular stability

The next step in emergency care is to ensure adequate cerebral perfusion. Sustained post-traumatic hypotension in adults frequently points to extracranial sources, although transient hypotension after head injury is not an infrequent occurrence (Miller *et al.*, 1978). In infants, intracranial hemorrhage, particularly if associated with subgaleal hemorrhage, can lead to hypovolemia. In adults, intracranial hematomas do not reach a volume sufficient to cause hypovolemic shock. Therefore, sustained hypotension in adults is due to either other systemic injuries or brainstem failure. The latter condition commonly is a terminal event.

Concomitant SCI may cause shock secondary to the loss of sympathetic innervation of vascular smooth muscle. This vasoparalysis results in a sudden increase in the vascular bed and pooling of a large portion of blood volume into the lower extremities. Elevating the legs above the heart level or using pneumatic anti-shock trousers is the management of choice. The anesthesiologist should be familiar with the mechanics of this latter device and its safe operation. Deflation begins with the abdominal section. The blood pressure is monitored while a small amount of air is allowed to escape. If the pressure drops more than 5 mmHg (0.66 kPa), deflation is stopped and fluid resuscitation resumed. After successful deflation of the abdominal segment, leg sections are released one at a time. Blood pressure must be continuously monitored.

Monitoring

In the patient who has sustained head and neck trauma when urgent surgery for cervical stabilization is indicated, monitoring of intracranial dynamics and systemic parameters are essential. The most important monitors are described further.

Intracranial pressure
Although quantitative assessment of cerebral blood flow can be made non-invasively, the technique is not yet in general use and thus reliance must be placed on stable intracranial pressure (ICP) as an indicator of non-progression of brain injury.

As a regulating mechanism, cerebral perfusion takes precedence over changes in ICP (cerebral perfusion pressure = mean arterial pressure − ICP). Thus, should ICP continue to increase beyond the point at which decrease in cerebral blood volume can compensate, blood pressure rises to maintain cerebral perfusion against increased extravascular pressure.

After the compensatory mechanisms are exhausted, any further mass increase causes a very rapid rise in ICP and marked deterioration in the patient's clinical condition. Intracranial pressure/volume relationships may be described by a compliance curve (Figure 5.1). Initial volume increases cause little pressure change; later increases cause rapid rise. The pressure reaction to volume (P/V) is defined as compliance. Steepness of the slope in clinical practice is expressed as 'tightness' of the intracranial contents. By plotting the pressure on a logarithmic axis against volume, the exponential pressure/volume can be converted to a linear function. The slope of this line is termed the pressure/volume index (PVI) (Marmarou, Shulman and LaMorgese, 1975). Practically, PVI is defined as the volume (milliliters) necessary to raise the CSF pressure by a factor of 10, i.e.:

$$PVI = \frac{V}{\log_{10} P_p/P_0}$$

where V is the volume injected into the lateral ventricle, P_p the peak ICP, and P_0 the initial ICP.

Adding to or withdrawing small quantities of fluid from the ventricular system and noting the pressure change permits easy calculation of PVI. As improvement in intracranial dynamics by therapeutic maneuvers is frequently manifested by improvement in compliance before actual decrease in pressure, this simple calculation is a useful guide.

Intracranial pressure monitoring may be performed by four methods (Table 5.1). Adequate measurements may be obtained after placement of various devices in the subarachnoid space (e.g. three-way stopcock, multi-orifice catheter, or hollow screw), which are then connected to an external pressure transducer. Normal pressure is 10–15 mmHg (1.3–2.0 kPa). Levels of 15–20 mmHg (2.0–2.7 kPa) are considered abnormal. Measurements should be obtained after fixation of the transducer at the level of the occiput. Intracranial pressure systems should be filled with fluid (normal saline, not heparinized solutions) and should not be connected to

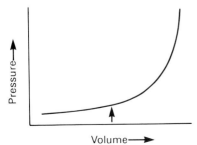

Figure 5.1 Pressure/volume compliance curve

Table 5.1 Methods of measuring intracranial pressure

Method	Advantages	Disadvantages
Subarachnoid bolt	Simple	Cannot drain CSF Compliance measurement difficult
Intraventricular catheter	CSF drainage possible Compliance measurements more accurate	Difficult if edema present
Implanted epidural transducer	Infection unlikely Simple	Cannot drain CSF Calibration may be more difficult to maintain
CT scan	Simple, non-invasive	One-time measurement only

Table 5.2 Therapy of intracranial hypertension

Surgical	Pharmacologic
Hyperventilation	Diuretics
Head elevation	Barbiturates
CSF drainage	Beta adrenergic blockade
Release of intracranial mass	

pressure systems or 'flushed' to ensure patency. Fluid should be gently withdrawn and no more than 0.5–1 ml added to re-establish a normal waveform. Therapy of intracranial hypertension is outlined in Table 5.2.

Hyperventilation acts within seconds to decrease cerebral blood flow and reduce ICP. After an initial decrease, ICP slowly rises and stabilizes after 3–5 h, usually at a lower level than in untreated patients. Less advantageous effects of hyperventilation include a shift of the oxygen dissociation curve to the left (oxygen is less available to the tissues), decreased systemic blood pressure, and reduced cerebral blood volume. Reduction of brain volume may also be achieved by administration of hypertonic solutions, diuretics, and steroids.

Electrophysiologic monitoring
Electroencephalographic and somatosensory evoked potential (SSEP) monitoring are used to assess function of the nervous system during anesthesia and surgery. Hopefully, early detection of neurological dysfunction will allow appropriate intervention to prevent or minimize damage. Somatosensory evoked potentials may be used during operations on the spine or cord, or to assess spinal cord function during surgery on other parts of the body. Although use of SSEP is well established (posterior tibial nerve and median nerve), the major postoperative neurological deficits involve motor rather than sensory changes. Means of detecting interference with motor pathways have not been well developed. To date, 'wake up' tests have been used with the risk of extubation, painful memories, or need for repeated induction of anesthesia. Electrical motor evoked potentials (MEPs) cause considerable discomfort and are not recommended for perioperative assessment. Magnetically induced MEPs avoid some of these complications and have been investigated for intraoperative monitoring (Barker *et al.*, 1987; Smith *et al.*, 1988). The initial results are promising and suggest further applications for this monitor.

Electrophysiologic markers have been used to assess depth of coma and predict outcome. The electroencephalogram (EEG) may be altered in several ways. Generalized alpha rhythm, unsuppressed by external stimulation, perhaps because of differential damage of the reticular system, sparing the mid-brain, has been demonstrated (Tomassen and Kamphuisen, 1986). In cases of 'alpha coma', etiology determines outcome. Drug intoxication has a benign prognosis. Electrophysiologic monitoring is reliable in an intensive care unit to follow the course of head injured patients (Nau and Rimfel, 1987). Evoked potential techniques allow differentiation between patients with drug-induced EEG changes and those with brain injury and evaluation of functional state and prognosis. Patients with raised intracranial pressure undergo characteristic alterations in flash and brainstem evoked potentials. Monitoring of spectral edge frequency allows an assessment of cerebral activity. Sudden decrease indicates lowered brain perfusion. Intraoperative therapy is rather restricted and includes advising the surgeon of the changes, inducing hypertension, stabilizing the temperature, ensuring normovolemia and decreasing anesthetic concentration. Emergency neurosurgical consultation is necessary if other changes occur (e.g. unilateral pupillary dilatation). Placement of a burr hole or computed tomography scan may be indicated.

Systemic monitoring
Standard monitoring in all patients with multiple trauma includes continuous blood pressure monitoring by intra-arterial cannula placement, pulse oximetry, capnography, temperature, continuous electrocardiography and fluid balance.

Patients in the acute phase of injury have a marginal capacity to respond to volume stress and are therefore prone to the development of pulmonary edema. Placement of a central venous catheter or pulmonary artery catheter is essential to assess optimal volume resuscitation during surgery. Urine output is a guide to volume administration and should be optimally maintained at 0.5–1.0 ml/kg per hour. Blood loss must be adequately replaced.

Neurological assessment

To compare initial findings of central nervous system responsiveness with results of subsequent examinations, the neurological examination must be succinct and reproducible. Assessment of level of consciousness, examination of the eye and assessment of brainstem function are of special importance. The level of consciousness is very important in evaluating the extent of injury. Duration and depth of unconsciousness correlates well with the depth of brain injury (Levin *et al.*, 1988). As popular expressions of degree of responsiveness indicate marked variation in appreciation of actual levels, a quantitative measure of neurological function is desirable for clinical and research needs. The Glasgow Coma Scale (GCS) was developed as a prognostic indicator of outcome after head injury and has been adopted as an indicator of efficacy of therapy of cerebral trauma (Table 5.3). The GCS consists of three components – eye opening, motor response and verbal response (Jennett *et al.*, 1973; Teasdale and Jennett, 1974; Teasdale *et al.*, 1979). Motor responses are the most sensitive and correlate best with the extent and outcome of severe injury (Overgaard *et al.*, 1973; Teasdale *et al.*, 1979). The correlation is highest in severe injuries.

Table 5.3 Glasgow Coma Scale

Best verbal response	
None	1
Incomprehensible sound	2
Inappropriate words	3
Confused	4
Oriented	5
Eyes open	
None	1
To pain	2
To speech	3
Spontaneously	4
Best motor response	
None	1
Abnormal extensor	2
Abnormal flexion	3
Withdraws	4
Localizes	5
Obeys	6
Total range	15–3

Abdominal injuries

As mentioned, in the patient with complete SCI and lack of sensory appreciation, diagnosis of abdominal injury may be delayed, especially if there is concomitant head injury and decreased consciousness. Systemic examination is necessary (Berman, 1988). Although attention may become focused on a particular injury, there must be a constant reappraisal of the patient's respiratory, circulatory and neurological status. Additional diagnostic and therapeutic measures include the following.

Urinary catheterization.   Low output of urine with a high specific gravity indicates the need for additional fluids. Anuria in the presence of normal blood pressure may signal renal obstruction or injury. Hemoglobinuria indicates pelvic injury. Myoglobinuria accompanies severe muscle destruction (crush injury or burn).

Central venous catheterization.   The central venous pressure serves as an indicator of the adequacy of volume replacement.

Nasogastric tube placement.   This relieves and prevents gastric distension. In the patient with facial trauma, the possibility of cribriform fracture exists, and the oral route should be used.

Peritoneal lavage.   This is useful in the diagnosis of occult intra-abdominal bleeding, especially in the patient with head injury, alcohol or drug overdose, or SCI. Blunt trauma to the liver carries a mortality rate of about 35%. Multiple trauma patients have a significantly higher mortality for each additional system seriously injured. Preoperative shock increases the death rate to 58% (Pretre *et al.*, 1988).

Fluid therapy

Traditional vital signs, such as blood pressure and pulse, may be of no value in assessing volume status in the patient with spinal cord transection.

Injury to the cord above the level of T6 results in vasodilatation and postural hypotension due to loss of sympathetic tone below the site of injury. Lesions in the region of T1–4 eliminate sympathetic innervation of the sinoatrial node and allow vagal effects to predominate on the heart rate.

The SCI patient presenting with hypotension may have hemorrhagic shock from concurrent multiple trauma. However, the presence of an abnormal heart rate is not reliable in differentiating the cause of hypotension. Although tachycardia usually accompanies hemorrhagic shock, bradycardia may indicate either neurogenic etiology or accompanying volume depletion.

Systolic blood pressure commonly stabilizes at 90–100 mmHg (12.0–13.3 kPa), which is considered adequate for cord perfusion in the supine position. However, loss of sympathetic tone and the compensatory mechanism for postural changes may jeopardize cord perfusion during repositioning and periods of operative blood loss. Spinal cord perfusion pressure should be adequately maintained with judicious volume loading using crystalloid or colloid solutions or blood replacement. Atropine 0.4 mg may be given to correct bradycardia.

If hypotension persists despite reasonable fluid administration, the judicious use of vasopressors to replace the loss of neurogenic vasoconstriction will usually promptly restore the blood pressure to normal.

Based on the supposition that head injured patients should be maintained 'dry', tradition has demanded establishment of a negative fluid balance.

The rationale for maintaining hypovolemia, ostensibly to decrease cerebral edema, has been questioned for several reasons:

1. Under experimental conditions cerebral water content decreases minimally despite complete fluid restriction (Jelsma and McQueen, 1967).
2. Hypotension associated with hypovolemia may decrease regional cerebral blood flow and increase hypoxia.
3. Hypovolemia may decrease oxygen transport to areas of the brain with normal autoregulation, and cause a reflex vasodilatation and increased ICP.
4. Preoperative hypovolemia increases the risk of an unstable anesthetic course.

The primary goal of fluid therapy is to maintain the balance between overhydration with the risk of cerebral edema, and dehydration contributing to cardiovascular instability, respiratory complications and further neurological damage.

In the head injured victim, once the skull is opened, reflex vasodilatation does not increase ICP and the emphasis must be on cardiovascular stability. Maintenance fluids should be given at a rate of 1.0–1.5 ml/kg per hour. Glucose-containing solutions should be avoided to decrease the size of infarct in compromised cerebral areas (Sieber *et al.*, 1987). Rapid fluid losses from hemorrhage or diuresis may compromise cardiovascular stability, and should be replaced as needed with balanced salt solutions, such as lactated Ringer's solution, or with 5% albumin or whole blood. Normally, the first 500–1000 ml of blood loss need not be replaced. Packed red blood cells are used less frequently because a mild degree of hemodilution, to a hematocrit between 28 and 32, has several theoretical advantages. The rheologic properties of blood (for example, viscosity) are improved at this level as compared with a hematocrit of 35–40. There is no significant difference in the oxygen delivery of blood at these two levels.

Finally, mild isovolemic hemodilution may enhance cortical blood flow to ischemic regions of brain. Experimentally, hemodilution with normal saline increases cerebral blood flow significantly and is associated with a moderate increase in ICP. Hypertonic lactated Ringer's solution also elevates cerebral blood flow but may decrease ICP (Wood, Snyder and Simeone, 1982; Todd, Tommasino and Moore, 1985; Prough et al., 1986). Rapid fluid replacement should be avoided, as sudden volume expansion may elevate ICP.

The patient in shock, whether it be spinal cord or due to multiple trauma, will present with some or all of the following clinical signs: hypotension, tachycardia, oliguria, pallor, coolness of the extremities, cyanosis, and low central venous pressure. In more severe cases (loss of 35% or more of circulating blood volume), the patient may be confused, restless and show signs of air hunger. Although signs of hypovolemia generally correlate with the degree of blood loss, geriatric patients, anemic patients and those taking various medications (diuretics, narcotics, phenothiazines) may exhibit signs out of proportion to the degree of blood loss. Patients receiving beta adrenergic blocking agents and calcium entry antagonists may not develop tachycardia.

The American College of Surgeons (1981) has developed a scheme to quantify and classify hemorrhagic shock (Table 5.4). Since no one sign is reliable in making a diagnosis, several of the parameters indicated should be used. Classification is intended as a guide to the type and volume of replacement required.

Class I hemorrhage is defined as acute loss of up to 15% of total circulating volume. Clinically, the diagnosis is potentially difficult to make, especially in the young and previously healthy adult. Pulse rate, blood pressure, respiration and even pulse pressure may appear to be within normal limits. Volume replacement may be with crystalloid or balanced salt solution (lactated Ringer's, Normosol[R]). Three milliliters of crystalloid is used to replace each milliliter of blood loss (3 : 1 rule).

Class II hemorrhage is loss of 20–25% of circulating blood volume (1000–1250 ml in the 70 kg patient) and will cause tachycardia of 100 beats/min or more, tachypnea and a narrowed pulse pressure. High spinal cord injury may mask these changes.

Table 5.4 American College of Surgeons classes of acute hemorrhage

	Class I	Class II	Class III	Class IV
Blood loss (ml)	<750	1000–1250	1500–1800	2000–2500
Blood loss (%)[a]	<15	20–25	30–35	40–50
Pulse rate[b]	72–84	>100	>120	>140
Blood pressure (mmHg)[c]	118/82	110/80	70/90/50/60	<50–60 systolic
Pulse pressure (mmHg)	36	30	20–30	10–20
Respiratory rate	14–20	20–30	30–40	>35
Urine output (ml/h)[d]	30–35	25–30	5–15	negligible
CNS – Mental status	slightly anxious	mildly anxious	anxious and confused	confused/lethargic
Fluid replacement (use 3 : 1 rule for fluid resuscitation)	crystalloid	crystalloid	crystalloid + blood	crystalloid + blood

[a] Percentage of blood volume in a 70 kg adult; [b] assume normal of 72/min; [c] assume normal of 120/80; [d] assume normal of 40–50 ml/h.

Urinary output begins to decline to less than 0.5 ml/kg per hour. Fluid therapy in these patients should be started with balanced salt solutions. The 3:1 rule for replacement should be used here, and the need for component therapy evaluated on an individual basis. Restoration of effective intravascular volume should not be delayed pending availability of blood or colloid.

Class III hemorrhage is the acute loss of 30–35% of intravascular volume (1500–1750 ml/70 kg). It produces the classical signs associated with hypovolemia in virtually all patients. In addition to a tachycardia usually greater than 120 beats/min, tachypnea of 30–40 breaths/min and a significantly narrowed pulse pressure, patients have altered mental status (confusion) and significant decreases in urine output due to inadequate cerebral and renal perfusion. Restoration of circulating volume requires blood therapy. Effective circulating volume and oxygen carrying capacity must be restored.

Class IV hemorrhage represents the extreme case of hemorrhagic blood loss (> 40%). Heart rate reaches 140 beats/min or more, and the pulse pressure tracing is narrowed to 10–20 mmHg (1.3–2.7 kPa). All signs seen with lesser degrees of shock are manifest to a greater degree. As in class III, blood therapy must be started immediately.

Positioning

Patients with multiple trauma, especially if they are neurologically intact or experiencing only transient paresis, must be maintained in neutral cervical positions. If cervical x-rays indicate fracture or there is decreasing neurological intactness in an alert patient or neck pain, then tongs and cervical traction should be applied. In an emergency situation, distraction of ruptured cervical fragments may be achieved by traction on hair or on surgical tape applied under the chin and along the cheeks. These patients are usually not good candidates for regional anesthesia (e.g. spinal, epidural block) because placement of the anesthetic generally requires a lateral position.

In cases of complete transection, a supine position is preferred, as a head-up tilt may cause hypotension. An interesting observation has been made in evaluating the effect of head injury and fracture healing (Spencer, 1987). Using a simple method of quantifying fracture healing, 53 patients who had limb fractures and also severe head injuries were studied and compared with 30 patients who had limb fractures but no head injury. Those with head injuries had a greater healing response and united more rapidly. Radiological and histological analyses revealed that the terms 'myositis ossificans' and 'heterotopic bone' may be more appropriate than 'fracture callus' to describe the healing response in these patients. Thus, in positioning of the multiple injured patient, the risk of causing further malalignment may be more quickly dissipated if head injury also co-exists.

Summary

Patients with multiple trauma including SCI are very difficult management cases. Systematic evaluation is essential. In cases of head injury, establishment of the airway and adequate oxygenation must take precedence – even at the risk of increasing neurological damage by laryngoscopy, a complication that is usually avoided by fiberoptic or awake intubation. Instrumentation of the nose should be avoided to decrease the risk of cerebral contamination in the patient with basal skull fracture.

Finally, as the cervical cord is probably only a microcosm of the brain, it also requires adequate fluid resuscitation and supplemental oxygen therapy at all times.

References

American College of Surgeons (1981) Advanced Trauma Life Support Course. ACS, Chicago

Bachulis, B.L., Long, W.B., Hynes, G.D. and Johnson, M.C. (1987) Clinical indications for cervical spine radiographs in the traumatized patient. *American Journal of Surgery*, **153**, 473–478

Barker, A.T., Eng, B., Freeston, I.L. Jalinous, R. and Jarratt, J.A. (1987) Magnetic stimulation of the human brain and peripheral nervous system: an introduction and the results of an initial clinical evaluation. *Neurosurgery*, **20**, 100–109

Bayless, P. and Ray, V.G. (1989) Incidence of cervical spine injuries in association with blunt head trauma. *American Journal of Emergency Medicine*, **7**(2), 139–142

Berman, J. (1988) *The Trauma Victim in Preanesthetic Assessment I* (ed. E. Frost), Birkhauser, Boston, pp. 10–20

Davidoff, G., Thomas, P., Berent, S., Dijkers, M. and Doljanac, R. (1988) Closed head injury in acute traumatic spinal cord injury: incidence and risk factors. *Archives of Physical Medicine and Rehabilitation*, **69**(10), 869–872

Eisenberg, H.M., Cayard, O., Papanicolou, A.C., Weiner, R., Franklin, D., Jane, J., Grossmann, R., Tabaddor, K., Becker, D.P., Marshall, L.F. and Kunitz, S. (1983) The effects of 3 potentially preventable complications on outcome after severe closed head injury. In *Intracranial Pressure V* (eds S. Ishii, H. Nagai and M. Brock), Springer Verlag, Berlin, pp. 549–553

Gbaanador, G.B., Fruin, A.H. and Taylor, C. (1986) Role of routine emergency cervical radiography in head trauma. *American Journal of Surgery*, **152**(6), 643–648

Gildenberg, P.L. and Makela, M.E. (1982) The effect of early intubation and ventilation in outcome following head trauma. In *Symposium on Neural Trauma* (Charlottesville, VA), Raven Press, New York

Grande, C. (1988) Airway management of the trauma patient in the resuscitation area of the trauma center. *Trauma Quarterly*, **5**(1), 30–49

Grande, C.M. and Barton, C.R. (1988) Appropriate techniques for airway management of emergency patients with suspected spinal cord injury. *Anesthesia and Analgesia*, **67**, 714–715

Hart, L.H. (1986) Hidden chest trauma in the head-injured patient. *Critical Care Nurse*, **6**(4), 51–57

Jelsma, L.F. and McQueen, J.D. (1967) Effect of experimental water restriction on brain water. *Journal of Neurosurgery*, **26**, 35–40

Jennett, B. (1988) Coma, intracranial pressure, intensive care, head injury and neoplasia. *Current Opinions in Neurosurgery and Neurology*, **1**(1), 1–2

Jennett, B., Teasdale, G., Galbraith, S. *et al*. (1973) Severe head injuries in three countries. *Journal of Neurology, Neurosurgery and Psychiatry*, **40**, 291–298

Levin, H., Williams, D., Crofford, M.J., High, W.M., Eisenberg, H.M., Amparo, E.G., Guinto, F.C. Jr, Kalisky, Z., Handel, S.F. and Goldman, A.M. (1988) Relationship of depth of brain lesions to consciousness and outcome after closed head injury. *Journal of Neurosurgery*, **69**, 861–866

Marmavou, A., Shulman, K. and LaMorgese, J. (1975) Compartmental analysis of compliance and outflow resistance of the cerebrospinal fluid system. *Journal of Neurosurgery*, **43**, 523–534

Mendelow, A.D. (1988) Head injuries. *Current Opinions in Neurosurgery and Neurology*, **1**(1), 37–45

Miller, J.D., Sweet, R.C., Narayan, R. and Becker, D.P. (1978) Early insults to the injured brain. *Journal of the American Medical Association*, **240**, 439–442

Nau, H.E. and Rimfel, J. (1987) Multimodality evoked potentials and electro encephalography in severe coma cases – clinical experiences in a neurosurgical intensive care unit. *Intensive Care Medicine*, **13**, 249–255

Overgaard, J., Hvid-Hansen, O., Land, A., Pedersen, K.K., Christensen, K.K., Haase, J., Hein, O. and Tweed, W.A. (1973) Prognosis after head injury based on early clinical examination. *Lancet* **2**, 631–635

Pfenninger, E., Ahnefeld, F.W., Kilian, J. and Dell, U. (1987) Blood gases at the scene of the accident and on admission to hospital following cranio-cerebral trauma. *Der Anaesthetist*, **36**, 570–576

Pretre, R., Mentha, G., Huber, O., Meyer, P., Vogel, J. and Rohner, A. (1988) Hepatic trauma: risk factors influencing outcome. *British Journal of Surgery*, **75**(6), 520–524

Prough, D.S., Johnson, J.C., Stump, D.A., Stullken, E.H., Poole, G.V. Jr. and Howard, G. (1986) Effects of hypertonic saline versus lactated Ringer's solution on cerebral oxygen transport during resuscitation from hemorrhagic shock. *Journal of Neurosurgery*, **64**, 627–632

Reid, D.C., Henderson, R., Saboe, L. and Miller, J.D.R. (1987) Etiology and clinical course of missed spine fractures. *Journal of Trauma*, **27**, 980–986

Shrago, G.G. (1973) Cervical spine injuries: association with head trauma: a review of 50 patients. *American Journal of Roentgenology*, **118**, 670–673

Sieber, F.E., Smith, D.S., Traystman, R.J. and Wollman, H. (1987) Glucose: a re-evaluation of its intraoperative use. *Anesthesiology*, **67**, 72–81

Singbartl, G. and Cunitz, G. (1987) Pathophysiology, emergency care and anesthesia in patients with severe head injury. *Anaesthesist*, **36**, 321–332

Smith, B.J., Conture, L.J., Shields, C.B., Paloheimo, M.P. and Edmonds, H.R. Jr. (1988) Cortical motor evoked potentials produced by magnetic stimulation: initial study. *Anesthesia and Analgesia*, **67**, S211

Spencer, R.F. (1987) The effect of head injury on fracture healing. A quantitative assessment. *Journal of Bone and Joint Surgery*, **69-B**(4), 525–528

Teasdale, G. and Jennett, B. (1974) Assessment of coma and impaired consciousness. A practical scale. *Lancet*, **2**, 81–84

Teasdale, G., Murray, G., Parker, L. and Jennett, B. (1979) Adding up the Glasgow Coma Score. *Acta Neurochirurgica* (Wien) (suppl.), **28**, 13–16

Todd, M.M., Tommasino, C. and Moore, S. (1985) Cerebral effects of isovolemic hemodilution with a hypertonic saline solution. *Journal of Neurosurgery*, **63**, 944–948

Tomassen, W. and Kamphuisen, H.A.C. (1986) Alpha coma. *Journal of Neurological Science*, **76**, 1–11

Wood, J.H., Snyder, L.L. and Simeone, F.A. (1982) Failure of intravascular volume expansion without hemodilution to elevate cortical blood flow in regions of experimental focal ischemia. *Journal of Neurosurgery*, **56**, 80–91

Chapter 6

Intensive care management of spinal cord injury

Patrick A. LaSala and Elizabeth A. M. Frost

Syndromes

Several distinct syndromes after spinal cord injury (SCI) may require short- or long-term intensive care.

Complete lesion
Fracture dislocations of vertebral bodies and knife or bullet wounds may cause a complete injury of the spinal cord. There is immediate loss of sensation and all voluntary movement below the lesion. Additionally, bladder and bowel control are lost. Upper cervical spinal cord transection may affect respiration. There is an initial period of 'spinal shock', where flaccidity and absent tendon reflexes exist below the lesion. Cardiovascular instability may be a concomitant feature due to disruption of the autonomic pathways. Spinal shock is a physiologic condition and does not imply that there is anatomical transection of the spinal cord. It occurs immediately after injury and may persist for weeks. With resolution of spinal shock, upper motor neuron signs emerge with increased reflexes. There is usually no return of motor or sensory function.

Incomplete lesion
The signs of partial transection are dependent upon the level of the involved segment and the mechanism of injury. In partial injuries some ascending or descending tracts may be spared, with consequent residual function below the level of the lesion. A common partial injury involves the anterior spinal cord at the cervical level and is associated with closed flexion. This results in the anterior spinal cord syndrome which presents with loss of motor function and of pain and temperature sensation below the level of injury. Posterior column function, i.e. position and vibration sense, is preserved. The cord damage may be related to a change in blood flow, with decreased flow from the anterior spinal artery supplying the anterior and lateral tracts, whereas the posterior columns or tracts are spared due to the separate supply from the two posterior spinal arteries.

Another partial lesion results in the Brown-Séquard syndrome, which is the result of physiologic or anatomic hemisection of the spinal cord. The functional loss consists of ipsilateral weakness and loss of position and vibration sense associated with contralateral loss of pain and temperature sensation. These injuries are usually associated with penetrating wounds from a gunshot or stabbing. Closed rotational injuries may also cause this syndrome.

Central cord syndrome is the result of a third partial lesion that causes neuronal loss involving the central gray matter with possible extension into the white matter. The central cord syndrome most commonly results from hyperextension involving the lower cervical segments in patients with pre-existing cervical spondylosis or stenosis (Marar, 1974). The functional deficits consist of motor and sensory loss that is greater in the upper extremities and is most severe in the distal upper extremity corresponding to lower cervical injury.

Pathophysiology

Some understanding of the pathophysiology of SCI is essential to appropriately manage these patients in an intensive care facility.

In the majority of cases, SCI is not associated with actual transection, but with contusion or compression of the cord substance. A series of events is established that leads to a progressive decrease in blood flow and subsequent hypoxic injury to the spinal cord. Allen (1914) has described the pathological changes that occur after blunt trauma. Hemorrhages involving the central gray matter occur first, followed by progressive breakdown and necrosis of the gray matter and, later, the adjacent white matter. Platelet thrombi accumulate in the injured vessels and water and protein are extravasated (Griffiths, 1975). Edema from the site of injury extends a short distance within the gray matter and to a larger extent along adjacent white matter tracts (Stewart and Wagner, 1979). In addition to the pathological changes in SCI, several metabolic changes have been described. These include local accumulation of biogenic amines (Zivin *et al.*, 1976; Brodner and Dohrmann, 1977), disturbances of energy metabolism (Anderson *et al.*, 1976, 1982), release of arachidonic acid (Hallenbeck, Jacobs and Faden, 1983; Demediuk *et al.*, 1985), changes in ion metabolism (Young and Flamm, 1982; Young, Yen and Blight, 1982; Young *et al.*, 1982), particularly calcium (Young, Yen and Blight, 1982; Stokes, Fox and Hollinden, 1983) and the formation of free radicals (Seligman *et al.*, 1977).

Despite the wealth of information concerning the pathologic and metabolic events in SCI, the loss of neurological function after injury remains poorly understood. Given the current level of understanding, the goals of therapy throughout the intensive care period include reversing the mechanical (compressive) disturbance and arresting the ongoing pathologic processes that lead to irreversible cord damage and permanent neurological deficits.

Intensive care management

The intensive care management of acute SCI has a twofold goal. The first is to maintain spinal cord patency and avoid additional spinal cord or nerve root injury. This is achieved by careful attention to external fixation often using a halo device or Gardner-Wells tongs. Complications from these devices are rare and usually consist of pin-site infection or pin loosening and pressure sores. Conscientious use of the log-rolling technique allows these patients to be nursed on standard beds, preventing pressure sores while avoiding further neurological compromise. The second goal is to monitor and treat secondary complications of SCI such as respiratory insufficiency, cardiovascular instability, gastrointestinal and urologic complications and sepsis. These complications may be life threatening and require vigorous management in the intensive care unit.

Respiratory complications

A frequent complication of SCI is respiratory insufficiency. The respiratory problems that develop depend on the level and extent of injury. Spinal cord injury involving the cervical segments C3–5 interrupts phrenic nerve function and may result in bilateral hemidiaphragmatic paralysis (Albin, 1984). Additionally, the intercostal musculature may be paralysed leaving only the strap muscles, sternocleidomastoid, trapezius, and scalene to perform the work of breathing. This situation results in a stereotypic breathing pattern referred to as abdominal paradox. With this pattern, the abdominal wall is sucked in due to a negative pressure gradient created by the raising of the hemidiaphragms by accessory muscle contraction. The activity cannot sustain adequate ventilation and respiratory failure develops rapidly. Lower cervical injury spares phrenic nerve function for the most part. However, the normal stabilizing effect of intercostal muscle contraction on the rib cage is lost, which makes diaphragmatic movement less effective. The net effect of unopposed diaphragmatic contraction is paradoxical inward motion of the upper and middle rib cage during inspiration.

Bedside assessment of pulmonary function includes, in addition to ventilatory rate and rib cage and abdominal wall movement, arterial blood gas determination of Pa_{O_2} and Pa_{CO_2} and measurement of vital capacity. Ventilatory failure ($Pa_{CO_2} > 50$ mmHg (6.6 kPa) and $Pa_{O_2} < 70$ mmHg (9.3 kPa)) requires mechanical support. In cervical injuries, the neck must remain immobilized, although endotracheal intubation can usually be carried out (see Chapter 5).

Despite being widely accepted, there is no scientific work to support the belief that nasotracheal intubation is better tolerated in the intensive care unit and that patients require less sedation (Hefner, 1988). Indeed, in one study, discomfort was found to be similar in patients intubated either by the oral or nasal route (Depoix *et al.*, 1987). Nasal bleeding was registered in 45.3% of patients intubated through the nose. Moreover, in 9.4% of these patients a positive culture was revealed just after intubation; only 2.3% of the patients intubated through the mouth had a positive blood culture. Another not entirely recognized, but serious complication of nasotracheal intubation is paranasal sinusitis followed by septicemia. In many centers, nasotracheal intubation has been discarded as a routine approach. If it is indicated, less than 5 days of use is recommended (Bindsher, 1989).

Tracheostomy as an emergency procedure is rarely necessary. In general, timing of tracheostomy should be determined by observing laryngeal abnormalities rather than by a predetermined length of tracheal intubation (Colice, Stukel and Dain, 1989). Increasing mucosal ulceration along the posteromedial aspects of the vocal cords and laryngeal edema and patients requiring support for more than 4 weeks are indications for tracheostomy. In this group, tracheostomy may bring about earlier resumption of eating and communication and make tracheopulmonary toilet easier.

In the spontaneously breathing quadriplegic patient, respiratory muscle function is maximized in the supine position (Luce and Culver, 1982). This position however makes aspiration of gastric contents more likely and interferes with early mobilization of patients. With these constraints, careful continued monitoring of pulmonary function is mandatory.

Intercostal and abdominal wall muscle paralyses prevent the normal development of raised intra-abdominal and intrathoracic pressure to handle secretions and leads to a higher frequency of mucus plugging and pneumonia. In addition to careful suctioning through the endotracheal tube, which can produce significant bradycardia in patients with autonomic hyperreflexia, quad coughing can be used to clear secretions. This maneuver requires a therapist to press forcibly on the abdomen to expel secretions.

Overall intensive respiratory monitoring after SCI includes respiratory rate, vital capacity, pulse oximetry, and arterial blood gas measurements. The results of the above parameters determine the need for supplemental oxygen or mechanical ventilation. Adequate ventilation may be, in part, position dependent and changes in position may alter respiratory function. In neck injuries, movement of the neck must be avoided. Maintaining adequate oxygenation, particularly in the immediate period after SCI, may help to minimize cord injury due to ischemia.

Mechanical ventilation
Mechanical ventilation may be required after SCI to maintain adequate ventilation in patients with intercostal or phrenic nerve damage or to allow sufficient oxygenation after aspiration or chest trauma. The main aims of ventilatory support are to maintain adequate gas exchange, to diminish barotrauma and to improve synchronization between patient and machine effort. Several modes of ventilation have been introduced, including high frequency ventilation (HFV), inverse ratio ventilation (IRV), positive end expiratory pressure (PEEP), intermittent mandatory ventilation (IMV), and negative end expiratory pressure (NEEP).

The efficacy of HFV remains largely unproven, mainly due to technical problems such as disconnection or kinking of the jet catheter, hypothermia, CO_2 retention and insufficient humidification (Berre *et al.*, 1987; Holzapeel *et al.*, 1987). Many patients do not demonstrate improved gas exchange until the mean airway pressure has been raised. Mean alveolar pressure has been shown to exceed airway pressure during high frequency oscillatory ventilation which indicates that the lung volume increases more than during static inflation (Smith, Frankel and Ariangno, 1988). However, a study of a patient with severe respiratory insufficiency showed that ventilation with a combination of high frequency positive pressure ventilation with low rate conventional mechanical ventilation yielded consistently better arterial oxygenation and lower pulmonary shunt at lower inspired oxygen fractions (Barzilay *et al.*, 1987).

The better results are ascribed to lower peak pressure, lower PEEP and a lower oxygen fraction whereby barotrauma and oxygen toxicity are minimized. Inverse ratio ventilation is a new approach to the improvement of gas exchange by minimizing peak inflation pressure. If PEEP is held constant, the increase in mean alveolar pressure provided by IRV may improve gas exchange without substantially increasing the risk of barotrauma. However, it is not yet clear whether IRV offers any advantages over conventional ventilation. Moreover, because IRV tends to cause air trapping, it is not recommended for patients with airflow obstruction.

Recently, NEEP has been reintroduced. In one laboratory study, the hemodynamic effects of NEEP compared favorably with those of PEEP (Skaburskis, Helal and Zidulda, 1987). NEEP, -9 cmH$_2$O (-0.9 kPa), produced the same increase in functional residual capacity (FRC) as did 10.8 cmH$_2$O (1.0 kPa) of PEEP. Gas exchange did not, however, differ significantly between the two modes, although cardiac output was 15.8% higher during NEEP than during PEEP, which was reflected in an increased mixed venous oxygen saturation.

Why cardiac output is reduced by PEEP remains unclear. A recent clinical study of patients with adult respiratory distress syndrome, a not uncommon complication of high cord injury, demonstrated decreased left and right ventricular end diastolic volumes, which were related to a preload reduction in both ventricles accompanied by a change in ventricular configuration caused by external compression (Potkin *et al.*, 1987). Furthermore, the right and left ventricular ejection fractions did not decline with progressive degrees of PEEP.

Another review of the effects of PEEP on hemodynamic changes during mechanical ventilation yielded different findings (Biondi *et al.*, 1988). A significant initial decline in right ventricular volume at low PEEP levels (0–5 cmH$_2$O; 0–0.5 kPa) was consistent with a decrease in right venticular preload. At higher PEEP levels (15–20 cmH$_2$O; 1.5–2 kPa) the right ventricle volume increased consistently with either an increase in right ventricular afterload or with a decline in the contractile state of the right ventricle. A concomitant decrease in the right ventricle ejection fraction and stroke volume index occurred. Perhaps decreased thoracic compliance in the first group blunted the hemodynamic changes, which may explain the discrepancies of ejection fractions, although laboratory studies have not confirmed the importance of different patient populations in this area. In animals made respiratorily insufficient and low in compliance by injection of N-nitroso-N-methyl methane, the fractional transmission of a given airway pressure to pleura and pericardium was directly related to pulmonary compliance (Venus, Cohen and Smith, 1988). However, the presence of low lung compliance did not blunt the hemodynamic consequences of PEEP, since a higher airway pressure was required to inflate the injured lungs.

Another study in a dog model indicated that most of the reduced alveolar perfusion caused by PEEP is a result of direct compression of the alveolar capillaries rather than a reduction of cardiac output (Nieman, Paskanik and Bredenberg, 1988).

PEEP, by distending the lungs, may compress the atria. Atrial natriuretic peptide (ANP) is released from the atrial cardiocytes during atrial distension and has natriuretic, vasorelaxant and aldosterone-inhibiting properties. During mechanical ventilation and PEEP, levels of ANP are significantly depressed, causing decreased cardiac index, urinary flow and urinary sodium excretion (Leithner *et al.*, 1987; Frass *et al.*, 1988). Thus urinary output should not be used as a guide to adequacy of volume replacement in the mechanically ventilated patient with SCI. Rather, measurements from a pulmonary artery catheter should be used as a more accurate indicator of volume status.

At present, the best method for maintaining adequate respiratory status in a patient with SCI who requires mechanical ventilation is with continuous positive airway pressure and intermittent mechanical ventilation at the lowest number required to maintain adequate oxygenation and prevent atelectasis.

Weaning
Weaning from respiratory support is an important aspect of intensive care. Since mechanical ventilation is likely to entail complications such as infection, tracheal injury, barotrauma, oxygen toxicity and cardiovascular compromise, discontinuation should be achieved as soon as possible.

Several problems are associated with weaning, and positive predication criteria have been established including minute ventilation of <10 liters, a maximum voluntary ventilation maneuver of double the minute ventilation, vital capacity >1 liter, maximal inspiratory pressure of less than -30 cmH$_2$O (-2.9 kPa), an alveolar–arterial oxygen tension difference of <350 mmHg (46.5 kPa) with $F_{IO_2} = 1.0$, V_D/V_T <0.6 and FRC >50% of predicted (Sporn and Morganroth, 1988). Other conditions that may compromise the ability to wean include infection, fever, hypervolemia, dysrhythmias, nutritional deficiencies, decreased levels of consciousness, pain and psychological impairment, all of which are particularly common in the quadriplegic patient. However, in general, adopting the above criteria, the failure rate is about 5.5% in elderly patients with progressive cardio-pulmonary dysfunction and almost negligible in young, previously healthy patients (Demling *et al.*, 1988). If head injury complicates the SCI, the need for reintubation is about 5%. On the other hand, the morbidity rate due to failed extubation is almost 50% in all groups. Whether weaning is achieved by T-piece or decreased continuous positive airway pressure (CPAP) does not affect the failure rate. Failure is more likely to occur in patients intubated for more than one week.

A recently introduced parameter, still under investigation, estimates the work of breathing (WOB) by indirect calorimetry, expressed as the percentage difference in oxygen consumption between spontaneous and mechanical ventilation. In a comparison of healthy volunteers and patients recovering from respiratory failure, the average WOB for healthy volunteers was 3.7%; for patients successfully weaned, 7.7%; and for those who were unable to maintain spontaneous respiration, 24.7% (Lewis *et al.*, 1988).

Cardiovascular complications

Acute phase
Cardiovascular complications of SCI are brought about by disturbances of the autonomic nervous system. Cardiovascular homeostasis is dependent upon an intact autonomic nervous system. SCI involving the cervical cord interrupts sympathetic innervation of the heart which exit the spinal cord in preganglionic fibers at the first through fourth thoracic levels (Clemente, 1985). Parasympathetic control is exerted through the vagus nerve which exists from the medulla oblongata well above the SCI. An autonomic imbalance favoring parasympathetic control is created. Lehmann *et al.* (1987) studied cardiovascular abnormalities accompanying acute SCI clinically. They concluded that the autonomic imbalance and unopposed parasympathetic tone is responsible for the frequently observed association of bradydysrhythmias with cervical but not thoracic or lumbar cord lesions, including the subnormal rise in heart rate with high dose atropine, the lack of heart rate response to propranolol after parasympathetic blockade, the prevention of bradydysrhythmias with low dose sympathomimetic agents and the ability of unopposed vagal tone to mimic many of the observed results, including bradycardia, sinus arrest, atrioventricular block and atrial fibrillation. Hypotension is another major cardiovascular complication of acute cervical cord injury (Meinecke, Rosenkranz and Durek, 1971; Mathias *et al.*, 1979). It is associated with a decrease in systemic vascular resistance and increased cardiac output (Meyer *et al.*, 1971). Vasodilatation is the likely primary disturbance, and can be explained by a loss of arteriolar sympathetic tone.

Several investigators have examined the effect of SCI on the cardiovascular system in the animal model (Alexander and Kerr, 1964; Greenhoot and Mauck, 1972; Greenhoot, Shiel and Mauck, 1972; Eidelberg, 1973; Evans, Kobrine and Rizzoli, 1980). These studies reveal an initial hyperadrenergic response, with a systemic pressor response and a widened pulse pressure lasting several minutes after injury (Greenhoot, Shiel and Mauck, 1972; Dro *et al.*, 1982). This initial response results from an acute activation of the sympathetic nervous system and adrenal medulla (Young *et al.*, 1980). It is rarely appreciated clinically, as the pressor response is presumed to have receded before the initial examination of the patient. The phase is followed within minutes by hypotension, bradycardia and cardiac rhythm changes (Greenhoot and Mauck, 1972; Tibbs *et al.*, 1978; Rawe and Perot, 1979). The absence of normal sympathetic function can persist for days to weeks after SCI causing cardiovascular instability requiring intensive care management. The time course for resolution of cardiovascular abnormalities parallels that of 'spinal shock' which is manifested by flaccid paralysis, areflexia and bowel and bladder atony (Mathias and Frankel, 1983).

Chronic phase
Eventually a chronic cord syndrome evolves which includes spasticity, involuntary muscle spasms and hyperreflexia. The autonomic nervous system develops a hyperactive state termed 'autonomic hyperreflexia' that is manifested by paroxysmal hypertension, sweating and cutis anserina triggered by cutaneous or visceral stimulation below the lesion (Shea *et al.*, 1973). This process of sympathetic dis-inhibition probably leads to the resolution of the bradydysrhythmias, hypotension and other cardiovascular abnormalities which develop shortly after injury (Lehmann *et al.*, 1987). The mechanism responsible for autonomic hyperreflexia is still incompletely understood. Possible mechanisms include a loss of reflex inhibitory sympathetic control from higher centers, and increase in adrenoceptor number or function, or an alteration in the metabolism of neurotransmitters (Naftchi *et al.*, 1974; Mathias *et al.*, 1976a).

Monitoring
In patients with severe cord injuries, cardiovascular abnormalities should be anticipated. Blood pressure is best measured continuously through a radial artery catheter or by finger plethysmography acutely. Heart rate is measured by electrocardiographic (ECG) monitoring. In patients with central venous access, cardiac output is measured through a pulmonary artery catheter.

Cardiovascular therapy
In previous studies (Piepmeier *et al.*, 1985; Lehmann *et al.*, 1987) bradydysrhythmias were present in all patients suffering severe cervical SCI. Other problems include supraventricular tachydysrhythmias and cardiac arrest. In a study of patients with severe cervical injury, 5 of 31 suffered cardiac arrest (Lehmann *et al.*, 1987). Severe bradydysrhythmias, marked hypotension, supraventricular and ventricular tachy-dysrhythmias and atrioventricular block were frequent antecedents to the arrest. These warning signs may be used to identify patients at risk. Transvenous pace-makers should be inserted (Botel, Schottky and Uhlenbruch, 1978).

Therapy for patients with cardiovascular abnormalities is divided into treatment for hypotension and for bradydysrhythmias. Fluid replacement is the first step for treatment of hypotension. Vasoconstricting agents are used when fluid replacement is ineffective. The usual agents are phenylephrine and dopamine (Christensen *et al.*, 1975; Mathias *et al.*, 1976b). Bradydysrhythmias are treated with intermittent injections of atropine. This is not always effective treatment, as the proposed mechanism for the slow heart rate is inadequate sympathetic rather than excessive parasympathetic tone. Isoproterenol infusions may reduce the rate of dysrhythmias and, possibly, cardiac arrest in this group of patients, although controlled trials have not yet been completed.

Gastrointestinal complications

Gastric and intestinal atony is common in SCI. If unrecognized it may lead to gastric aspiration or to abdominal distension. Abdominal distension can cause ventilatory compromise by creating upward pressure on the diaphragms. Early nasogastric tube placement lowers the risk for both complications. Peptic ulceration with hemorrhage or perforation is a relatively infrequent but potentially dangerous complication. The usual signs of perforated viscus – abdominal guarding, rigidity and tachycardia – may be absent in patients with SCI. A lateral decubitus abdominal film will reveal free air. Acid/base monitoring of gastric contents and maintaining pH above 4.0 may reduce the risk of peptic ulceration. Pancreatitis may also complicate SCI. If it develops, patients are kept on nasogastric suction and fed intravenously until amylase levels return to normal. Oral feedings are withheld until evidence of intestinal function returns. Intravenous hyperalimentation is utilized for patients with prolonged atony.

After severe SCI the bladder is initially distended due to acute denervation. The lack of sensation results in overdistension and urinary stasis. Urinary complications can be avoided with the use of intermittent catheterization in the acute phase. Eventually many patients develop reflex emptying of the bladder, reducing the risk of infection and calculi.

Infection

Sepsis is a major problem in the intensive care of the patient with high SCI. More than 80% of patients admitted to an intensive care unit for 5 or more days develop an infection (Dobb, 1989). In 60–100% of patients with prolonged tracheal intubation, the tracheobronchial tree is colonized either by *Pseudomonas* sp., enteric Gram-negative bacilli, or by *Staphylococcus aureus*. More than 50% of these patients develop pneumonia (Bartlett, 1987). The risk of sepsis is greatest in the traumatized patient – approaching 50% (Potgieter *et al.*, 1987). One factor promoting Gram-negative overgrowth of the stomach and subsequent retrograde pharyngeal colonization is the increase in the pH of gastric contents caused by antacids or H_2-histamine receptor blockers. These drugs are commonly given to critically ill patients as prophylaxis against stress-induced upper gastrointestinal bleeding. Significantly lower concentrations of Gram-negative organisms in gastric aspirates, pharyngeal swabs and tracheal aspirates may be achieved by using sucralfate instead of antacids and/or H_2-receptor blockers (Driks *et al.*, 1987). Also, the risk of pneumonia is reduced by 50%. Sucralfate maintains the gastric acid barrier and provides prophylaxis against upper gastrointestinal bleeding.

The prophylactic use of antibiotics has long been advocated (Dobb, 1989). In laboratory studies, topically applied polymyxin B and gentamicin, combined with intravenous penicillin, has been shown to be beneficial in reducing the incidence of pneumonia and maintaining lobar sterility (Johanson *et al.*, 1988a). Similar findings have been obtained in patients who received 50 mg polymyxin B, 80 mg gentamicin dissolved in 10 ml saline 0.9% and instilled every 6 h into the nose, oropharynx and stomach (Unertl *et al.*, 1987). Amphotericin B was also used locally to decrease yeast colonization. Other studies have successfully used an oral paste of non-absorbable antibiotics, Orabase[R] (Squibb) containing 2% polymyxin E, 2% tobramycin, and 2% amphotericin B in combination with intravenous cefotaxime and a gastric mixture of polymyxin E, tobramycin and amphotericin B (Van Uffelen, Rommes and Van Saene, 1987). Still other clinical studies have indicated equally beneficial effects from nebulized tobramycin (Vogel, Krauscrill and Rommelsheim, 1988). Other prospective studies have concluded that although the frequency of pneumonias may be reduced, should respiratory infection develop it is due to selection of resistant bacteria, treatment is difficult and mortality is high (Baumgartner and Glauser, 1987). This local antiseptic approach, although not yet proven effective in large clinical trials, is a promising therapeutic intervention.

All these prophylactic regimens have been shown to reduce the frequency of oropharyngeal and/or gastric colonization with potentially pathogenic organisms. Most likely an antibiotic scheme such as selective parenteral and enteral antisepsis regimen (SPEAR) reduces the risk of nasocomial pneumonia in intensive care unit patients (Anonymous, 1988; Ledingham *et al.*, 1988).

Sepsis from catheter
Vascular catheterization is employed in almost 100% of patients in intensive care units. The risk of catheter-related sepsis is reduced by adhering to strict protocols for insertion and care. The exact relation between incidence of infection and duration of catheter insertion, use of multilumen catheter and other infective foci is unknown. One large study indicated that femoral catheters were colonized more than twice as frequently as subclavian catheters (Collignon *et al.*, 1988). Generally, catheter colonization is low with arterial (0–1.8%) and central venous cannulae (1.2%), and much higher for pulmonary artery catheters (5.9%) and intra-arterial balloon pumps (14.3%) despite duration of insertion (Hudson-Civetta *et al.*, 1987; Damen, 1988; Ducharme *et al.*, 1988; Rose *et al.*, 1988). Frequent changing of triple lumen catheters over a guidewire every 3 days has not been shown to reduce the rate of colonization (Powell *et al.*, 1988).

Sampling for infection
Inaccuracy in the assessment of routine sputum cultures and of tracheal aspiration through endotracheal or tracheostomy tubes is problematic. Tracheal aspirates reveal up to 78% of all lung organisms, but have a high false-positive rate. Bronchoalveolar lavage reveal 74% of organisms, with a much lower false-positive rate (Martin *et al.*, 1987; Johanson *et al.*, 1988b).

Although endotoxemia may be predictive of septicemia, it does not identify the source of the organism. In ICU patients this is often a nasocomial pneumonia which can be difficult to diagnose in intubated patients because bacterial isolates may be caused by colonization rather than infection, and pulmonary infiltrates can have a non-infective cause. The presence of elastin fibres with many bacteria on examination of Gram-stained sputum (>1 organism per 1000× microscope field) is highly predictive of infection rather than colonization (Salata *et al.*, 1987).

Therapy of sepsis
A study of human volunteers has assessed the effect of ibuprofen, a cyclo-oxygenase inhibitor, on the response to an endotoxin infusion (Revhaug *et al.*, 1988). Ibuprofen reduced the fever, tachycardia and the increase in the metabolic rate and stress hormone response to endotoxin infusion, but did not affect the leucocytosis or increase in C-reactive protein concentration, perhaps due to inhibition of prostaglandin synthesis. However, the febrile response to sepsis may enhance the killing of infecting organism, and cyclo-oxygenase inhibitors can precipitate renal failure.

Two recent multi-center prospective studies have shown that steroid administration to patients with sepsis not only provides no benefit but may actually increase morbidity and mortality by increasing secondary infection (Bone *et al.*, 1987; Veterans Administration, 1987). Thus, although steroids are still often employed in the care of patients with central nervous system injury, their use has not been associated with improved outcome.

Naloxone, although improving hemodynamic variables in animals, has given inconsistent results in clinical studies (Roberts *et al.*, 1988).

Therapy of infection remains mainly supportive, with administration of appropriate antibiotics. The infective source must be identified and treated, by surgical means if indicated (e.g. excision of thrombosed veins and decubitus ulcers). Cryoprecipitate infusions have been used to normalize plasma fibronectin concentrations during septicemia and appear to improve organ function (Hesselvik *et al.*, 1987). Fibronectin, a major opsonin that facilitates the clearance of organisms and other particles from the blood by monocytes and fixed macrophages, is often reduced in patients with severe sepsis (Hesselvik, 1987).

Sedation

Sedative drugs may be hazardous in patients with respiratory insufficiency due to SCI or concomitant head injury (Bingham and Hinds, 1987). However, appropriate sedation and pain relief is essential to reduce the stress response, lower intracranial pressure, decrease the distress caused by procedures such as endotracheal suctioning, allay anxiety, encourage sleep and facilitate controlled ventilation (Willatts *et al.*, 1988).

The depth of sedation should be assessed regularly, aiming for a comfortable, cooperative patient who is easily aroused. Physiologic variables are remarkably unreliable in the SCI patient. Linear analogue scores are subjective and do not give a reproducible response between observers. The EEG and power spectral analyses have proved valuable in assessing sedation (Veselis *et al.*, 1988). Further development is required before this technique is routinely used in the intensive care unit. Lower esophageal contractility is affected by so many drugs that it cannot, as yet, be used as a reliable indicator of sedation (Evans, Bithell and Vlachonikolis, 1987).

Ideally, a sedative drug should have a short half-life, inactive metabolites, no adverse systemic effects, no drug interactions or organ toxicity and be excreted independently of renal or hepatic function (Willatts, 1989). Although administering drugs by continuous infusion is advantageous, in the critically ill patient changes in organ perfusion and impaired metabolism require constant attention to the rate of administration. Opioids produce drowsiness, euphoria and analgesia, but also nausea and vomiting, truncal rigidity, prolonged ventilatory depression, impaired intestinal absorption and, perhaps, tolerance. Gastric emptying is also reduced and may compound the delays already caused by SCI. Morphine is extensively taken up by the tissues but, because it is relatively lipid insoluble, it crosses the blood brain barrier slowly. In hypotensive patients, liver blood flow is reduced and thus clearance of the drug is reduced. Morphine excretion is also reduced by sepsis, inotropic therapy and renal failure. Fentanyl in high dosage reduces the stress response to trauma. It is highly fat soluble and single doses have a short duration of action. However, after prolonged administration, clearance depends solely on metabolism. Profound respiratory depression occurs. Alfentanil is short acting, with an elimination half-life of 100 min. It is a potent analgesic with a lack of cardiovascular effects (Cohen and Kelly, 1987). Studies have compared sedation caused by propofol and midazolam combined with morphine, given by continuous infusion in intubated patients, and found easier control and faster weaning with propofol (Grounds *et al.*, 1987). However, heart rate and blood pressure may be reduced more by propofol, limiting its use in the SCI patient (Newman *et al.*, 1987).

Diazepam is a useful sedative, anticonvulsant and amnesic agent. Its metabolite, desmethyl-diazepam is also a sedative, accounting for prolonged somnolence. Midazolam, a water-soluble benzodiazepine derivative, has a wide variation in effective dose (Oldenhof *et al.*, 1988). Antagonism with opioids may occur. In the critically ill patient, the half-life of midazolam is unpredictably increased. Hepatic clearance is reduced in the presence of cimetidine.

Conclusions

Spinal cord injury continues to be an important cause of morbidity, particularly in young adults in their maximally productive years. There has been much improvement in minimizing the complications associated with SCI and in providing effective rehabilitation programs once the acute management is completed. Current intensive care management in the acute setting of injury focuses on the cardiovascular complications of dysrhythmia and hypotension, preserving renal functions and avoiding sepsis, as well as preventing gastrointestinal and thromboembolic complications.

References

Albin, M.S. (1984) Acute spinal cord trauma. In *Textbook of Critical Care* (eds W.C. Shoemaker, W.L. Thompson and P.R. Holbrook), W.B. Saunders Co., Philadelphia, pp. 928–936

Alexander, S. and Kerr, F.W.L. (1964) Blood pressure responses in acute compression of the spinal cord. *Journal of Neurosurgery*, **21**, 485–491

Allen, A.R. (1914) Remarks on the histopathological changes in the spinal cord due to impact An experimental study. *Journal of Nervous and Mental Diseases*, **41**, 141

Anderson, D.K., Means, E.D., Waters, T.R. and Green, E.S. (1982) Microvascular perfusion and metabolism in injured spinal cord after methylprednisolone treatment. *Journal of Neurosurgery*, **56**, 106–113

Anderson, D.K., Prockop, L.D., Means, E.D. and Hartley, L.E. (1976) Cerebrospinal fluid lactate and electrolyte levels following experimental spinal cord injury. *Journal of Neurosurgery*, **44**, 715–722

Anonymous (1988) Microbial selective decontamination in intensive care patients. *Lancet*, **i**, 803

Bartlett, J.G. (1987) Diagnosis of bacterial infections of the lung. *Clinical Chest Medicine*, **8**, 119–134

Barzilay, E., Lev, A., Ibrahim, M. and Lesmes, C. (1987) Traumatic respiration insufficiency: comparison of conventional mechanical ventilation to high-frequency positive pressure with low-rate ventilation. *Critical Care Medicine*, **15**, 118–121

Baumgartner, J.D. and Glauser, M.P. (1987) Antibiotics for prevention of bacterial pneumonia in an intensive care unit. *Schwiezerische Medizinische Wochenschrift*, **117**, 707–711

Berre, J., Ros, A.M., Vincent, J.L., Dufaye, P., Brimioulle, S. and Kahn, R.J. (1987) Technical and psychological complications of high-frequency jet ventilation. *Intensive Care Medicine*, **13**, 96–99

Bindsher, L. (1989) Respiratory care. *Current Opinion in Anesthesiology*, **2**, 173–177

Bingham, R.M. and Hinds, C.J. (1987) Influence of bolus doses of phenoperidine on intracranial pressure and systemic arterial pressure in traumatic coma. *British Journal of Anaesthesia*, **59**, 592–595

Biondi, J.W., Schulman, D.S., Soufer, R., Matthay, R.A., Hines, R.L., Kay, H.R. and Barash, P.G. (1988) The effect of incremental positive end-expiratory pressure on right ventricular hemodynamics and ejection fraction. *Anesthesia and Analgesia*, **67**, 144–151

Bone, R.C., Fisher, C.J. Jr, Clemmer, T.P., Slotman, G.J., Metz, C.A. and Balk, R.A. (1987) A controlled clinical trial of high-dose methylprednisolone in the treatment of severe sepsis and septic shock. *New England Journal of Medicine*, **317**, 653–658

Botel, U., Schottky, H. and Uhlenbruch, K. (1978) Die Anwendung von Herzschrittmachern wegen unfallbedingter, rezidvierender Herzstillstande bei hohen Halsmarklahmungen. *Hefte zur Unfallheilkunde*, **132**, 370–373

Brodner, R.A. and Dohrmann, G.J. (1977) Norepinephrine, dopamine and serotine in experimental spinal cord trauma: current status. *Paraplegia*, **15**, 166–71

Christensen, N.J., Frankel, H.L., Mathias, C.J. and Spalding, J.M.K. (1975) Enhanced pressor response to noradrenaline in human subjects with chronic sympathetic decentralization. *Journal of Physiology*, **252**, 39P–40P

Clemente, C.D. (ed.) (1985) Visceral nervous system. In *Gray's Anatomy of the Human Body*. Lea and Febiger, Philadelphia, pp. 1247–1272

Cohen, A.T. and Kelly, D.R. (1987) Assessment of alfentanil by intravenous infusion as long-term sedation in intensive care. *Anaesthesia*, **42**, 545–556

Colice, G.L., Stukel, T.A. and Dain, B. (1989) Laryngeal complications of prolonged intubation. *Chest*, **96**, 877–884

Collignon, P., Soni, N., Pearson, I., Sorrell, T. and Woods, P. (1988) Sepsis association with central venous catheters in critically ill patients. *Intensive Care Medicine*, **14**, 227–231

Damen, J. (1988) The microbiologic risk of invasive hemodynamic monitoring in open heart patients requiring prolonged ICU treatment. *Intensive Care Medicine*, **14**, 156–162

Demediuk, P., Saunders, R.D., Clenendon, N.R., Means, E.D., Anderson, D.K. and Korrocks, L.A. (1985) Changes in lipid metabolism in traumatized spinal cord. *Progress in Brain Research*, **63**, 1–16

Demling, R.H., Read, T., Lind, L.J. and Flanagan, H.L. (1988) Incidence and morbidity of extubation failure in surgical intensive care patients. *Critical Care Medicine*, **16**, 573–577

Depoix, J.P., Malbezin, S., Videcoq, M., Hazebroucq, J., Barbier-Bohm, G., Gauzit, R. and Desmonts, J.M. (1987) Oral intubation versus nasal intubation in adult cardiac surgery. *British Journal of Anaesthesia*, **59**, 167–169

Dobb, G.J. (1989) Sepsis. *Current Opinion in Anesthesiology*, **2**(2), 185–191

Driks, M.R., Craven, D.E., Celli, B.R., Manning, M., Burke, R.A., Garving, M., Kunches, L.M., Farber, H.W., Wedel, S.A. and McCabe, W.R. (1987) Nosocomial pneumonia in intubated patients given sucralfate as compared with antacids or histamine type 2 blockers: the role of gastric colonization. *New England Journal of Medicine*, **317**, 1376–1382

Dro, P., Gschaedler, R., Dollfus, P., Komminoth, R. and Florange, W. (1982) Clinical and anatomical observation of a patient with a complete lesion at C1 with maintenance of a normal blood pressure during 40 minutes after the accident. *Paraplegia*, **20**, 169–173

Ducharme, F.M., Gauthier, M., Lacroix, J. and Lafleur, L. (1988) Incidence of infection related to arterial catheterization in children – a prospective study. *Critical Care Medicine*, **16**, 272–276

Eidelberg, E.E. (1973) Cardiovascular response to experimental spinal cord compression. *Journal of Neurosurgery*, **38**, 326–331

Evans, D.E., Kobrine, A.I. and Rizzoli, H.V. (1980) Cardiac arrhythmias accompanying acute compression of the spinal cord. *Journal of Neurosurgery*, **52**, 52–59

Evans, J.M., Bithell, J.F. and Vlachonikolis, I.G. (1987) Relationship between lower oesophageal contractility, clinical signs and halothane concentration during general anaesthesia and surgery in man. *British Journal of Anaesthesia*, **59**, 1346–1355

Frass, M., Popvic, R., Hartter, E., Auinger, C., Woloszcauk, W. and Leithner, C. (1988) Atrial natriuretic peptide decrease during spontaneous breathing with continuous positive airway pressure in volume-expanded healthy volunteers. *Critical Care Medicine*, **16**, 831–835

Greenhoot, J.H. and Mauck, H.P. (1972) The effects of cervical cord injury on cardiac rhythm and conduction. *American Heart Journal*, **83**, 659–662

Greenhoot, J.H., Shiel, F.O.M. and Mauck, H.P. (1972) Experimental spinal cord injury: electrocardiographic abnormalities and fuchsinophilic myocardial degeneration. *Archives of Neurology*, **26**, 524–529

Griffiths, I.R. (1975) Vasogenic edema following acute and chronic spinal cord compression in the dog. *Journal of Neurosurgery*, **42**, 155

Grounds, R.M., Lalor, J.M., Lumley, J., Royston, D. and Morgan, M. (1987) Propofol infusion for sedation in the intensive care unit: preliminary report. *British Medical Journal*, **294**, 397–400

Hallenbeck, J.M., Jacobs, T.P. and Faden, A.I. (1983) Combined PGI2, indomethacin and heparin improves neurologic recovery after spinal trauma in cats. *Journal of Neurosurgery*, **58**, 749–754

Hefner, J.E. (1988) Tracheal intubation in mechanically ventilated patients. *Clinical Chest Medicine*, **9**, 23–35

Hesselvik, J.F. (1987) Plasm fibronectin levels in sepsis – influencing factors. *Critical Care Medicine*, **15**, 1092–1097

Hesselvik, F., Brodin, B., Carlsson, C., Cedergren, B., Jorfeldt, L. and Lieden G. (1987) Cryoprecipitate infusion fails to improve organ function in septic shock. *Critical Care Medicine*, **15**, 475–483

Holzapeel, L., Robert, D., Perrin, F., Gaussorques, P. and Giudicelli, D.P. (1987) Comparison of high-frequency jet ventilation to conventional ventilation in adults with respiratory distress syndrome. *Intensive Care Medicine*, **13**, 100–105

Hudson-Civetta, J.A., Civetta, J.M., Martinez, O.V. and Hoffman, T.A. (1987) Risk and detection of pulmonary artery catheter-related infection in septic surgical patients. *Critical Care Medicine*, **15**, 29–34

Johanson, W.G., Seidenfeld, J.J., De Los Santos, R., Coalson, J.J. and Gomez, P. (1988a) Prevention of nosocomial pneumonia using topical and parenteral antimicrobial agents. *Amercian Review of Respiratory Diseases*, **137**, 265–272

Johanson, W.G., Seidenfeld, J.J., Gomez, P., De Los Santos, R. and Coalson, J.J. (1988a) Bacteriologic diagnosis of nosocomial pneumonia following prolonged mechanical ventilation. *American Review of Respiratory Diseases*, **137**, 259–264

Ledingham, I.McA., Alcock, S.R., Eastway, A.T., McDonald, J.C., McKay, I.C. and Ramsay, G. (1988) Triple regimen of selective decontamination of the digestive tract, systemic cefotaxime, and microbiological surveillance for prevention of acquired infection in intensive care. *Lancet*, **i**, 785–789

Lehmann, K.G., Lane, J.G., Piepmeir, J.M. and Batsford, W.P. (1987) Cardiovascular abnormalities accompanying acute spinal cord injury in humans: incidence, time course and severity. *Journal of the American College of Cardiologists*, **10**, 46–52

Leithner, C., Frass, M., Pacher, R., Hartter, E., Pesl, H. and Woloszczuk, W. (1987) Mechanical ventilation with positive end-expiratory pressure decreases release alpha-atrial natriuretic peptide. *Critical Care Medicine*, **15**, 484–488

Lewis, W.D., Chwals, W., Benotti, P.N., Lakshman, K., O'Donnell, C., Blackburn, G.L. and Bistrian, B.R. (1988) Bedside assessment of the work of breathing. *Critical Care Medicine*, **16**, 117–122

Luce, J.M. and Culver, B.H. (1982) Respiratory muscle function in health and disease. *Chest*, **81**, 82

Marar, B.C. (1974) The pattern of neurological damage as an aid to the diagnosis of the mechanism in cervical spine injuries. *Journal of Bone and Joint Surgery*, **56-A**, 1648–1654

Martin, W.J. II, Smith, T.F., Sanderson, D.R., Brutinel, W.M., Cockerill, F.R. III and Douglas, W.W. (1987) Role of bronchoalveolar lavage in the assessment of opportunistic pulmonary infections: utility and complication. *Mayo Clinic Proceedings*, **62**, 549–557

Mathias, C.J., Christensen, N.J., Corbett, J.L., Frankel, H.L. and Spalding, J.M.K. (1976a) Plasma catecholamines during paroxysmal neurogenic hypertension in quadriplegic man. *Circulation Research*, **39**, 204–208

Mathias, C.J., Christensen, N.J., Frankel, H.L. and Spalding, J.M.K. (1979) Cardiovascular control in recently injured tetraplegics in spinal shock. *Quarterly Journal of Medicine*, **48**, 273–287

Mathias, C.J. and Frankel, H.L. (1983) Clinical manifestations of malfunctioning sympathetic mechanisms in tetraplegia. *Journal of the Autonomic Nervous System*, **7**, 303–312

Mathias, C.J., Frankel, H.L., Christensen, N.J. and Spalding, J.M.K. (1976b) Enhanced pressor response to noradrenaline in patients with cervical spinal cord transection. *Brain*, **99**, 757–770

Meinecke, F.W., Rosenkranz, K.A. and Durek, C.M. (1971) Regulation of the cardiovascular system in patients with fresh injuries to the spinal cord: preliminary report. *Paraplegia*, **9**, 109–112.

Meyer, G.A., Berman, I.R., Doty, D.B., Mosely, R.V. and Guitierrez, V.S. (1971) Hemodynamic responses to acute quadriplegia with or without chest trauma. *Journal of Neurosurgery*, **34**, 168–177

Naftchi, N.E., Wooten, G.F., Lowman, E.W. and Axelrod, J. (1974) Relationship between serum dopamine-β-hydroxylase activity, catecholamine metabolism and hemodynamic changes during paroxysmal hypertension in quadriplegia. *Circulation Research*, **35**, 850–861

Newman, L.H., McDonald, J.C., Wallace, P.G.M. and Ledingham, I.McA. (1987) Propofol infusion for sedation in intensive care. *Anaesthesia*, **42**, 929–937

Nieman, G.F., Paskanik, A.M. and Bredenberg, C.E. (1988) Effect of positive end-expiratory pressure on alveolar capillary perfusion. *Journal of Thoracic and Cardiovascular Surgery*, **95**, 712–716

Oldenhof, H., De Jong, M., Steenhoek, A. and Janknegt, R. (1988) Clinical pharmacokinetics of midazolam in intensive care patients, a wide interpatient variability. *Clinical Pharmacology and Therapeutics*, **43**, 263–269

Piepmeier, J.M., Lehmann, E.B. and Lane, J.G. (1985) Cardiovascular instability following acute cervical spinal cord trauma. *CNS Trauma*, **2**(153), 60

Potgieter, P.D., Linton, D.M., Oliver, S. and Forder, A.A. (1987) Nosocomial infections, **15**, 495–498

Potkin, R.T., Hudson, L.D., Weaver, L.J. and Trobaugh, G. (1987) Effect of positive end-expiratory pressure on right and left ventricular function in patients with the adult respiratory distress syndrome. *American Review of Respiratory Diseases*, **135**, 307–311

Powell, C., Kudsk, K.A., Kulich, P.A., Mandelbaum, J.A. and Fabri, P.J. (1988) Effect of frequent guidewire changes on triple lumen catheter sepsis. *Journal of Parenteral and Enteral Nutrition*, **12**, 462–464

Rawe, S. and Perot, P. (1979) Pressor response resulting from experimental contusion injury to the spinal cord. *Journal of Neurosurgery*, **50**, 58–63

Revhaug, A., Michie, H.R., Manson, J.McK., Watters, J.M., Dinarello, C.A., Wolff, S.M. and Wilmore, D.W. (1988) Inhibition of cyclo-oxygenase attenuates the metabolic response to endotoxin in humans. *Archives of Surgery*, **123**, 162–170

Roberts, D.E., Dobson, K.E., Hall, K.W. and Light, R.B. (1988) Effects of prolonged naloxone infusion in septic shock. *Lancet*, **ii**, 699–701

Rose, S.G., Pitsch, R.J., Karrer, F.W. and Moor, B.J. (1988) Subclavian catheter infections. *Journal of Parenteral and Enteral Nutrition*, **12**, 511–512

Salata, R.A., Lederman, M.M., Shlaes, D.M., Jacobs, M.R., Eckstein, E., Tweardy, D., Toossi, A., Chmielewski, R., Marino, J., King, C.H., Graham, R.C. and Ellner, J.J. (1987) Diagnosis of nosocomial pneumonia in intubated, intensive care unit patients. *American Review of Respiratory Diseases*, **135**, 426–432

Seligman, M.L., Flamm, E.S., Goldstein, B.D., Poser, R.G., Demopoulos, H.B. and Ransohoff, J. (1977) Spectrofluorescent detection of malonaldehyde as a measure of lipid free radical damage in response to ethanol potentiation of spinal cord trauma. *Lipids*, **12**, 945–950

Shea, J.D., Gioffre, R., Carrion, H. and Small, M.P. (1973) Autonomic hyperreflexia in spinal cord injury. *South Medical Journal*, **66**, 869–872

Skaburskis, M., Helal, R. and Zidulda, A. (1987) Hemodynamic effects of external continuous negative pressure ventilation compared with those of continuous positive pressure ventilation in dogs with acute lung injury. *American Review of Respiratory Diseases*, **136**, 886–891

Smith, D.W., Frankel, L.R. and Ariangno, R.L. (1988) Dissociation of mean airway pressure and lung volume during high-frequency oscillatory ventilation. *Critical Care Medicine*, **16**, 531–535

Sporn, P.H.S. and Morganroth, M.L. (1988) Discontinuation of mechanical ventilation. *Clinical Chest Medicine*, **9**, 113–126

Stewart, W.B. and Wagner, F.C. (1979) Vascular permeability changes in contused feline spinal cord. *Brain Research*, **169**, 163–167

Stokes, B.T., Fox, P. and Hollinden, G. (1983) Extracellular calcium activity in the injured spinal cord. *Experimental Neurology*, **80**, 561–572

Tibbs, P., Young, B., McAllister, R., Brooks, W. and Tackett, L. (1978) Studies of experimental cervical spinal cord transection. *Journal of Neurosurgery*, **49**, 558–562

Unertl, K., Ruckdeschel, G., Selbmann, H.K., Jensen, U., Frost, H., Lenhart, F.P. and Peter, K. (1987) Prevention of colonization and respiratory infection in long-term ventilated patients by local antimicrobial prophylaxis. *Intensive Care Medicine*, **13**, 106–113

Van Uffelen, R., Rommes, J.H. and Van Saene, H.K.F. (1987) Preventing lower airway colonization and infection in mechanically ventilated patients. *Critical Care Medicine*, **15**, 99–102

Venus, B., Cohen, L.E. and Smith, R.A. (1988) Hemodynamics and intrathoracic pressure transmission during controlled mechanical ventilation and positive end-expiratory pressure in normal and low compliant lungs. *Critical Care Medicine*, **16**, 686–690

Veselis, R.A., Long, C.W., Shah, N.K. and Bedford, R.F. (1988) Increased EEG activity correlates with clinical sedation. *Critical Care Medicine*, **16**, 383

Veterans Administration Systemic Sepsis Cooperative Study Group (1987) Effect of high-dose glucocorticoid therapy on mortality in patients with clinical signs of systemic sepsis. *New England Journal of Medicine*, **317**, 659–665

Vogel, F., Krauscrill, P. and Rommelsheim, K. (1988) Prevention of pneumonias in artificially ventilated patients. *Atemweg Lungenkrank*, **14**, 108–112

Willatts, S.M. (1989) Sedation. *Current Opinion in Anesthesiology*, **2**, 202–205

Willatts, S.M., Kong, K.L., Prys-Roberts, C., Harvey, J. and Irish, M.J. (1988) Plasma catecholamine concentrations during sedation for ventilated patients requiring intensive therapy. *British Journal of Anaesthesia*, **59**, 502P

Young, W., Decrescito, V., Tomashula, J. and Ho, V. (1980) The role of the sympathetic nervous system in pressor responses induced by spinal injury. *Journal of Neurosurgery*, **52**, 473–481

Young, W. and Flamm, E.S. (1982) Effect of high-dose corticosteroid therapy on blood flow, evoked potentials and extracellular calcium in experimental spinal injury. *Journal of Neurosurgery*, **57**, 667–673

Young, W., Koreh, I., Yen, V. and Lindsay, A. (1982) Effect of sympathectomy on extracellular potassium ionic activity and blood flow in experimental spinal cord contusion. *Brain Research*, **253**, 115–124

Young, W., Yen, V. and Blight, A. (1982) Extracellular calcium ionic activity in experimental spinal cord contusion. *Brain Research*, **253**, 105–113

Zivin, J.A., Doppman, J.L., Reid, J.L., Tappaz, M.L., Shavedra, J.M., Kopin, I.J. and Jacobowitz, D.M. (1976) Biochemical and histochemical studies of biogenic amines in spinal cord trauma. *Neurology*, **26**, 99–107

Chapter 7

Anaesthetic care for spinal injuries: parenteral nutrition

Olli Kirvelä and Jeffrey Askanazi

Introduction

The outcome of any injury depends on the severity of the trauma and on the therapeutic support given to optimize recovery. Nutritional support is a fundamental part of this therapy. If adequate nutrition is not provided, the patient has to mobilize his or her own energy stores, which may severely impair recovery. Nutritional support can be given either enterally or parenterally. The enteral route is the more natural way of giving artificial nutrition, although in some circumstances parenteral nutrition is required or recommended. This chapter will concentrate on parenteral nutrition.

Little is known about the acute metabolic requirements of patients with spinal cord injury (SCI). Such patients are usually fed enterally, but there are situations in the acute period when parenteral nutrition is needed. Spinal cord injuries are often complicated by other traumas. This often results in prolonged delays in oral or enteral feeding, until gastrointestinal function returns; consequently, attempts to achieve nitrogen balance with enteral feeding in the early postoperative or post-trauma period in complicated neuorsurgical patients have been largely unsuccessful (Haider *et al.*, 1975; Savitz *et al.*, 1978; Rapp *et al.*, 1983). Poor tolerance for enteral feeding has been observed in the first 14 days following head injury (Twyman *et al.*, 1985; Norton *et al.*, 1988); increased gastric residuals, prolonged paralytic ileus, abdominal distension, aspiration pneumonitis, and diarrhea may delay initiation of enteral alimentation for as long as 3 weeks (Young *et al.*, 1987; Norton *et al.*, 1988). It is therefore suggested that parenteral nutritional support be utilized following SCI until enteral nutrition can be tolerated.

Parenteral nutrition may decrease morbidity and mortality in critically ill neurosurgical patients; several studies have shown that parenteral support has a favorable effect on outcome in severely brain injured patients (Rapp *et al.*, 1983; Waters, Dechert and Bartlett, 1986; Young *et al.*, 1987). When no complicating factors are present, however, enteral feeding should be preferred in patients with SCI.

The design of optimal metabolic and nutritional support programs for spinal cord injured patients relies on an understanding of the metabolic responses and nutritional complications that occur with SCI. These issues will therefore be reviewed briefly.

General principles

Body composition

The body is composed of fat and lean body mass (LBM). The latter is subdivided into extracellular fluid (ECF), body cell mass (BCM) and extracellular supportive structures such as skeleton, cartilage and tendons. The sum of the LBM and adipose tissue is equal to total body weight (TBWt). Fat functions as the energy storage area. It is a relatively anhydrous mass, with water representing only about 5% by weight, whereas in skeletal muscle the total water content is 80% by weight. Since fat provides 9.5 cal/g and fat tissue is only 5% water, this is a very compact storage area. Metabolic use of 1 g of fat results in 9000 kcal, whereas 1 kg of skeletal muscle yields only 800 kcal.

Extracellular mass consists of plasma, interstitial water, transcellular water – cerebral spinal fluid (CSF), pericardial fluid, and fluid in the joint spaces – and the supporting structures, such as skeleton, tendons and cartilage. Body cell mass is the metabolically active portion of the LBM. It consists of skeletal muscle (60%), viscera (30%) and the cells of the supporting structure of the extracellular mass, such as red blood cells and the cellular component of adipose tissue. The standard 70 kg man contains about 20 kg of fat and about 50 kg of LBM, about equally divided by weight as ECF and BCM. These parameters vary with sex, body build and age. Females tend to have decreased LBM and increased adipose tissue. The ratio of LBM to TBWt also decreases with age. Very muscular individuals will have a greater than normal ratio of LBM : TBWt. These relationships remain constant as long as caloric intake equals expenditure. Excess energy is stored as fat; there are no storage deposits of protein, and glycogen cannot be stored in any significant amount.

Fuel stores

To maintain adequate metabolism during periods of increased energy needs or reduced dietary intake, expenditure of endogenous tissue stores is required. The energy available from circulating substrates is negligible. Carbohydrate is stored as glycogen in liver and muscle. The average healthy adult stores 200–300 g of carbohydrate, which can provide approximately 900 kcal. This can fulfill energy requirements for only 8–10 h; thus the glycogen stores become depleted within the first 24 h of starvation.

Fat contributes about 15–30% of body weight. The average adult male has about 140 000 kcal stored as fat. This constitutes 85% of the total body energy stores and is the major energy source during periods of prolonged starvation. Fat is stored as triglyceride.

Protein is present in lean body tissue, the major part in skeletal muscle and visceral organs. Fourteen to 20% of body weight is protein, giving a total available amount of some 24 000 kcal. Although protein breakdown provides some energy, this is by no means its main function. Some loss of function always accompanies the use of LBM for the generation of energy.

An individual's total caloric storage could potentially sustain life for 2 months; in practical terms, however, most persons would be at the point of death upon burning approximately 140 000 kcal, or about 75% of their fat and 50% of their protein. This occurs in approximately 60 days during a complete unstressed fast, but metabolic stress due to injury or surgery may dramatically speed up depletion of the body's energy stores.

Body composition, trauma and spinal cord injury

Changes in body composition in post-trauma patients result from various combinations of starvation, injury, infection, different substrate infusions, and other factors that may be less well defined.

The rate of LBM loss increases with the severity of surgical trauma (Kinney *et al.*, 1968). Both surgical and accidental trauma will often necessitate the administration of large quantities of fluid, causing an acute increase in the ECF compartment (Ariel and Kreman, 1950; Elwyn, Bryan-Brown and Shoemaker, 1975). These fluids are not usually retained in normal patients, but underlying complications, such as sepsis, may cause a failure in diuresis. After initial fluid resuscitation, sepsis has been shown to be associated with further increases in ECF volume and decreases in serum sodium concentration (Insel and Elwyn, 1986).

Infusions of glucose alone will cause an absolute and relative increase in ECF. One week of carbohydrate feeding can produce the fully developed kwashiorkor syndrome (marked expansion of ECF with pitting edema, ascites, and anasarca) in an undernourished child (Viteri *et al.*, 1969). In adults the normal 5% dextrose infusion (100 g glucose/day) results in marked sodium retention with little effect on potassium losses; i.e. administration of carbohydrate as the only nutrient exacerbates the increased ECF : BMC ratio (Gamble, 1946–47). The use of 5% dextrose-saline has been found to abolish the sodium loss completely, while potassium loss exceeds that of a complete fast, thus resulting in a greater ECF : BCM ratio than total starvation. Carbohydrates can also increase ECF when given in great excess, even if protein is given simultaneously (Schutz *et al.*, 1982).

An expanded ECF volume is generally considered undesirable. It is correlated with postoperative complications and undesirable effects on pulmonary and cerebral function (Elwyn, Bryan-Brown and Shoemaker, 1975; Savitz *et al.*, 1978). Adequate nutrition will result in a relative decrease of ECF when water retention has occurred for nutritional reasons alone. However, if the expanded ECF is the result of trauma or sepsis, nutritional support alone may not be sufficient.

Protein depletion will affect the protein content of all organs. The liver and gut are rapidly depleted, while the brain is affected less than other organs. In severe protein depletion, the gut may be unable to tolerate or digest food, presumably because protein is needed to produce digestive enzymes. Skeletal muscle is most affected and may lose as much as 70% of its protein.

Spinal cord injury has some unique effects of major clinical importance on fluid and electrolyte balance. It results in lowered salt tolerance. Hyperphosphatemia and hypermagnesemia are also frequent in early SCI, and there is increased urinary excretion of bone minerals in early phases. Sustained stimulation of the juxtaglomerular apparatus and increased plasma renin activity (PRA) may result from the removal of descending inhibition on the sympathetic nervous system (Claus-Walker and Halstead, 1982). Plasma renin activity has no direct physiologic effect on the body, but it stimulates angiotensin II formation, which has a hyper-tensive effect and also promotes synthesis of aldosterone.

Skeletal muscle paralysis is the major consequence of the partial isolation of the somatic nervous system (Geiser and Trueta, 1958; Downey and Darling, 1971; Sutton, 1973). This paralysis leads to various metabolic changes. Progressive weight loss, an increased proportion of body fat (Cardus, Spencer and McTaggart, 1969), and a decreased lean body mass (Cardus and McTaggart, 1972) are a constant finding in these patients. Decreased urine creatinine per unit of body weight occurs in early

SCI, due to a reduction of creatinine phosphorylation to phosphocreatinine and hydrolysis to creatinine in muscle, accompanied by high blood and urine creatinine (Lindan, 1967; Cardus, Spencer and McTaggart, 1969; Cardus and McTaggart, 1972). Hyperuricosuria without hyperuricosemia has been observed in early SCI, possibly due to a loss of intracellular purines. Fluid compartment volumes are in the normal range, but there is a relative increase of the ECF to intracellular volume. Fluid balance is strongly negative for the first month post-injury (Claus-Walker *et al.*, 1977–78a). Relatively high urine potassium ion observed in early SCI is probably due to losses of intracellular material (Claus-Walker *et al.*, 1977, 1977–78b). This is followed by low exchangeable potassium ion and relatively low serum potassium ion later (Cardus, Spencer and McTaggart, 1969; Claus-Walker *et al.*, 1977, 1977–78a).

Low normal serum Na^+ and variable urine Na^+ have been reported in early SCI (Claus-Walker, 1977–1978b), with very low urine Na^+ in late SCI and high exchangeable Na^+, which was probably stored in the relatively increased ECF (Cardus, Spencer and McTaggart, 1969). Spinal cord injury is followed by the histochemical appearance of atrophied muscle fibers which contain fewer enzymes and more connective tissue, lipids, and water than normal fibers (Lindan, 1967; Cardus, Spencer and McTaggart, 1969; Grimby *et al.*, 1976; Herbison, Jaweed and Ditunno, 1978).

Energy generation

By metabolism of carbohydrate, lipid and protein, energy is released for mechanical work, synthesis, membrane transport and thermogenesis. Under different circumstances, glucose, amino acids, fatty acids, triglycerides, lactate and ketones all play a role in energy generation. Glucose metabolism generally occurs along the glycolysis and the oxidative phosphorylation pathway. Glycolysis produces a small amount of adenosine triphosphate as compared to oxidative phosphorylation, since it proceeds anaerobically; however, it becomes important during anoxic and hypoxic conditions. Fatty acids and amino acids are metabolized aerobically and use slightly more oxygen per kilocalorie of energy generated than does glucose.

Metabolic response to spinal cord injury and surgery

Classically the metabolic response to trauma is divided into the early 'ebb' or shock phase and the subsequent 'flow' phase (Cuthbertson, 1942). The shock phase is associated with an early period of weight gain due to fluid sequestration. The metabolic rate is depressed, body temperature is lowered, and the circulating blood volume reduced. It is followed after a day or two by the catabolic flow phase, in which metabolic activity is increased. In this stage, body energy stores are mobilized to meet increased needs. Weight is lost as the retained fluid is mobilized along with fat and lean body mass. Maximal nitrogen loss generally occurs between the 4th and 8th day after injury. Nitrogen excretion and resting energy expenditure (REE) are increased as a function of the severity of the trauma (Cuthbertson and Tilstone, 1969; Kinney *et al.*, 1970). The catabolic phase is followed by the anabolic or recovery phase. The degree of the catabolic response depends on the severity and duration of the trauma or stress.

The catabolic response can be viewed as a mobilization of body stores of glycogen, protein, and fat to ensure adequate circulatory levels of substrate (glucose, fatty acids and amino acids) when dietary intake is limited. The increased available amino acid pool occurs predominantly at the expense of skeletal muscle. These amino acids may be oxidized directly for fuel, but are mainly used for gluconeogenesis; this process also makes more precursors available for synthesis of visceral protein and the proteins of tissue repair.

In response to injury, gluconeogenesis is increased despite the high circulating levels of glucose (Long *et al.*, 1971). This hyperglycemia, referred to as the 'diabetes of injury', reflects the urgent nature of glucose requirements for the healing tissues (Chen and Postlewait, 1964). Fat is mobilized to obtain high circulating levels of fatty acids, and is used for the energy needs of cardiac, skeletal and respiratory muscles; this allows glucose to be spared for tissues that specifically require it, such as the central nervous system, the cellular immune system and the healing wound. There is an increased body metabolism in response to trauma which is characterized by fever and enhanced oxygen consumption. The hormonal changes include increased release of adrenal glucocorticoid, glucagon and catecholamines. These changes contribute to the mobilization of energy stores and provision of gluconeogenic substrates.

The metabolic response to SCI is to some extent similar to what occurs after general body trauma. However, there are some important differences. Several factors, such as steroids, nutritional support, and barbiturates, modify the metabolic response to spinal cord trauma. The level of injury and transection are also decisive for the response. The presence of other injuries and tissue damage will increase the extent of metabolic response in these patients.

The extent of metabolic response to SCI has been poorly defined. Metabolic changes in SCI are affected by the denervation of the area below transection and are unique because of the muscle atrophy that results from paralysis. The atrophy results in protein breakdown, which may provide a reservoir of amino acids that can supply not only the nitrogen but also the caloric needs of the patients. All of this leads to altered body composition.

The decrease in metabolic needs can be very significant. In one study of the caloric needs of 5 acute quadriplegics, actual mean energy expenditure was only 67% of the expected energy expenditure (Kearns *et al.*, 1983). In chronic patients after spinal transection, the calorie requirements are generally diminished in relation to the level of injury (Mollinger *et al.*, 1985).

Another important factor is that many patients with SCI are treated with glucocorticoids. Clearly, steroids are harmful to protein metabolism, causing increased catabolism and impairing the resistance to infection, which, when it occurs, increases metabolic demands (Kaktis and Pitts, 1980).

The diminished metabolic response can be seen as a consequence of spinal cord transection. This causes some of the differences in metabolic response compared to other types of trauma. Serial measurements of catecholamines and their metabolites and blood dopamine beta-hydroxylase (an enzyme which increases the formation of norepinephrine (noradrenaline) in nerve endings, needed for formation of norepinephrine (noradrenaline) from dopamine in nerve endings) demonstrated that immediately after trauma, plasma epinephrine (adrenaline) and norepinephrine (noradrenaline) and their urinary metabolites were usually in low normal range. As long as there was no stimulation, catecholamines and their metabolites remained low thereafter (Claus-Walker and Halstead, 1982). Low normal values were also found for dopamine beta-hydroxylase blood levels (Claus-Walker and Halstead, 1982). This results also in reduction of hemodynamic control and unpredictable circulatory responses to stress. In patients with added chest injuries, vascular spaces may become overexpanded by intravenous infusion, leading to pulmonary edema.

Altered glucose metabolism has been found in this patient group during stress and non-stress conditions. The rate of changes in blood sugar are slower than normal, and stress response can be inappropriate in certain types of stress. These alterations in glycogenolysis may contribute in part to a temporary decrease in glucose available to the brain, which has been observed in these patients (Claus-Walker and Halstead, 1982). Evaluation of blood glucose during stress discloses frequent inappropriate increases during surgery.

Goals and indications for parenteral nutrition

Goals of parenteral nutrition

Optimal parenteral nutrition provides the organism with all the substrates it needs in well-balanced amounts, so that there will be no further deterioration to the metabolic profiles. It has three main goals. The first is to maintain body tissue; this is a prophylactic support in which total parenteral nutrition (TPN) is given to prevent the development of malnutrition. The second is to replete body tissues in the already malnourished patient. The third is the prevention and correction of specific micronutrient deficiencies (vitamins, trace elements, etc.).

The first step in planning any nutritional regimen is to identify the need for intervention. The next step is to determine the route of delivery. The last step is to prescribe the required amounts of macronutrients and micronutrients based on the clinical setting and nutritional assessment of the patient.

Indications for parenteral nutrition

To determine whether a patient needs parenteral nutrition, numerous questions have to be answered. Does the period and degree of metabolic derangement jeopardize the patient's recovery from SCI? Is it possible to meet the patient's caloric and protein needs with enteral or oral feeding or is parenteral nutrition required? Will aggressive nutritional therapy improve the patient's recovery?

Patients who are well nourished and have no complicating factors should receive conventional hypocaloric fluid therapy and enteral or oral feeding. However, if the patient is depleted prior to injury, more aggressive nutritional therapy may be needed.

Severe metabolic abnormalities are observed after multiple injuries and surgery. Such patients are hypercatabolic and are at high risk of rapidly developing malnutrition, even though their pre-morbid nutritional status was adequate. In these patients, TPN has been shown to improve outcome and decrease morbidity and mortality. Enteral nutrition may not be well tolerated and its use may seriously delay the initiation of adequate nutritional support; therefore, parenteral nutrition is required until enteral nutrition can be tolerated.

Practical aspects of parenteral nutrition

Nutritional requirements

Requirements for different nutrients vary greatly depending on the type of injury and underlying status.

Energy
Energy expenditure should be estimated by some method to prevent insufficient caloric intake as well as overfeeding. Under ordinary circumstances, the basal energy expenditure can be calculated from the Harris-Benedict equation. The equation is based on the patient's sex, weight (W), height (H) and age (A):

$$\text{Female: } 655 + 9.6(W) + 1.7(H) - 4.7(A) = \text{kcal/day}$$
$$\text{Male: } 66 + 13.7(W) + 5(H) - 6.8(A) = \text{kcal/day}$$

In SCI these calculations are only of limited value. There are too many factors to be considered: the extent of trauma, level of SCI, respiratory support, possible infection and fever, etc. The metabolic needs also fluctuate heavily from day to day. All this makes accurate prediction of energy expenditure impossible in complicated cases. Energy requirements can also be established using indirect calorimetry. The introduction of new, smaller and easy to use machines has made this method available for clinical practice. Bedside metabolic charts and monitors are now readily available and are capable of measuring daily energy expenditures to within 10%. In patients with SCI, measurement of energy expenditure is by far preferable to estimates of energy expenditure and is therefore recommended. Failure to provide full replacement of expended calories will result in consumption of body protein to a marked degree. Avoidance of underfeeding through nutritional assessment may reduce the mortality and morbidity associated with coma of acute onset. Although extremes of underfeeding may have complications, so may overfeeding; overfeeding, particularly with glucose, may lead to hypermetabolism, hyperglycemia and hyperosmolality, hepatic steatosis, increased intracranial pressure and elevated CO_2 production.

Nitrogen balance is sensitive to protein intake as well as to total energy (calories) consumed; for comparative caloric amounts, the effect of protein exceeds that of non-protein calories. Optimal nutritional support first maximizes protein intake and only then adds sufficient calories in the form of glucose and fat to cover the energy requirements (Blackburn *et al.*, 1977). A positive nitrogen balance cannot be achieved by giving amino acids alone. Non-protein calories can reduce nitrogen excretion, but only to a minimal level in the absence of protein intake (Calloway and Spector, 1954). Thus both protein and non-protein energy are required. However, the effects of nitrogen and energy intake on nitrogen balance are not independent of one another; their interaction is complex. If nitrogen intake is adequate, zero nitrogen balance is achieved when caloric intake meets caloric expenditure. Similarly, increasing caloric intake above requirements increases nitrogen retention and results in net positive nitrogen balance (Cuthbertson, McCutcheon and Munro, 1937). Changes in body composition that occur with hyperalimentation have been found to consist of approximately two parts fat to one part lean body mass (Keys, Anderson and Brozek, 1955), but will depend on the precise composition of the nutritional regimen.

The large nitrogen loss that occurs during the first 6 days of fasting can be halved by daily ingestion of as little as 100 g of glucose. The nitrogen-sparing effect of a relatively small (400 kcal/g) caloric load occurs only with carbohydrates, since fat does not produce the same suppression of nitrogen excretion during fasting (Cathcart, 1909). On the other hand, restriction of either fat or carbohydrate in the diet increases nitrogen output, although nitrogen loss is greater with carbohydrate restriction (Werner *et al.*, 1949), while restoring either improves nitrogen retention (Munro, 1964). The ability of fat as compared to glucose to spare nitrogen has been studied extensively. At low dosages, glucose is clearly superior to fat. When carbohydrate is administered in amounts of more than 600 kcal/day, the nitrogen-sparing effects of fat and carbohydrate are equal (Munro, 1964), while fat has only a small nitrogen-sparing effect in the absence of 600 kcal/day of carbohydrates (Brennan *et al.*, 1975; Long *et al.*, 1977).

However, no differences in nitrogen balances have been detected in studies comparing groups receiving the non-protein calories in form of glucose ('glucose system') with those whose non-protein calories were supplied as half fat and half glucose ('lipid system') (MacFie, Smith and Hill, 1981; Nordenström *et al.*, 1983). When the lipid system is administered, a lesser calorigenic response and a decreased norepinephrine (noradrenaline) excretion have been found compared to the glucose system (Nordenström *et al.*, 1981). A reduction in carbon dioxide production has also been observed in patients receiving the lipid system, which may be of critical importance in patients with reduced pulmonary reserves or in weaning patients from respirators (Askanazi *et al.*, 1981). Liver function tests have shown fewer abnormalities when lipid was used to replace one-third of the glucose calories (Meguid *et al.*, 1984). These studies provide evidence of the efficacy of 20% fat emulsion as a concentrated nutrient source that allows provision of calories without overhydration and hemodilution. General use of fat as a calorie source in TPN in the USA has developed only gradually, despite the fact that fat emulsions represent a logical alternative to glucose loading. This is especially true in patients with an exaggerated caloric requirement and a diminished ability to clear exogenous glucose, as is the case with critically ill neurosurgical patients, as well as those with hepatic or pulmonary dysfunction.

In patients with SCI, nitrogen balance will be inevitably negative in the acute period because of denervation of large masses of muscle. Therefore the use of nitrogen balance as a method of assessing the effectiveness of nutritional support in these patients is senseless. Furthermore, zero nitrogen balance cannot be the goal of nutritional support.

Normally, carbohydrates contribute 40–60%, protein 10–15% and fat 30–40% of the total energy intake. The amount of the protein intake used for energy varies, since some of the amino acids are used for protein synthesis. The non-protein calories can be provided by carbohydrates or fat. A minimum of approximately 500 kcal/day should be administered as glucose to supply carbohydrate for the brain, bone marrow and injured tissue. On the other hand, fat should be given to provide sufficient essential fatty acids (linoleic and linolenic acid). Essential fatty acid deficiency syndrome (EFAD) has been reported in patients who received fat-free intravenous nutrition.

Once the minimal intake for glucose and fat are met, additional non-protein calories may be provided as either of these substrates. The optimum balance of fat and glucose has not yet been determined. Total parenteral nutrition systems with 50% of non-protein calories delivered as fat are as effective in maintaining nitrogen balance as those using 100% glucose, and seem to minimize metabolic complications.

Protein
Negative nitrogen balance is associated with resorption and positive nitrogen balance with deposition of cellular protoplasm. In healthy adults, nitrogen equilibrium is established when daily protein intake is about 1.0 g/kg per day. Surgical stress and possible postoperative complications increase nitrogen requirements; protein intake has to be increased accordingly to prevent loss of cellular protoplasmic mass (with the reservations made above for this patient group). As a simple guide, to make up for the increased protein needs after major surgery and postoperative complications, protein must be increased in proportion to energy (calorie/nitrogen ratio) to about 100–125 kcal/g nitrogen. When a nutritional program is aimed at repleting lean body mass, protein intake must be increased above maintenance protein requirements. However, nitrogen intakes exceeding 20 g/day are not generally considered to be beneficial.

Electrolytes, trace elements, and vitamins are important in maintaining normal metabolic functions. They are essential nutrients and therefore have to be supplied as part of nutritional therapy (Tables 7.1 and 7.2). Electrolytes, however, should be closely monitored and administered according to observed changes in electrolyte levels. Changes in electrolytes, discussed above, will occur.

Table 7.1 Recommended daily intakes (RDI) of electrolytes and micronutrients by parenteral route (After Shenkin, 1986, by permission)

Electrolyte/micronutrient	RDI	Unit
Natrium	1.0–1.4	(mmol/kg)/day
Kalium	0.7–0.9	(mmol/kg)/day
Calcium	0.11	(mmol/kg)/day
Phosphorus	0.15	(mmol/kg)/day
Magnesium	0.04	(mmol/kg)/day
Iron	20	μmol
	1.1	mg
Zinc	100	μmol
	6.4	mg
Copper	20	μmol
	1.3	mg
Iodine	1.0	μmol
	127	mg
Manganese	5	μmol
	0.27	mg
Fluoride	50	μmol
	0.95	mg
Chromium	0.2	μmol
	0.01	mg
Selenium	0.4	μmol
	0.03	mg
Molybdenum	0.2	μmol
	0.02	mg

Table 7.2 Recommended daily intakes (RDI) of vitamins in parenteral nutrition (From Shenkin, 1986, by permission)

Vitamin	RDI		Unit
	American Medical Association	Glasgow Royal Infirmary	
Retinol	1000	1000	μg
	3300	3300	IU
Ergocalciferol	5	5	μg
	200	200	IU
α-Tocopheryl	10	10	mg
Vitamin K	–	150	μg
Ascorbic acid	100	100	mg
Thiamine	3.0	3.0	mg
Riboflavin	3.6	3.6	mg
Pyridoxine	4.0	4.0	mg
Niacin	40	40	mg
Vitamin B_{12}	60	60	μg
Pantothenic acid	15	15	mg
Biotin	60	60	μg
Folic acid	400	400	μg

Administration of nutrients

Several systems have been developed for the administration of parenteral nutrition. It is separated into two subgroups, according to the route of administration: peripheral and central parenteral nutrition.

Peripheral parenteral nutrition
Short-term intravenous nutrition can be administered by peripheral vein. The limiting factor in peripheral nutrition is the osmolality of the solution, since peripheral veins do not tolerate hyperosmolal liquids. Blackburn et al. (1973) suggested a regimen consisting of a diluted amino acid solution alone. Unfortunately this kind of treatment is still widely used, even though it has been shown to be both ineffective and expensive (Elwyn et al., 1978). In Central European countries the use of diluted amino acid solutions, together with either fructose, sorbitol or xylitol as the non-protein caloric source, is widespread in postoperative nutritional support. These products usually contain electrolytes and even trace elements in varying compositions and are meant to be used as basic postoperative fluid therapy. A commercial mixture of glycerol and amino acids with electrolytes is also available. It is meant for nutritional maintenance in the postoperative period and may have some advantages over conventional solutions in diabetic patients (Lev-Ran et al., 1987). All the therapies presented here are essentially hypocaloric if given in near iso-osmolal concentrations and therefore cannot contain enough calories to cover postoperative needs. Consequently, their use is mainly restricted to patients recovering from uneventful surgery, or needing only supplemental nutrition.

When lipids are added to peripheral nutrition, the caloric content can be substantially increased without raising the osmolality of the solution. An example of such a mixture would be 500 ml of a 20% fat emulsion, 1000 ml of 8.5% amino acid solution and 1000 ml of 10% dextrose. This provides nearly 1800 kcal/day when infused at 100 ml/h. The use of an 'all-in-one system' makes this procedure very simple and safe. The final concentration of dextrose is less than 5%, hence the phlebitis rate is quite low and comparable with that observed with 5% dextrose and saline solution. The results observed with this kind of nutritional support are good because the amounts of nutrients are sufficient for most patients recovering from uncomplicated spinal injury. The therapy can be started on the first postoperative day with full concentration. The water load of the regimen is enough to cover most patient needs. In patients with fluid restriction the use of more concentrated solutions via the central route is recommended. The peripheral vein puncture site should be rotated every 2–3 days to avoid thrombophlebitis.

Parenteral nutrition via central venous route
A central venous line is still the most commonly used route for administration of parenteral nutrition. Many patients who require nutritional support have a central venous line for other reasons and the use of this line for delivering nutrition is then a rational approach. In cases of long-term TPN, however, a separate line for nutrients is recommended. The central line is necessary if high concentrations of glucose or other carbohydrates, amino acids, or electrolytes are needed.

Initiation of TPN with a high concentration of glucose should be gradual. On the first postoperative day we recommend the use of a mixture similar to that used in peripheral parenteral nutrition ('all-in-one'). On subsequent days, glucose concentration can be increased according to blood glucose levels. If blood glucose levels cannot be controlled by changing the glucose concentration, insulin can be given with the mixture.

Delivery of nutrients   Cyclic administration of nutrients has been suggested, alternating dextrose-containing with dextrose-free solutions. This method has the theoretical advantage of avoiding prolonged hyperinsulinemia and allowing release of endogenous fatty acids from adipose tissue and may also optimize visceral protein preservation and avoid alterations in hepatic function (Miani *et al.*, 1976).

Mixing all the components for TPN in one mix ('three-in-one system') before administration simplifies procedures for the nursing personnel and may also reduce the risk of infection. Until now the most common mode of delivery has been to give separate infusions of amino acids, fat and carbohydrate and add vitamins and trace elements into the solutions before infusion ('bottle system'). With this system, the nursing personnel has to mix the components, monitor infusion rate of more solutions given at the same time and change bottles several times during the day. In addition to the work involved for the nursing staff, the mixing of solutions in the ward may not be satisfactory from a hygienic point of view, since it requires considerable manipulation of infusion sets and connections.

Complications   The most common metabolic complications of TPN are hyperglycemia and glucosuria. These depend on the rate of infusion and the carbohydrate source. Frequent monitoring of glucose in urine and serum is required during TPN. If a patient becomes hyperglycemic (blood glucose 250 mg/dl), the infusion rate of glucose should be reduced (Wolfe *et al.*, 1986). Insulin may be administered to the solution if the blood glucose levels cannot be controlled by reducing the amount of glucose infused. The requirement for insulin often decreases rapidly when the patient's stress resolves and the patient shifts from the catabolic to the anabolic state. The need for insulin should be re-evaluated daily by close monitoring of blood and urinary sugars. The tendency towards hyperosmolarity can be prevented if the plasma osmolarity, sodium, blood urea nitrogen, acid/base balance and blood sugar

**Table 7.3 Mechanical catheter-related
complications of total parenteral nutrition**

Central venous catheter
  Malposition
  Catheter embolism
  Air embolism
  Thrombosis and thromboembolism
  Sepsis
  Cardiac dysrhythmias
  Myocardial perforation

Subclavian or internal jugular venipuncture
  Arterial puncture
  Pneumothorax, hemothorax, chylothorax
  Brachial plexus injury
  Mediastinal hematoma

Peripheral venipuncture
  Pain
  Hematoma
  Thrombosis
  Phlebitis
  Extravasation

are carefully monitored. Another frequent metabolic complication is hyper-chloremic acidosis, which can be prevented by decreasing the ratio of chloride to acetate in the TPN (Wolfe *et al.*, 1986). Rapid infusions of amino acid solutions have been associated with nausea, headache, and a warm sensation. When the patient begins to become anabolic, large amounts of K^+ and phosphate shift into the

**Table 7.4 Suggested monitoring schedule during total parenteral nutrition
(From Robin and Gregg, 1986, by permission)**

Parameter	Suggested frequency	
	Early	After stability
Volume in (intravenous and oral)	Daily	Daily
Volume out (urine and drainage)	Daily	Daily
Body temperature	Daily	Daily
Urine S & A	q.i.d.	b.i.d.
Electrolytes	Daily	Biweekly
BUN/creatinine	Biweekly	Biweekly
Ca^{2+}, P, Mg^{2+}	Biweekly	Weekly
CBC, platelets	Weekly	Weekly
Glucose	Daily	Biweekly
PT, PTT	Weekly	Weekly
Triglycerides, cholesterol	Weekly	Weekly
Liver profile	Biweekly	Weekly
ABGs, urine electrolytes, drainage analysis, blood cultures, serum insulin, ketones, plasma amino acids, plasma fatty acids	Variable	Variable
Weight	Biweekly	Biweekly

S & A, sugar and acetone; BUN, blood urea nitrogen; CBC, complete blood count; PT, prothrombin
time; PTT, partial thromboplastin time; ABGs, arterial blood gases.

intracellular space; to avoid a deficit of these, supplementation will be needed. Hepatic dysfunction has been reported. However, replacement of part of the TPN glucose calories with fat leads to better glucose tolerance and fewer hepatic complications (Meguid *et al.*, 1984).

The mechanical catheter-related complications are outlined in Table 7.3. Of these complications, sepsis requires special mention. Strict antiseptic conditions should prevail during catheter placement; if possible, the catheter should be used only for infusion of TPN. The frequency of induction of sepsis is increased with the use of multilumen catheters for TPN (Parsa *et al.*, 1972).

The ability of SCI patients to handle large fluid loads is diminished due to decreased vascular responses; therefore, they are prone to complications caused by overhydration.

Patient monitoring   Table 7.4 gives guidelines for monitoring the patient for the development of infection or metabolic complications. When the patient is stable and tolerating a particular regimen, most of these determinations can be performed less frequently.

Weight should be measured daily; acute changes reflect changes in water and sodium.

New horizons

Spinal cord injury affects ventilation, depending on the level of transection; prolonged ventilatory support may sometimes be necessary. The role of the diaphragm in respiration usually increases in these situations. Diaphragm muscle fatigue has been demonstrated in humans (Juan *et al.*, 1984) and may be responsible for some of the symptoms experienced by patients with respiratory diseases (Aldrich, Arora and Rochester, 1982), especially upon exertion (Aldrich *et al.*, 1983). Diaphragmatic fatigue refers to the inability of the muscle to maintain an expected force with continued or repeated contraction (Roussos and Moxham, 1985). Studies have also demonstrated that there is an increased incidence of ventilatory fatigue under conditions of undernutrition (Arora and Rochester, 1982).

An alteration in plasma amino acids may play a role in neurotransmission and fatigue (Newsholme and Leech, 1983). Tryptophan is a precursor of 5-hydroxy-tryptamine (5-HT) and serotonin and the resulting decrease in brain serotonin activity may be responsible for the central effects observed with branched chain amino acids (BCAA) enriched infusions on fatigue, ventilation, food intake and gastric emptying. Elevated plasma levels of BCAA may decrease the transport of tryptophan across the blood brain barrier (BBB). In experimental animals the brain serotonin content is related to the brain content of its precursor, tryptophan (Fernstrom and Wurtman, 1971), and tryptophan competes with other large neutral amino acids of the same transport system into the brain (Fernstrom, Larin and Wurtman, 1973). An increased rate of transport of tryptophan across the BBB increases the rate of synthesis of 5-HT in the brain, so increasing the cerebral concentration of 5-HT. There is evidence that an increase in this latter neuro-transmitter can result in sleep, so that it might also cause a decrease in mental alertness and/or cause fatigue. In a recent study in healthy volunteers during sustained exercise, the plasma levels of BCAA decreased significantly, whereas there was no change in total tryptophan (Blomstrand, Celsing and Newsholme,

1988). The plasma concentration of free tryptophan was found to rise 2.4-fold during prolonged exercise (1.5 h). This increase is probably due to pronounced elevation in the concentration of plasma free fatty acids during exercise, since these are known to displace tryptophan from albumin. The observed increase in plasma tryptophan concentration, together with the decrease in plasma concentration of branched chain amino acids, gives rise to a marked increase in the plasma concentration ratio of free tryptophan/branched chain amino acids. This should lead to an increase in the rate of transport of tryptophan across the BBB and hence to an increase in the rate of synthesis of 5-HT in the brain. An elevated concentration of 5-HT in specific areas of the brain may be responsible, at least in part, for the development of physical and/or mental fatigue during prolonged exercise.

Increasing the amino acid content of TPN increases the ventilatory demand by increasing both oxygen consumption and ventilatory drive (Askanazi et al., 1984). The study of Takala et al. (1988), where 85% BCAA solution was compared to standard amino acid solution, showed that not only the quantity of amino acids but also the composition of the amino acid solution affects the ventilatory response. There was a major increase in the ventilatory response to CO_2 inhalation during administration of the BCAA solution which did not occur with the standard solution. Serotonin and its precursors depress both resting ventilation and the ventilatory responses to carbon dioxide in experimental animals, evidently via serotoninergic activation in the brain (Armijo and Florez, 1974; Lunberg, Mueller and Breese, 1980). If the same is true for human beings, an increase in the plasma ratio of the large neutral amino acids to tryptophan may well contribute to increasing respiratory drive during the high supply of branched chain amino acids. The accentuation of the respiratory effects of amino acids by BCAA may have important clinical relevance. Increasing respiratory drive will further increase the work of breathing and make fatigue of respiratory muscles more likely to ensue. On the other hand, recovery of normal ventilatory responsiveness may be enhanced in patients with decreased ventilatory drive due to anesthesia, medication, prolonged administration of 5% dextrose or apneas of different origins. The combined effect of decreasing central fatigue in respiratory muscles and increasing ventilatory drive may prove to be beneficial in SCI patients. However, no clinical data is yet available and therefore no proposals for their clinical use can be made.

It may be possible to increase appetite and food intake by giving BCAA-enriched amino acid solutions. In a recent study we found that TPN with standard amino acid solutions reduces appetite and food intake by an amount that closely compensates for the infused calories (Gil et al., 1990a). This loss in appetite and food intake may prolong the transition from intravenous to oral feeding in patients who need nutritional support. The reduction in food intake previously seen when TPN is administered does not seem to occur or at least is less pronounced when an amino acid solution high in BCAA is given (Gil et al., 1990b). If this regimen really decreases the TPN-related reduction in appetite and food intake, BCAA-enriched solutions may prove useful in the transition from TPN to oral feeding or to increase the total (intravenous + oral) calorie intake.

Aspiration of gastric contents remains a major cause of morbidity and mortality in clinical anesthesia. The use of parenteral nutrition as an adjunct to oral feeding in surgical patients increases the risk of aspiration by further delaying gastric emptying (MacGregor et al., 1979). The recent observation (N. D'Attellis, unpublished data) that an increased BCAA : AA ratio during TPN (as compared to standard amino acid solution) results in stimulation of gastric emptying may have clinical significance. In patients for whom parenteral nutritional support is an essential part of therapy, a BCAA-enriched amino acid solution could offer one possibility of decreasing the risk of aspiration during transition to enteral feeding.

References

Aldrich, T.K., Adams, J.M., Arora, N.S. *et al.* (1983) Power spectral analysis of the diaphragm electromyogram. *Journal of Applied Physiology,* **54**, 1579–1584

Aldrich, T.K., Arora, N.S. and Rochester, D.F. (1982) The influence of airway obstruction and maximal voluntary ventilation in lung disease. *American Review of Respiratory Diseases,* **126**, 195–199

Ariel, I.M. and Kremen, A.J. (1950) Compartmental distribution of sodium chloride in surgical patients pre- and post-operatively. *Annals of Surgery,* **132**, 1009–1026

Armijo, J.A. and Florez, J. (1974) The influence of increased brain 5-hydroxytryptamine upon the respiratory activity of cats. *Neuropharmacology,* **13**, 977–986

Arora, N.S. and Rochester, D.F. (1982) Respiratory muscle strength and maximal voluntary ventilation in undernourished patients. *American Review of Respiratory Diseases,* **126**, 5–8

Askanazi, J., Nordenström, J., Rosenbaum, S.H. *et al.* (1981) Nutrition for the patient with respiratory failure: glucose vs fat. *Anesthesiology,* **54**, 373–377

Askanazi, J., Weissman, C., LaSala, P.A. *et al.* (1984) Effect of protein intake on ventilatory drive. *Anesthesiology,* **60**, 106–110

Blackburn, G.L., Bistrian, B.R., Miani, B.S. *et al.* (1977) Nutritional and metabolic assessment of the hospitalized patient. *Journal of Parenteral and Enteral Nutrition,* **1**, 11–22

Blackburn, G.L., Flatt, J.P., Glowes, G.H.A. *et al.* (1973) Peripheral intravenous feeding with isotonic amino acid solutions. *American Journal of Surgery,* **125**, 447–454

Blomstrand, E., Celsing, F. and Newsholme, E.A. (1988) Changes in plasma concentrations of aromatic and branched chain amino acids during sustained exercise in man and their possible role in fatigue. *Acta physiologica scandinavica,* **133**, 115–121

Brennan, M.F., Fitzpatrick, G.F., Cohen, K.H. *et al.* (1975) Glycerol: major contributor to the short term protein sparing effect of fat emulsions in normal man. *Annals of Surgery,* **182**, 386–394

Calloway, D.H. and Spector, H. (1954) Nitrogen balance as related to calorie and protein intake in active young men. *American Journal of Clinical Nutrition,* **2**, 405–412

Cardus, D. and McTaggart, W.G. (1972) Total creatinine in patients with extensive muscular paralysis estimated by radioisotope tracer method. Baylor College of Medicine, Social and Rehabilitation Services Project R122, Project Report 11, Houston, Texas

Cardus, D., Spencer, W.A. and McTaggart, W.G. (1969) Study of gross composition of body of patients with extensive muscular paralysis. Baylor College of Medicine, Social and Rehabilitation Project RD-1871-M, Final Report, Houston, Texas

Cathcart, E.D. (1909) The influence of carbohydrates and fats on protein metabolism. *Journal of Physiology (London),* **39**, 311–330

Chen, R.W. and Postlethwait, R.W. (1964) The biochemistry of wound healing. *Monographs in the Surgical Sciences,* **1**, 215–276

Claus-Walker, J., Cardus, D., Griffith, D. *et al.* (1977–78a) Metabolic effects of sodium restriction and thiazides in tetraplegic patients. *Paraplegia,* **15**, 3–10

Claus-Walker, J., Carter, R.E., DiFerrante, N.M. *et al.* (1977–78b) Immediate endocrine and metabolic consequences of traumatic quadriplegia in young women. *Paraplegia,* **15**, 202–208

Claus-Walker, J., and Halstead, L.S. (1982) Metabolic and endocrine changes in spinal cord injury: II (Section 2). Partial decentralization of the autonomic nervous system. *Archives of Physical Medicine and Rehabilitation,* **63**, 576–580

Claus-Walker, J., Spencer, W.A., Carter, R.E. *et al.* (1977) Electrolytes and renin-angiotensin-aldosterone axis in traumatic quadriplegia. *Archives of Physical Medicine and Rehabilitation.* **58**, 283–286

Cuthbertson, D.P. (1942) Post-shock metabolic response. *Lancet*, **1**, 433–437
Cuthbertson, D.P., McCutcheon, A. and Munro, H.N. (1937) A study of the effect of overfeeding on the protein metabolism of man. *Biochemical Journal*, **31**, 681–693
Cuthbertson, D.P. and Tilstone, W.J. (1969) Metabolism during the post injury period. *Advances in Clinical Chemistry*, **12**, 1–55
Downey, J.A. and Darling, R.C. (eds) (1971) *Physiological Basis of Rehabilitation Medicine*, Saunders, Philadelphia
Elwyn, D.H., Bryan-Brown, C.W. and Shoemaker, W.C. (1975) Nutritional aspects of body water dislocations in postoperative and depleted patients. *Annals of Surgery*, **182**, 76–85
Elwyn, D.H., Gump, F.E., Iles, M. *et al.* (1978) Protein and energy sparing of glucose added in hypocaloric amounts to peripheral infusions of amino acids. *Metabolism*, **27**, 325–331
Fernstrom, J.D., Larin, F. and Wurtman, R.J. (1973) Correlations between brain tryptophan and plasma neutral amino acid levels following food consumption in rats. *Life Sciences*, **13**, 517–524
Fernstrom, J.D. and Wurtman, R.J. (1971) Brain serotonin content: physiologic dependence on plasma tryptophan levels. *Science*, **173**, 149–152
Gamble, J.L. (1946–47) Physiological information gained from studies on the life raft ration. *Harvey Lectures*, **42**, 247–273
Geiser, M. and Trueta, J. (1958) Muscle action, bone refraction, and bone formation: experimental study. *Journal of Bone and Joint Surgery*, **40-A**, 282–311
Gil, K., Skeie, B., Askanazi, J. *et al.* (1990a) Effect of intravenous nutrition on voluntary food intake (submitted)
Gil, K., Skeie, B., Kvetan, V. *et al.* (1990b) Effect of branched chain amino acid enriched parenteral nutrition on oral food intake (submitted)
Grimby, G., Broberg, C., Krotkiewska, I. *et al.* (1976) Muscle fiber composition in patients with traumatic cord lesion. *Scandinavian Journal of Rehabilitation Medicine*, **8**, 37–42
Haider, W., Lockner, F., Schlick, W. *et al.* (1975) Metabolic changes in the course of severe acute brain damage. *European Journal of Intensive Care Medicine*, **1**, 19–26
Herbison, G.J., Jaweed, M.M. and Ditunno, J.F. (1978) Muscle fiber atrophy after cast immobilization in rat. *Archives of Physical Medicine and Rehabilitation*, **59**, 301–305
Insel, J. and Elwyn, D.H. (1986) Body composition. In *Fluid and Electrolyte Management in Critical Care* (eds J. Askanazi, P. Starker and C. Weissman), Butterworths, London, pp. 3–31
Juan, G.P., Calverley, C., Talamo, J. *et al.* (1984) Effect of carbon dioxide on diaphragmatic function in human beings. *New England Journal of Medicine*, **310**, 874–879
Kaktis, J.V. and Pitts, L.H. (1980) Complications associated with use of megadose corticosteroids in head-injured adults. *Journal of Neurosurgery*, **12**, 166–171
Kearns, P.J., Jr, Pipp, T.L., Qurik, M. *et al.* (1983) Nutritional requirements in quadriplegics. Presented at the Meeting of American Society for Parenteral and Enteral Nutrition, Washington, DC, 23–26 January
Keys, A., Anderson, J.T. and Brozek, J. (1955) Weight gain from single overeating. Character of tissue gained. *Metabolism*, **4**, 427–432
Kinney, J.M., Duke, J.H., Jr, Long, C.L. *et al.* (1970) Tissue fuel and weight loss after injury. *Journal of Clinical Pathology* (suppl. 23), **4**, 65–72
Kinney, J.M., Long, C.L., Gump, F.E. *et al.* (1968) Tissue composition of weight loss in surgical patients. *Annals of Surgery*, **168**, 459–474
Lev-Ran, A., Johnsson, M., Hwang, D.L. *et al.* (1987) Double-blind study of glycerol vs glucose in parenteral nutrition of postsurgical insulin-treated diabetic patients. *Journal of Parenteral and Enteral Nutrition*, **11**, 271–274
Lindan, O. (1967) Metabolism and pathophysiology of spinal cord injury. Final Report, Grant RD 1144, May, Cleveland, Ohio
Long, C.L., Spencer, J.L., Kinney, J.M. *et al.* (1971) Carbohydrate metabolism in man: effect of elective operations and major surgery. *Journal of Applied Physiology*, **31**, 110–116
Long, J.M. III, Wilmore, D.W., Mason, A.D. Jr *et al.* (1977) Effect of carbohydrate and fat intake on nitrogen excretion during total intravenous feeding. *Annals of Surgery*, **185**, 417–422
Lunberg, D.B., Mueller, R.A. and Breese, G.R. (1980) An evaluation of the mechanism by which serotonergic activation depresses respiration. *Journal of Pharmacology and Experimental Therapeutics*, **212**, 397–404

MacFie, J., Smith, R.C. and Hill, G.L. (1981) Glucose or fat as a nonprotein energy source. *Gastroenterology*, **80**, 103–107

MacGregor, I.L., Wiley, Z.D., Lavigne, M.E. *et al.* (1979) Slowed rate of gastric emptying of solid food in man by high caloric parenteral nutrition. *American Journal of Surgery*, **138**, 652–654

Meguid, M.M., Akahoshi, M. Jeffers, S. *et al.* (1984) Amelioration of metabolic complications of conventional TPN: a prospective randomized study. *Archives of Surgery*, **119**, 1294–1298

Miani, B., Blackburn, G.L., Bistrian, B.R. *et al.* (1976) Cyclic hyperalimentation: an optimal technique for preservation of visceral protein. *Journal of Surgical Research*, **20**, 515–525

Mollinger, L.A., Spurr, G.B., El Ghatit, A.Z. *et al.* (1985) Daily energy expenditure and basal metabolic rates of patients with spinal cord injury. *Archives of Physical Medicine and Rehabilitation*, **66**, 420–426

Munro, H.N. (1964) General aspects of the regulation of protein metabolism by diet and by hormones. In *Mammalian Protein Metabolism*, Vol. 1 (eds H.N. Munro and J.B. Allison), Academic Press, New York, pp. 381–481

Newsholme, E.A. and Leech, A.R. (1983) *Biochemistry for the Medical Sciences*, John Wiley, New York, pp. 801–803

Nordenström, J., Askanazi, J., Elwyn, D.H. *et al.* (1983) Nitrogen balance during total parenteral nutrition: glucose vs. fat. *Annals of Surgery*, **197**, 27–33

Nordenström, J., Jeevanandam, M., Elwyn, D.H. *et al.* (1981) Increasing glucose intake during total parenteral nutrition increases norepinephrine excretion in trauma and sepsis. *Clinical Physiology*, **1**, 525–534

Norton, J.A., Ott, L.G., McClain, C. *et al.* (1988) Intolerance to enteral feeding in the brain-injured patient. *Journal of Neurosurgery*, **68**, 62–66

Parsa, M.H., Habif, D.V., Ferrer, J.M. *et al.* (1972) Intravenous hyperalimentation: indications, technique and complications. *Bulletin of the New York Academy of Medicine*, **48**, 920–942

Rapp, R.P., Young, B., Twyman, D. *et al.* (1983) The favorable effect of early parenteral feeding on survival in head-injured patients. *Journal of Neurosurgery*, **58**, 906–912

Robin, A.P. and Gregg, P.D. (1986) Basic principles of intravenous nutritional support. *Clinics in Chest Medicine*, **7**, 29–40

Roussos, C. and Moxham, J. (1985) Respiratory muscle fatigue. In *The Thorax* (eds C. Roussos and P.T. Maklem), Marcel Dekker, New York, pp. 829–870

Savitz, M.H., Bryan-Brown, C.W., Elwyn, D.H. *et al.* (1978) Postoperative nutritional failure and chronic cerebral edema in neurosurgical patients. *Mount Sinai Journal of Medicine*, **45**, 394–401

Schutz, Y., Acheson, K., Bessard, T. and Jequier, E. (1982) Effects of a 7-day carbohydrate hyper-alimentation on energy metabolism in healthy individuals. *Journal of Parenteral and Enteral Nutrition*, **6**, 351 (Abstract)

Shenkin, A. (1986) Vitamin and essential trace element recommendations during intravenous nutrition: theory and practice. *Proceedings of the Nutrition Society*, **45**, 383–390

Sutton, N.G. (1973) *Injuries of the Spinal Cord: The Management of Paraplegia and Tetraplegia*, Butterworths, London

Takala, J., Askanazi, J., Weissman, C. *et al.* (1988) Changes in respiratory control induced by amino acid infusions. *Critical Care Medicine*, **16**, 465–469

Twyman, D., Young, B., Ott, L. *et al.* (1985) High protein enteral feedings: a means of achieving positive nitrogen balance in head injured patients. *Journal of Parenteral and Enteral Nutrition*, **9**, 679–684

Viteri, F., Behar, M., Arroyave, G. and Scrimshaw, N.S. (1969) Clinical aspects of protein malnutrition, In *Mammalian Protein Metabolism*, Vol. 2 (eds H.N. Munro and J.B. Allison), Academic Press, New York, pp. 325–390

Waters, D.C., Dechert, R. and Bartlett, R. (1986) Metabolic studies in head injury patients: a preliminary report. *Surgery*, **100**, 531–534

Werner, S.C., Habif, D.V., Randall, H.T. *et al.* (1949) Postoperative nitrogen loss; comparison of effects of trauma and of caloric readjustment. *Annals of Surgery*, **130**, 668–702

Wolfe, B.M., Ryder, M.A., Nishikawa, R.A. *et al.* (1986) Complications of parenteral nutrition. *Americal Journal of Surgery*, **152**, 93–99

Young, B., Ott, L., Twyman, D. *et al.* (1987) The effect of nutritional support on outcome from severe head injury. *Journal of Neurosurgery*, **67**, 668–676

Chapter 8

Chronic care of spinal cord injury

J. D. Alderson

Introduction

Following complete transection of the spinal cord there is an initial period of spinal shock, lasting for approximately 1–3 weeks. This is characterized by complete loss of visceral and somatic sensation and flaccid paralysis below the level of the lesion, together with loss of tendon jerks and abdominal reflexes. There is a zone of hyperaesthesia immediately above the level of the lesion.

After approximately 1–3 weeks the acute spinal shock is replaced by a chronic phase of reflex activity which remains with the patient throughout his or her later life. The first reflex to appear is usually the Babinski sign. The reflex phase affects all dermatomes supplied by the spinal cord below the level of the injury. Muscular reflexes or spasms are predominantly flexor in nature, and initially can only be provoked by major stimuli. As the reflex phase develops, these reflexes are provoked by mild cutaneous stimuli. Extensor reflexes may return later, and can be associated with clonus. Occasionally the flexor reflexes may be associated with evacuation of the bowel and bladder, erection of the penis and seminal emission (Riddoch, 1917). Severe muscle spasm may cause serious incapacity during rehabilitation and may need long-term control.

Cardiovascular problems

Autonomic hyperreflexia

Of particular interest to the anaesthetist is the development of autonomic hyperreflexia. In this condition a reflex initiated in the area supplied by spinal nerves exiting below the level of the spinal cord injury (SCI) causes sympathetic discharge. This results in generalized vasoconstriction in this area which may cause serious hypertension. In high SCI, i.e. cervical, there is a functional separation of the whole of the sympathetic nervous system from the controlling influence of the nuclei in the brain stem and hypothalamus. The lower the level of the injury to the spinal cord, the more of the sympathetic outflow is above the level of the injury and therefore under the control of the higher centres. If there is a part of the sympathetic nervous system arising above the level of the injury and under the control of the higher centres, then it produces vasodilatation in the area it supplies. This can counteract the vasoconstriction occurring in vessels supplied by the sympathetic nerves below the injury and hence minimize any change in blood pressure. The demarcation line for troublesome autonomic hyperreflexia is about T6, and 85% of patients with chronic spinal cord injury at T6 and above will exhibit this reflex during routine activities (Kurnick, 1956). Why 15% of injuries above T6 do not experience this syndrome is not known, nor why some lower injuries do experience autonomic hyperreflexia.

During autonomic hyperreflexia the sudden rise in blood pressure produced by the vasoconstriction is detected by the baroreceptors in the aortic arch and carotid sinus, and relayed to the vasomotor centre by the glossopharyngeal (IX) and vagal (X) cranial nerves. The vasomotor centre sends inhibiting stimuli via the vagus to the cardiac sinoatrial node leading to bradycardia. Thus, classically the hypertension produced by autonomic hyperreflexia in a high SCI is accompanied by bradycardia. The hypertension may be severe, causing retinal, cerebral or subarachnoid haemorrhage, and may be fatal. Although the reflex may be set off by cutaneous stimuli below the level of spinal cord damage, visceral stimulation such as produced by distension of the bladder or rectum is a very potent stimulus, and the cardiovascular response is commonly proportional to the strength of the stimulus (Head and Riddock, 1917).

Surgery can be a very potent stimulus to autonomic hyperreflexia, especially when viscera are distended (e.g. cystoscopy). Studies in patients with cervical cord transections having autonomic hyperreflexic episodes have demonstrated not only hypertension and bradycardia, but also marked vasoconstriction with decrease in hand and calf blood flow (Corbett, Frankel and Harris, 1971). Constriction of peripheral capacitance vessels causes the central venous pressure to rise. Cardiac output, stroke volume, systemic vascular resistance and pulmonary arterial pressures have been shown to rise by Corbett et al. (1975), but Barker et al. (1985) suggest that the compensatory bradycardia may lead to a reduction in cardiac output if stroke volume does not increase. There is a rise in circulating plasma noradrenaline (norepinephrine), but not adrenaline (epinephrine) or renin, suggesting that the hypertension is purely due to sympathetic overactivity (noradrenaline is the sympathetic nervous system transmitter) and not the release of vasopressor hormones (Mathias et al., 1976; Frankel and Mathias, 1979).

The awake patient experiencing autonomic hyperreflexia may experience facial tingling, nasal obstruction, severe headache, dyspnoea, nausea and blurred vision (Head and Riddoch, 1917; Schumacher and Guthrie, 1951; Kurnick, 1956). Examination could reveal hypertension and bradycardia, arrhythmias (Kendrick et al., 1953), sweating (List and Pimenta, 1944), cutis anserina (goose flesh), cutaneous vasodilatation above and vasoconstriction below the level of the injury, loss of consciousness and convulsion (Johnson et al., 1975). Preoperative assessment must always include questions about the signs and symptoms of autonomic hyperreflexia.

Daily management of autonomic hyperreflexia
Autonomic hyperreflexia has a sudden onset and equally sudden regression. Thus before and after the reflex is initiated, the blood pressure may be normal, suddenly rising for a few seconds or minutes during the reflex to a dangerous level. This makes control difficult for daily activities.

Treatment begins with the assessment of the severity of autonomic hyperreflexia. Such reflexes may be deliberately produced by bladder catheter clamping during attempts to produce automatic bladder function. Patients should be taught to recognize the syndrome, and how to instigate appropriate treatment by removing the stimulus (unblock catheter, remove cutaneous irritation, etc.)

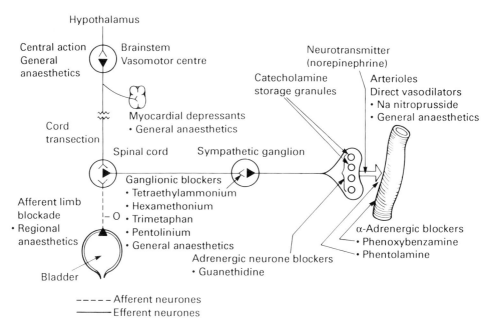

Figure 8.1 Sites of action of agents used for control of hypertension of autonomic hyperreflexia (From Schonwald, Fish and Perkash, 1981, by permission)

Various methods have been suggested to control the autonomic hyperreflexia (Figure 8.1). Therapeutic methods must act at sites throughout the body, and agents acting centrally or on the vasomotor centre of the brainstem are not usually effective. Ganglion blockers, alpha adrenergic blockers, catecholamine depleters and direct vasodilators all have their supporters (Schonwald, Fish and Perkash, 1981). One problem is that the resting blood pressure in tetraplegic patients is commonly low (Frankel *et al.*, 1972); therefore there is the danger of any therapeutic regimen pathologically lowering yet further the resting blood pressure (Figure 8.2). Orthostatic hypotension is also prone to occur in tetraplegics, thus yet further complicating treatment (Mathias *et al.*, 1980). Plasma levels of prostaglandin E have been shown to rise during autonomic hyperreflexia (Mathias *et al.*, 1975b) and are believed to help moderate the hypertension. Infusions of prostaglandin E have been used to control the hypertension of autonomic hyperreflexia (Johnson *et al.*, 1975). Oral clonidine has been shown to reduce the hypertensive effect of autonomic hyperreflexia and has the advantage of not reducing the resting blood pressure (Reid *et al.*, 1977; Mathias *et al.*, 1979). Guanethidine has also proved successful in preventing the hypertensive effects of autonomic hyperreflexia, but can cause postural hypotension (Brown, Carrion and Politano, 1979). The use of transdermal glyceryl trinitrate is being used successfully in at least one centre (G. Ravichandran, personal communication).

Management of autonomic hyperreflexia during surgery
Surgical procedures such as distension of the bladder or bowel are significant stimuli for the production of autonomic hyperreflexia, and provision must be taken to prevent this life-threatening condition occurring during surgery. Preoperative

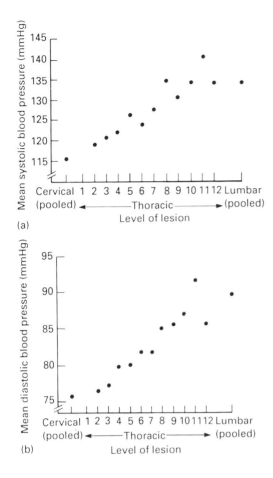

(a)

(b)

Figure 8.2 Blood pressure in paraplegic males: (a) mean systolic blood pressure/level of spinal cord lesion; (b) mean diastolic blood pressure/level of spinal cord lesion (From Frankel *et al.*, 1972, by permission)

assessment must be undertaken of those patients at risk (i.e. SCI of T6 and above).

Patients should be asked as to whether they get headaches, sweating or other signs of autonomic hyperreflexia, of which severe throbbing headache is the most significant. Fifteen per cent of patients with lesions above T6 are unaffected by autonomic hyperreflexia. Baseline pulse and blood pressure should be noted, bearing in mind the normal low resting blood pressure of high SCI.

Many SCI patients have no anxiety about surgical operations. They are aware of the fact that most procedures will be completely painless, unless the operation site encroaches on dermatomes supplied from above the SCI. It is important in the preoperative assessment to be aware of the sensory innervation of skin and viscera to be operated upon, and to be able to advise the patient as to the necessity or otherwise of anaesthesia for those areas supplied by nerves above the level of the SCI.

Transurethral urology and autonomic hyperreflexia.   Distension of the bladder is probably the major stimulus to autonomic hyperreflexia and many papers relate specifically to this procedure. Complete SCI patients at risk of autonomic hyper-reflexia, i.e. with spinal cord lesion above T6, will have no sensation from the operating site. However, distension of the bladder will be a potent stimulus for autonomic hyperreflexia. Most of these patients feel no apprehension of trans-urethral surgery in the knowledge that it will be painless, and therefore may deliberately wish not to receive general anaesthesia or sedation, so that they are able to discuss operative findings at the time with the urologist. In such cases, a method of control of autonomic hyperreflexia that does not interfere with the conscious state is preferable.

Spinal subarachnoid anaesthesia.   The use of regional anaesthesia to prevent the reflexes occurring has found favour with many. Spinal subarachnoid anaesthesia has been frequently used. Ciliberti, Goldfein and Rovenstine (1954) reported the use of spinal subarachnoid anaesthesia in 13 patients with injuries of T5 and above and claimed complete absence or hypertension or headache. The technique used was not described. Broecker, Hranowsky and Hackler (1979) described the use of low spinal anaesthesia using 25–50 mg of 5% hyperbaric lignocaine (lidocaine) given at the L3–4 or L4–5 interspace in 25 SCI patients with SCI above T7, this technique being completely successful. Schonwald, Fish and Perkash (1981) used either spinal amethocaine (tetracaine) 1% in doses from 8 mg to 14 mg or spinal lignocaine (lidocaine) 5% in doses from 50 mg to 75 mg. The only failure was in the lignocaine group, and this was put down to regression of the block before the completion of surgery.

Desmond (1970) has suggested that spinal anaesthesia in these patients may be hazardous, with technical problems in performing lumbar puncture, and more importantly unpredictability in control of the level of the anaesthetic block due to distortion of the vertebral column potentially leading to severe hypotension. Schonwald, Fish and Perkash (1981) believe the technical difficulties to have been overemphasized, especially in patients with high injuries, and Broecker, Hranowsky and Hackler (1979) reported no difficulties with their series of low spinals. Barker *et al.* (1985) used 1.2 ml hyperbaric cinchocaine (nupercaine), given at L2–3 or L3–4, and reported very stable cardiovascular parameters, with minimal fall in blood pressure (Figure 8.3). They suggested there was sufficient evidence to validate the uses of spinal anaesthesia to control autonomic hyperreflexia. Personal experience using either 1.2 ml 0.5% hyperbaric cinchocaine or 1.5–2 ml 0.5% hyperbaric bupivacaine (7.5–10 mg) confirms the stability of the cardiovascular system during initiation of the block, and during transurethral surgery, and it is now the method of choice for this work in this centre.

Spinal extradural anaesthesia.   The use of epidural (spinal extradural) anaesthesia to control autonomic hyperreflexia in transurethral surgery is more controversial. Johnson *et al.* (1975) reported the technique to be unpredictable, and this was confirmed by Broecker, Hranowsky and Hackler (1979), who injected 100 mg of mepivacaine into the L2–3 epidural space in 3 patients, two of whom suffered autonomic hyperreflexia. Schonwald, Fish and Perkash (1981) reported 4 cases, one of whom developed a total spinal anaesthetic as a result of inadvertent subarachnoid injection – a test dose proving useless in assessing correct location of the epidural space because of the patient's paraplegia. Despite these reports, several centres have been using epidural anaesthesia with complete satisfaction (Anonymous, 1975).

Other regional techniques.   Topical application of local anaesthetic agents to the urethral and bladder mucosa has been reported as producing many failures, probably because topical anaesthesia does not block the bladder muscle proprioceptors

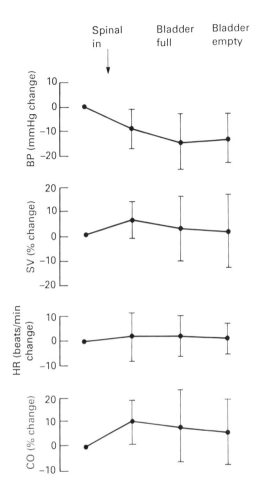

Spinal   Bladder   Bladder
in   full   empty

Figure 8.3 Cardiovascular parameters of patients liable to autonomic hyperreflexia following spinal anaesthesia (BP, blood pressure; SV, stroke volume; HR, heart rate; CO, cardiac output) (From Barker *et al.*, 1985, by permission)

stimulated by bladder distension (Texter, Reece and Hranowsky, 1976). Some workers find this technique useful (Comarr, 1959) especially in incomplete SCI, using 20 ml 2% lignocaine jelly (Rao *et al.*, 1977), or suggest the use of transacral anaesthesia of the sacral roots (Editorial Comment, 1979). Bilateral paravertebral sympathetic blocks have been found inadequate to prevent autonomic hyperreflexia (Thompson and Witham, 1948).

General anaesthesia.   Although most spinal injury patients undergoing trans-urethral procedures will prefer to be fully conscious, there will always be some who have a particular fear of theatre, or who, for other reasons, it is thought should be sedated or unconscious. In particular, it may be unreasonable to subject children to such procedures without general anaesthesia. The review by Ciliberti, Goldfein and Rovenstine (1954) of 27 patients with SCI above T5 found a 42.5% incidence of autonomic hyperreflexia. A wide range of techniques had been used, including sodium thiopentone, nitrous oxide, cyclopropane, ether and trichlorethylene. The authors commented that the deepening of anaesthesia was helpful in combating autonomic hyperreflexia. Drinker and Helrich (1963) demonstrated the use of halothane (with nitrous oxide and oxygen) to control autonomic hyperreflexia in a patient with C6 transection of the spinal cord, and recommended the use of this agent. It is assumed from their paper that respiration was spontaneous.

In 1975, the Sheffield spinal injury unit presented its experiences using nitrous oxide, oxygen and halothane with spontaneous respiration (after sodium thiopentone induction) on 45 spinal injury patients, of which 24 were cervical injuries (Alderson and Thomas, 1975). Twenty-one patients developed a rise in blood pressure consistent with autonomic hyperreflexia. The greatest rise though was of 40 mmHg (5.3 kPa) systolic, and in no case did the blood pressure rise above 160 mmHg (21.3 kPa) systolic. Of these 21 patients, 19 were cervical injuries and the other two T4 and T6. In 12 of these 21 patients, cardiac dysrhythmias were observed during the blood pressure rise, comprising supraventricular and ventricular ectopics, and 7 patients were treated with beta blockers. Although the blood pressure control was adequate, the cardiac dysrhythmias caused some concern. Similar cardiac dysrhythmias have previously been reported on a neurologically normal patient (Eggers and Baker, 1969). Cessation of the stimulus (bladder distension) allowed normal cardiac rhythm to return.

Schonwald, Fish and Perkash (1981) published their results confirming that halothane was effective in controlling autonomic hyperreflexia. No cardiac dysrhythmias were noticed and this was attributed to normocarbia being maintained by assisted or controlled ventilation. Enflurane was also found to be effective in controlling autonomic hyperreflexia. Welply, Mathias and Frankel (1975) also found halothane to be effective, the more so when combined with controlled ventilation. They postulated that the abnormal circulatory responses to the Valsalva reflex in SCI (Johnson, Smith and Spalding, 1969) (i.e. absence of overshoot of the blood pressure when intrathoracic pressure returns to normal) gives greater reduction of blood pressure than in neurologically normal patients with intact reflexes, controlled ventilation being regarded as a series of Valsalva manoeuvres.

Non-anaesthetic management.   The acute treatment of autonomic hyperreflexia during transurethral urology requires potent remedies. Historically, the long-acting ganglion blockers hexamethonium and pentolinium have been used (Ciliberti, Goldfein and Rovenstine, 1954; Kurnick, 1956; Texter, Reece and Hranowsky, 1976), but are no longer commercially available and may be too long acting to cope with the abrupt onset and cessation of autonomic hyperreflexia during cystoscopies. The short-acting ganglion blocker trimetaphan (Arfonad) has proved successful when given by intravenous infusion (Hassan, 1974; Thorn-Alquist, 1975; Wedley, 1976; Snow et al., 1977) (250 mg in 500 ml dilutant) titrated against the blood pressure (Figure 8.4).

The alpha adrenergic receptor blocking agent phentolamine has not been so successful in this application (Kurnick, 1956; Neider, O'Higgins and Aldrete, 1970) and large doses were required (Sizemore and Winternitz, 1970). Vandam and Rossier (1975) have suggested that sodium nitroprusside, being a direct vasodilator, might be of value. Sublingual glyceryl trinitrate can be helpful for more modest autonomic hyperreflexia (G. Ravichandran, personal communication).

Autonomic hyperreflexia and other surgical procedures.   Although transurethral urology is perhaps the most potent stimulus to autonomic hyperreflexia, the reflex can be produced by other cutaneous, visceral and somatic stimulation. Several

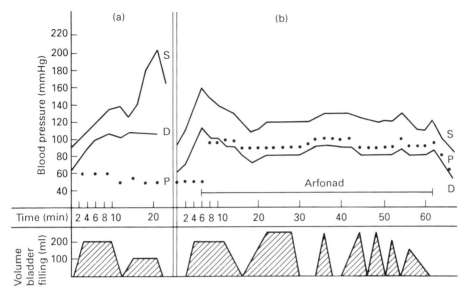

Figure 8.4 Course of events during cystoscopy and lithotripsy without (a) and with (b) intravenous drip of trimetaphan (Arfonad) (S, systolic blood pressure; D, diastolic blood pressure; P, pulse rate) (From Thorn-Alquist, 1975, by permission)

authors have commented on the use of anaesthesia or drugs to control or prevent autonomic hyperreflexia occurring during other surgical operations than those requiring bladder distension. However, it is important to realize that autonomic hyperreflexia might not have been produced during all of these procedures, and therefore results may be difficult to interpret in comparison with the more potent stimulus of cystoscopy. Neider, O'Higgins and Aldrete (1970) used epidural anaesthesia for nephrectomy, but needed to add an infusion of 0.1% trimetaphan (Arfonad) for manipulation of the kidney. The patient was awake throughout the 3½-hour operation, and complained of nausea during intestinal manipulation (normal vagal sensation).

Nitrous oxide, opiate general anaesthesia, was used by Schonwald, Fish and Perkash (1981) for 9 patients, two of whom developed intraoperative hypertension. One was during transurethral urology and the other during upper arm tendon transfers, the latter not responding to phentolamine but being controlled by the addition of 1% halothane. However, Hassan (1974) claimed that use of a relaxant technique using curare, nitrous oxide and oxygen, with intermittent positive pressure ventilation, prevented intraoperative hypertension in 12 patients. His paper did not mention the levels of SCI or the operations performed. The present writer has successfully used a relaxant technique using nitrous oxide and halothane for nephrectomy in a small number of patients without problem, and has also combined spinal anaesthesia with a relaxant sequence for the same operation, again uneventfully.

Some centres prefer to pretreat patients at risk of autonomic hyperreflexia with the alpha adrenergic blocker phenoxybenzamine. This long-acting agent can cause tachycardia, and anaesthetists should be aware of this intraoperatively. The use of adrenaline (epinephrine) to treat cardiovascular collapse in a patient who has received phenoxybenzamine is inappropriate, as the alpha blockage causes this mixed alpha and beta stimulant to act as a beta stimulant producing vasodilatation and tachycardia and making resuscitation impossible. Noradrenaline (norepinephrine) or phenylephrine should be used as vasopressors. The caveat against using adrenaline (epinephrine) in patients on phenoxybenzamine also applies to the addition of this drug to local anaesthetic infiltration to secure haemostasis.

Extracorporeal shock wave lithotripsy.   Spinal cord injury patients are at high risk of developing renal stones, having recurrent urinary tract infections. The use of extracorporeal shock wave lithotripsy provides a non-invasive effective method of treating complicated renal disease in the quadriplegic. Neuwirth, Royce and Chaussy (1986) used epidural or spinal anaesthesia to obviate the risk of autonomic hyperreflexia with satisfaction. More recently, Spirnak *et al.* (1988) claimed that the syndrome of autonomic hyperreflexia does not occur during extracorporeal shock wave lithotripsy; however, they noted peroperative elevation of blood pressure, which required treatment with hydralazine in 2 of the 5 patients. They suggest that this hypertensive phenomenon is an exaggeration of the normal physiological response of increased right atrial and systemic arterial pressures following the shift of peripheral blood volume into central vascular compartments following immersion (Arborelius *et al.*, 1972; Weber *et al.*, 1986). They recommend close monitoring during therapy by an anaesthetist.

Autonomic hyperreflexia and postoperative recovery.   Following surgery, it is important to realize that autonomic hyperreflexia may occur in the postoperative period, especially in susceptible patients recovering from transurethral urological surgery. Schonwald, Fish and Perkash (1981) recorded four of their episodes of autonomic hyperreflexia in the recovery room out of a total of 11 such episodes. It is important that bladder drainage catheters are regularly checked for patency.

Other cardiovascular problems

Reference has earlier been made to the lower resting blood pressure of SCI patients, the greatest reduction being seen in the highest SCIs (Frankel *et al.*, 1972).

The abnormal response to the Valsalva manoeuvre has also been mentioned. The neurologically normal patient responds to increased intrathoracic pressure with a well-documented response (Ganong, 1989). With the rise in intrathoracic pressure, the blood pressure increases because this intrathoracic pressure is added to the normal blood pressure. There is then a fall in blood pressure due to a reduction in venous return caused by the high intrathoracic pressure. The baroreceptors then respond to the reduction in blood pressure by producing vasoconstriction and tachycardia. Once the high intrathoracic pressure is removed, there is a short rise in blood pressure to above normal as blood now returns to the heart from the vasoconstricted periphery. Rapidly the baroreceptors correct this rise to normal and produce a bradycardia. In paraplegics, the increase in intrathoracic pressure causes a continuous fall of blood pressure with no tendency to level off (presumably therefore no compensatory vasoconstriction). When the intrathoracic pressure is released there is no overshoot of blood pressure or bradycardia, but just a gradual recovery of blood pressure and pulse rate to former levels (Welply, Mathias and Frankel,

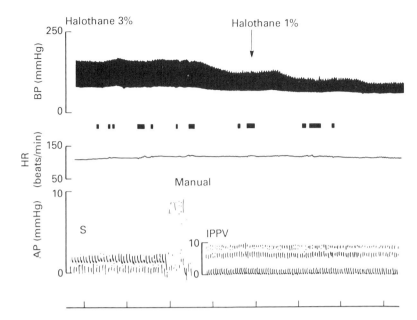

Figure 8.5 Effect of halothane and intermittent positive pressure ventilation (IPPV) on the blood pressure (BP) and heart rate (HR) of a tetraplegic during urological surgery. The blocks below the BP indicate bladder stimulation by diathermy. Airway pressure (AP) has been recorded during spontaneous respiration (S), manual controlled ventilation and IPPV (From Welply, Mathias and Frankel, 1975, by permission)

1975). This has important consequences for the use of positive pressure ventilation in SCI patients, and may lead to a greater reduction in blood pressure than anticipated when controlled ventilation is combined with myocardial depressants (e.g. halothane) (Figure 8.5).

Intubation can be hazardous in chronic tetraplegics, and cardiac arrests have occurred (Welply, Mathias and Frankel, 1975). In neurologically normal patients, intubation is associated with tachycardia and hypertension, thought to be due to stimulation of the sympathetic nervous system. In quadriplegics, with total sympathetic denervation a vagovagal reflex can predominate and cause asystole. This can be prevented by intravenous atropine 0.6 mg prior to induction and intubation (Welply, Mathias and Frankel, 1975). This problem is probably most likely to occur during the spinal shock phase of SCI.

Orthostatic hypotension can be a major problem for acute cervical SCI patients, but chronic SCI patients commonly develop improved tolerance of the upright posture, the mechanism being unclear (Krebs, Ragnarrson and Tuckman, 1983; Figoni, 1984). Neurologically intact man responds to the upright posture by an increase in systemic arteriolar resistance (Krebs, Ragnarrson and Tuckman, 1983). An increase in renal resistance can readily be measured in neurologically normal man. In quadriplegics, a rise is also measurable in renal resistance (Krebs, Ragnarrson and Tuckman, 1983), as is a rise in plasma renin (Mathias *et al.*, 1980), and a lesser rise in noradrenaline (norepinephrine) (Mathias *et al.*, 1975a). This suggests the possibility of a renal vascular receptor mechanism responsible for renin release and also perhaps increased sympathetic activity from the isolated spinal cord, supporting the concept of a spinal sympathetic vasomotor reflex pathway responsive to posture. Orthostatic training is an integral part of rehabilitation, as it allows early mobilization. The possibility of inadequate cardiovascular posture reflexes must always be considered during the positioning of patients for anaesthesia and surgery. If possible, upright posture should be avoided and particular emphasis placed on avoiding dependent venous pooling.

A study on blood volumes in chronic quadriplegics has shown a wide range of values, some patients having less than 60 ml/kg total blood volume (Desmond and Laws, 1974). In view of the unpredictable nature of this value, it has been suggested that blood volume measurements should be part of preoperative work-up.

Naftchi et al. (1978) have estimated a reduction in blood volume of 5–9% during the vasoconstriction of autonomic hyperreflexia, this occurring at the expense of plasma volume, which dropped by 10–15%, giving a corresponding increase in haematocrit. The absence or otherwise of autonomic hyperreflexia is obviously important, therefore, when measuring blood volume.

The variability of blood volume may make these patients intolerant of blood loss, in common with other types of neurological disease. Central venous pressure measurement may be helpful in fluid replacement therapy.

Respiratory system problems

With more aggressive treatment of urinary stasis and infection, cardiopulmonary problems now outrank renal disease as the most common cause of death in SCI patients, both during the acute phase and in later years (Carter, 1987). The level of spinal cord transection will directly affect respiratory function. If transection is below C6, then the diaphragm will be intact but ventilation reduced because of intercostal paralysis. Transection at C4 will cause major loss of diaphragmatic innervation and grossly impair alveolar ventilation (Quimby, Williams and Greifenstein, 1973).

The acute management of respiratory problems is dealt with in earlier chapters, the major goal being the production of normal blood gases with avoidance of hypoxia and ensuing vagal-produced cardiac arrest. It has been recommended that high SCI patients should receive serial vital capacity measurements until they are out of danger of respiratory failure and are able to average 1400–1500 ml (Carter, 1987). Once the SCI is stabilized, isometric exercises to neck muscles and strengthening of the accessory muscles of respiration are instituted to improve respiratory muscle function. Atelectasis must be vigorously treated with physiotherapy, and if necessary intermittent positive pressure ventilation instituted.

Cervical SCI patients may prove difficult to wean off ventilation. It has been shown that the diaphragm may become fatigued due to reduced muscle strength and a reduction in endurance in quadriplegics, which may lead to acute respiratory failure (Gross et al., 1980), but inspiratory muscle training (breathing through an inspiratory resistance for two 15-min episodes per day) helps prevent this. Weaning from ventilation should be gradual to prevent this fatigue syndrome occurring.

High SCI patients may take many weeks before they regain sufficient respiratory function to be weaned from ventilation (Table 8.1). Even those with C3 injuries, who are apnoeic at the time of injury, but may be resuscitated as a result of increased awareness of cardiopulmonary resuscitation among the general public, ambulance

Table 8.1 Effects of cervical spinal cord injury on respiratory vital capacity and subsequent recovery (From Carter, 1987, by permission)

Classification	No. patients	Average initial VC* (ml)	Average final VC (ml)	Average gain in VC (ml)	Average duration initial to final VC (days)
C3 (with return)	6	100	1180	1080	–
C4 (initial VC < 1000 ml)	26	670	1837	1167	75.5
C4 (initial VC > 1000 ml)	19	1550	2672	1122	57
Unilateral diaphragmatic paralysis					
A. Transient	16	1019	2151	1132	76
B. Permanent	6	1070	1862	792	56

* VC, vital capacity.

staff and paramedics, can recover sufficient respiratory function to avoid long-term ventilation (Carter, 1987).

In those patients in whom it is not possible to achieve long-term freedom from ventilation, short periods of time off the ventilator are encouraged as a safety margin for mechanical failure, and also for psychological well-being (Dingemans and Hawn, 1978). The use of halo-vest immobilization allows early resumption of the upright position within 1 month of injury and helps reduce respiratory complications. The aim of spinal injury units should be to rehabilitate the patient into the community. Dingemans and Hawn (1978) recommend the provision of three ventilator systems for discharge – a bedside unit, a portable ventilator and a self-inflating bag (Ambu bag), along with portable suction apparatus. Adequate family training has helped reduce the mortality from high injuries, and independent electric wheelchairs capable of carrying ventilator and suction equipment have helped rehabilitate these patients.

In the 1960s the Yale University School of Medicine began the use of phrenic nerve pacemakers – a system developed by William Glenn and colleagues in association with Avery Laboratories, Farmingdale, New York. By 1975, 37 patients with quadriplegia could be reviewed. Thirteen were on full-term pacing, with no other ventilatory support, and 10 other patients received paced ventilation for at least 50% of the time (Glenn *et al.*, 1976). The other 14 patients were unable to receive paced ventilatory support for up to 50% of the time, injury to one or both phrenic nerves being the major cause of failure.

The equipment consists of an external battery-powered transmitter, an aerial (antenna) placed on the skin, a receiver placed subcutaneously beneath the aerial, and platinum electrodes surrounding and stimulating the phrenic nerves. Surgery for implantation of the pacemaker was delayed for at least 2–3 months after injury to allow for possible return of diaphragmatic function. Local anaesthesia is used for the 4 in (100 mm) incision, 1 in (25 mm) above and parallel to the clavicle, the phrenic nerve isolated and a stimulating cuff attached where it crosses scalenus anterior muscle. Each side is implanted at a separate operation with a two-week gap between operations to reduce the risk of infection. The receiver is implanted subcutaneously in the mid or anterior axillary line at the costal margin, and the silastic-covered wires which are tunnelled from the cuff electrode and receiver are joined at a third subcutaneous incision at the level of the 4th rib in the mid-clavicular line. Stimulation begins at 5 min each hour on each side and is gradually increased. With good response it may be possible to stimulate each side alternately for 12-hourly periods for complete independence from mechanical ventilation. Stimulation of each phrenic nerve for longer than 16 h is not recommended. The tracheostomy should remain open, even with full pacing, for occasional suctioning, since these patients cannot cough effectively, and also for ventilation in case of pacemaker failure.

Carter *et al.* (1987) reviewed phrenic nerve ventilation (electrophrenic respiration, EPR) and mechanical ventilation. They found that the vast majority of both groups could be discharged home, and mortality rates were similar, although EPR patients appeared to live longer.

The anaesthetist faced with SCI patients must carefully consider and assess respiratory function. High SCI patients will have reduced vital capacity, and those with high cervical injuries will have reduced diaphragmatic activity. Intra-abdominal distension and faecal impaction can have marked effects on respiratory function, leading to respiratory depression, atelectasis and pneumonia (Desmond, 1970).

The use of anaesthetic drugs with respiratory depressant actions should be avoided if spontaneous respiration is wanted. Consideration should be given to the effect of surgical positioning on respiration (e.g. head-down positions), and mechanical ventilation instituted if respiratory function is likely to be embarrassed. The use of muscle relaxants poses the problem of postoperative reversal, and of recurarization. The use of atracurium, with its reversal not dependent on the use of anticholinesterases, may be preferred to other non-depolarizers.

Intubation should be performed as aseptically as possible, as should bronchial suction which may be necessary for prolonged procedures. The humidification of inspired gases should be considered. The use of simple tidal volume and vital capacity measurements have much to commend it when assessing when to extubate after surgery. Respiratory function and blood gas analysis may need monitoring well into the postoperative period after major procedures, and physiotherapy, including postural drainage, is important for the prevention of postoperative atelectasis.

Temperature regulation

Gardiner and Pembrey (1912) drew attention to the inability of paraplegics to maintain their central temperature in different environmental temperatures, and indicated that they were virtually poikilothermic. Thus a fall in ambient temperature causes a drop in body temperature, and a rise in ambient temperature causes a rise in body temperature. Work by Johnson (1971) confirmed that these patients have lost the ability to produce heat by shivering below the level of spinal injury, and that the mechanisms for heat loss are also disrupted below the level of the injury (sweating and vasodilatation). Pilo-erection, some vasodilatation and some vasoconstriction can occur in response to changes in ambient temperature. Johnson concluded that patients with transection of the spinal cord run the risk of hypothermia or hyperpyrexia.

It is important in surgery to attempt to keep the body temperature normal. Electrical warming mattresses maintained at body temperature are required for long procedures, and infusion and irrigation fluids should be brought to body temperature before use. Preoperative and postoperative care should include the provision of adequate clothing and blankets and monitoring of body temperature. The patients should never be left in a scanty operating gown in a cold room! Rocco and Vandam (1959) suggest the use of air-conditioned wards and theatres.

Ohry, Heim and Rozin (1983) have also described a hypothermic response to sepsis in young quadriplegics in association with leukopenia and mental deterioration, mimicking a similar syndrome in neurologically intact geriatrics. The anaesthetist should be aware of such abnormal thermoregulatory responses.

Genitourinary system

Advances in the understanding of urodynamics and of the neuro-urology of paraplegics has revolutionized the survival of these patients. Urinary complications have become less frequent and urological pathology is no longer the most important cause of death following SCI (Wyndaele, 1987). During the period of spinal shock the bladder becomes atonic and areflexic, but as the reflex phase is entered there is a return of detrusor muscle activity, with uninhibited detrusor contraction (detrusor hyperreflexia). These contractions may be poorly sustained, preventing full bladder emptying, and commonly the external sphincter also contracts during detrusor contraction (detrusor sphincter dyssynergia) (Thomas, 1986). Medical and surgical treatment to prevent upper tract dilatation and improve bladder emptying reduces the risk of renal damage and ascending infection which, over several years, may lead to renal failure from pyelonephritis, from renal stones or from renal amyloid disease. Detrusor activity can be reduced by anticholinergics, just as troublesome bladder spasm can be relieved by intravenous atropine during cystoscopy.

Clearly, assessment of renal function is important prior to anaesthesia, and the choice of anaesthetic drugs in impaired renal function should be made with knowledge of the amount of renal metabolism of the drugs. The problem and management of autonomic hyperreflexia have been discussed earlier in this chapter with relation to urology. Transurethral instrumentation, or even preoperative cleaning of the penis, can also provoke penile erections in SCI male patients, mediated through a spinal reflex. This author finds spinal anaesthesia useful as a prophylaxis against this occurrence.

In a study of neurologically normal male volunteers given intramuscular morphine as a controlled group, an increased incidence of involuntary erections has been reported (Rawal et al., 1983). It would seem reasonable, therefore, to avoid morphine-containing drugs as premedicants in paraplegic men awaiting transurethral procedures. Papaverine has been used therapeutically by injection into the corpora cavernosa to produce erections in paraplegic men for intercourse (Brindle, 1986). As papaveretum contains this drug it also should be avoided prior to transurethral procedures. Ketamine has been described to prevent penile erection occurring and to treat such erections in neurologically normal patients (Gale, 1972). The author of this chapter has found short-acting benzodiazepines (triazolam or temazepam) satisfactory for male patients requiring premedication prior to transurethral procedures.

Haemopoiesis

Anaemia is a common finding in SCI patients. Perkash and Brown (1982) reported that 52.3% had a mild to moderate anaemia, i.e. less than 13.6 g/100 ml, but Naftchi *et al.* (1978) have shown that autonomic hyperreflexia is associated with an acute reduction in plasma volume giving a rise in haematocrit. Therefore, interpretations of just one blood sample is difficult and it may be necessary to take several samples over different time intervals for the results to be meaningful. In the survey by Perkash and Brown (1982) most cases of anaemia are anaemias of chronic disorder associated with the condition : decubitus ulcer (83%) or urinary tract infection (41%). Removal of the cause allows the body to correct the anaemia.

Musculoskeletal system

Spinal cord injury is followed by a rapid bone resorption below the level of the injury. It is suggested that the alteration produced to the autonomic nerve supply by SCI produces circulatory disturbances, including arteriovenous shunts and vascular hyperplasia, and also vasomotor paralysis with interosseous venous stasis. These changes lead to bone blood gas changes and acidosis (Chantraine, 1978). There is hypercalciuria, but only rarely does hypercalcaemia occur, usually in rapidly growing adolescents suffering acute SCI (Steinberg, Birge and Cooke, 1978). Collagen formation, too, is abnormal (Chantraine, 1978). The end result is osteoporosis, with bones that are easily fractured, and previous reviews have emphasized the care that must be taken in positioning patients to prevent skeletal damage (Desmond, 1970).

Following SCI, new bone sometimes develops in the soft tissues around paralysed joints, possibly as a result of local trauma to those areas. Maturity of this new bone can take 18 months, and any surgical excision should be delayed until this new bone is mature, otherwise surgery may provoke further new bone formation, thus compounding the original condition.

Kyphoscoliosis can occur in young paraplegics, espcially with asymmetrical or incomplete SCI with imbalanced vertebral muscle tone. Tricot (1975) has reported cases of contractures and stiffness of the vertebral column following SCI. This may make the use of spinal subarachnoid and spinal extradural anaesthesia difficult or impossible.

Associated with bone atrophy is muscle atrophy and skin atrophy below the level of the lesion. The skin is prone to ulceration, and again considerable care during positioning of the patient will help to prevent decubitus ulceration. The incidence of pressure sores has been reported as being twice as high in tetraplegics as paraplegics (Bors, 1956).

Venepuncture may prove difficult in atrophied areas, which have fragile, small veins. The anaesthetist should be aware of the level of hyperaesthesia at the upper limit of the dermatomes involved in the SCI, necessitating local anaesthesia before venepuncture in this area, or avoidance of the area completely. Many cervical SCI patients have limited but important functional usage of the upper limb. The placement of intravenous lines should always take into account the possible inconvenience of the site to the patient.

Spasticity

Spinal cord injury patients develop spasticity when intact spinal reflex arcs exist below the level of the lesion that are isolated from higher centres. These reflexes develop during the first few weeks following injury, and may be so severe as to throw the patient from the wheelchair; or in the operating theatre to impede certain types of surgery, as surgery itself may provoke the reflex. Damage can occur to limbs from the violent spasms, and limb protection is important in operating theatres.

Patients with incomplete injuries tend to have more severe spasticity and it may be found that this spasticity prevents walking in patients with otherwise good muscle power. However, spasticity also aids the prevention of osteoporosis, improves venous return and reduces muscle wasting, so treatment is only required when spasticity proves handicapping to daily living.

Treatment should initially be directed to removing any obvious cause, such as pressure sore, urinary bladder stone, ingrowing toenail, etc., as commonly spasms are initiated by such irritative foci. Passive physiotherapy to stretch muscles helps reduce the incidence of spasm and contractures, as does encouraging mobility.

Baclofen acts at a spinal level, and can be given orally, with up to 90 mg/day being required. Certain centres are now giving baclofen by intrathecal infusion fed via sophisticated pumps implanted on the anterior chest wall. Directly placing the drug onto the spinal cord greatly reduces the required dosage; normally between 50 μg and 200 μg/day is adequate (G. Ravichandran, personal communication). Dantrolene sodium is also useful, but benzodiazepines are now less popular because of the undesired sedation and addictive effects.

Localized spasticity can be treated by surgical neurectomy if a diagnostic nerve block with bupivacaine confirms the value of the procedure. Intrathecal neurolytic agents such as 6% aqueous phenol are occasionally indicated for severe lower limb spasm, but will convert the lesion from upper to lower motor neurone, and may therefore alter not only spasticity but also bladder and bowel control, and sexual function.

In the operating theatre, regional local anaesthesia (e.g. spinal subarachnoid block) will remove spasticity and spasm, and this technique is particularly useful if this is associated with autonomic hyperreflexia. General anaesthesia with muscle relaxation will also remove spasticity, but just as with regional anaesthesia obviously has no effect on contractures. Intravenous benzodiazepines can be given to reduce spasticity intraoperatively, but the conscious level of the patient should be carefully monitored if this technique is used. Limbs should always be well protected with padding and well secured to the operating table stirrups as appropriate for the proposed operative procedure.

Psychological problems

It is generally assumed that SCI patients will be depressed, but Howell *et al.* (1981) found only a 22.7% incidence of minor depressive disorders (using research diagnostic criteria) in traumatic spinal cord injuries of less than 3 months duration. This should be compared with a general community survey of approximately 6% depression. High cervical injuries (C4 and above) face severe problems. Faced with possible ventilator dependence, and inability to use the upper limbs, the patient becomes virtually totally dependent on his family and rehabilitation team. The patient will have to adapt his only remaining resources, namely the mind and the ability to communicate, to this state. He will undergo a marked regression of physical and emotional well-being, and is faced with having to realign ego parameters. The focal point of the patient, the family and the rehabilitation team is the months of rehabilitation and social reintegration. Family involvement is essential (Burnham and Werner, 1979).

Those SCI patients with low cervical level of injury and below are usually fairly independent, and usually adjust very well.

Acute abdomen

Juler and Eltorai (1985) presented a review of 36 SCI patients with visceral disease. The response to visceral disease was shown to depend on the level of SCI, whether the cord lesion was complete or incomplete, and whether reflex arcs were intact below the level of injury. They described spinal injuries above the level of the splanchnic outflow (T8) as high, and below as low. Of the 10 patients with appendicitis, the two with low injuries were able to localize abdominal pain to the right lower quadrant early in the disease as in neurologically normal patients, and early surgery avoided perforation of the appendix. Of the 8 with high lesions, all but one eventually developed pain localized to the right lower quadrant but also associated with symptoms of autonomic hyperreflexia. All of these 8 patients had perforated appendixes with walled-off abscesses at operation, suggesting delay in surgical recognition of the disease process.

In the group of 11 patients operated on for perforated viscus, all 8 patients with high injuries developed autonomic hyperreflexia and shoulder tip pain, but only one could localize abdominal pain to the upper abdomen. The 3 patients with low injuries did not develop autonomic hyperreflexia and presented as in the neurologically normal patient.

Of the 16 patients undergoing emergency laparotomy for small bowel obstruction, those with high lesions presented with autonomic hyperreflexia but poor localization of abdominal pain.

It is thus important that the symptoms of autonomic hyperreflexia are recognized as a possible result of visceral disease and surgical advice sought. The impaired motor, reflex and sensory functions of SCI patients may otherwise lead to delays in surgical management, and mortality rates of 10–15% have been quoted.

Anaesthesia for the acute abdomen in SCI patients would clearly require consideration of autonomic hyperreflexia. The rapid-sequence induction used in neurologically normal patients for such surgery may need modifying in these patients. Increased sensitivity to sodium thiopentone has been noted in SCI patients, causing precipitous drops in blood pressure (Desmond and Laws, 1974), and therefore should be used cautiously in such patients, and particular attention made preoperatively to correction of fluid and electrolyte imbalance including dehydration. The use of suxamethonium is hazardous in the period extending from 3 days after SCI until approximately 8–9 months later, as it can cause a massive release of potassium into the circulation, with resultant cardiac arrest (Fraser and Edmonds-Seal, 1982).

Obstetrics

In neurologically normal patients, the onset of labour is associated with the perception of increasing abdominal discomfort and later often frank pain related to uterine contractions. The sensory pathway is via the sympathetic nervous system, with central connection with the 11th and 12th thoracic nerve roots. During delivery, descent of the baby into the vagina stimulates the pudendal and pelvic nerves, with sensory input at S2, 3, 4.

Patients with SCI above T10 should theoretically be unaware of any sensation of labour or delivery; however, Wanner, Rageth and Zach (1987) in their review found that all their patients perceived labour, usually in the form of strong abdominal spasms. More importantly, high SCI patients developed autonomic hyperreflexia during uterine contractions. This reflex can also occur during insertion of vaginal specula.

There is a tendency to premature labour, and labour may be rapid; consequently, unattended deliveries can occur. It has been recommended that pregnant paraplegic

---

Suggested checklist for anaesthesia in patients with chronic spinal cord injury

1. Is sensory abolition at operation site necessary? – note sensory level
                                                  – complete or incomplete
                                                  – sensory loss
                                                  – surgical field
2. How long since spinal cord injury? – reflex phase (if earlier spinal shock, different problem)
                                        – able to use suxamethonium (avoid 3 days to 9 months)
3. How high is spinal cord injury?
    (a) below T6
    (b) above T6 – ?susceptible to autonomic hyperreflexia
                 If yes, formulate – monitoring of CVS
                                   – treatment plan – ?spinal anaesthesia
                                                     – ?epidural anaesthesia
                                                     – ?GA with halothane or enflurane
                                                     – ?potent i.v. hypotensive agents
    (c) cervical – ?susceptible to autonomic hyperreflexia (see 3b)
                 – respiratory function
                 – intubation or tracheal suction arrest (treat with atropine)
                 – Valsalva (IPPV)
4. Anaemic? Blood volume and reaction to blood loss
5. Positioning – muscle spasm? securely locate limbs
                – risk of fractures
                – osteoporosis and joint stiffness
6. Temperature control – theatre temperature
                        – warm infusion and irrigation fluids to body temperature
                        – patient warming blanket?
7. Infection ?control
8. Renal function and drugs?
9. Drug interactions – antispasmodics
                      – anticholinergics
10. Psychiatric state and suitability for operation?
11. Prophylaxis against deep venous thrombosis?
12. Premedication – necessary?
                  – urology – avoid morphine/papaverine in males
13. Induction agent and BP ↓
14. Postoperative recovery and assessment ?intensive care

Figure 8.6

patients are examined at antenatal clinic visits from 28 weeks' gestation onwards, and hospitalized if cervical dilatation is occurring, or hospitalized at 32 weeks' gestation at the latest (Robertson, 1972).

Anaemia is common, increasing the likelihood of pressure sores, and may require blood transfusions (Aminoff, 1978). There is an increased susceptibility to venous thrombosis in paraplegics, which is exacerbated in pregnancy (Oppenheimer, 1971).

The hypertension produced by autonomic hyperreflexia in labour can easily be misdiagnosed as due to pre-eclampsia. However, oedema and proteinuria will be absent, and the hypertension is intermittent and related to contractions. Ravichandran, Cummins and Smith (1981) attempted to control the hypertension of autonomic hyperreflexia with sodium nitroprusside infusion, but control proved difficult and a lumbar epidural with bupivacaine (10 ml 0.25% bupivacaine 1–2 hourly) was instituted with success. Epidural bupivacaine is recommended as the method of choice, although general anaesthesia has also been used successfully to control this hypertension (Wanner, Rageth and Zach, 1987). The method of general anaesthesia is not stated, however.

Baraka (1985) has reported the successful use of a single injection of epidural pethidine (meperidine) 100 mg to control autonomic hyperreflexia for the 2 h prior to delivery in a 25-year-old T6 paraplegic parturient. Abouleish, Hanley and Palmer (1989), however, found that an epidural infusion of fentanyl (10 μg/h following a 75 μg loading dose) failed to control autonomic hyperreflexia in a 30-year-old C4/5 quadriplegic, and changed to epidural bupivacaine with complete success. Although epidural bupivacaine appears well proven as a method of controlling autonomic hyperreflexia in labour, the use of epidural opiates requires further work.

Vaginal delivery is usually possible, although mid-cavity forceps delivery may be required due to paralysis of the muscles involved in expulsion.

Figure 8.6 gives a suggested checklist for anaesthesia in patients with chronic spinal cord injury.

References

Abouleish, E.I., Hanley, E.S. and Palmer, S.M. (1989) Can epidural fentanyl control autonomic hyperreflexia in a quadriplegic parturient? *Anaesthesia and Analgesia*, **68**, 523–526

Alderson, J.D. and Thomas, D.G. (1975) The use of halothane anaesthesia to control autonomic hyperreflexia during trans-urethral bladder surgery in spinal cord injury patients. *Paraplegia*, **13**, 183–188

Aminoff, M.J. (1978) Neurological disorders and pregnancy. *American Journal of Obstetrics and Gynaecology*, **132**, 325–335

Anonymous (1975) Discussions on Proceedings of the Annual Scientific Meeting of the International Medical Society of Paraplegia. *Paraplegia*, **13**, 189–190

Arborelius, M. Jr., Balldin, V.I., Lilja, B. and Lundgren, C.E.G. (1972) Haemodynamic changes in man during immersion with the head above water. *Aerospace Medicine*, **43**, 592–598

Baraka, A. (1985) Epidural meperidine for control of autonomic hyperreflexia in a paraplegic parturient. *Anesthesiology*, **62**, 688–690

Barker, I., Alderson, J., Lydon, M. and Franks, C.I. (1985) Cardiovascular effects of spinal subarachnoid anaesthesia. A study in patients with chronic spinal cord injuries. *Anaesthesia*, **40**, 533–536

Bors, E. (1956) The challenge of quadriplegia. *Bulletin of Los Angeles Neurological Society*, **21**, 105–123

Brindle, G.S. (1986) Maintenance treatment of erectile impotence by cavernosal unstriated muscle relaxant injection. *British Journal of Psychiatry*, **149**, 210–215

Broecker, B.H., Hranowsky, N. and Hackler, R.H. (1979) Low spinal anaesthesia for the prevention of autonomic dysreflexia in the spinal cord injury patient. *Journal of Urology*, **122**, 366

Brown, B.T., Carrion, H.M. and Politano, V.A. (1979) Guanethidine sulphate in the prevention of autonomic hyperreflexia. *Journal of Urology*, **122**, 55–57

Burnham, L. and Werner, G. (1979) The high level tetraplegic: psychological survival and adjustment. *Paraplegia*, **16**, 184–192

Carter, R.E. (1987) Respiratory aspects of spinal cord injury management. *Paraplegia*, **25**, 262–266

Carter, R.E., Donovan, W.H., Halstead, L. and Wilkerson, M.A. (1987) Comparative study of electrophrenic nerve stimulation and mechanical ventilatory support in traumatic spinal cord injury. *Paraplegia*, **25**, 86–91

Chantraine, A. (1978) Actual concept of osteoporosis in paraplegia. *Paraplegia*, **16**, 51–58

Ciliberti, B.J., Goldfein, J. and Rovenstine, E.A. (1954) Hypertension during anaesthesia in patients with spinal cord injuries. *Anesthesiology*, **15**, 273–279

Comarr, A.E. (1959) The practical urological management of the patient with spinal cord injury. *British Journal of Urology*, **31**, 1–46

Corbett, J.L., Debarge, O., Frankel, H.L. and Mathias, C.J. (1975) Cardiovascular responses in tetraplegic man to muscle spasm, bladder percussion, and head up tilt. *Clinical and Experimental Pharmacology and Physiology*, suppl. 2, 189–193

Corbett, J.L., Frankel, H.L. and Harris, P.J. (1971) Cardiovascular changes associated with skeletal muscle spasm in tetraplegic man. *Journal of Physiology (London)*, **215**, 381–393

Desmond, J. (1970) Paraplegia, problems confronting the anesthesiologist. *Canadian Anaesthetists Society Journal*, **17**, 435–451

Desmond, J.W. and Laws, A.K. (1974) Blood volume and capacitance vessel compliance in the quadriplegic patient. *Cardiac Anaesthetic Society Journal*, **21**, 421–426

Dingemans, L.M. and Hawn, J.M. (1978) Mobility and equipment for the ventilator-dependent tetraplegic. *Paraplegia*, **16**, 175–183

Drinker, A.S. and Helrich, M. (1963) Halothane anaesthesia in the paraplegic patient. *Anesthesiology*, **24**, 399–400

Editorial Comment (1979) *Journal of Urology*, **122**, 366

Eggers, G.W.N. and Baker, J.J. (1969) Ventricular tachycardia due to distension of the urinary bladder. *Anesthesia and Analgesia*, **48**, 963–967

Figoni, S.F. (1984) Cardiovascular and haemodynamic responses to tilting and to standing in tetraplegic patients: a review. *Paraplegia*, **22**, 99–109

Frankel, H.L. and Mathias, C.J. (1979) Cardiovascular aspects of autonomic dysreflexia since Guttmann & Witteridge (1947). *Paraplegia*, **17**, 46–51

Frankel, H.L., Michaelis, L.S., Golding, D.R. and Beral, V. (1972) The blood pressure in paraplegia. *Paraplegia*, **10**, 193–198

Fraser, A. and Edmonds-Seal, J. (1982) Spinal cord injuries. A review of the problems facing the anaesthetist. *Anaesthesia*, **37**, 1084–1098

Gale, A.S. (1972) Ketamine prevention of penile turgescence. *Journal of the American Medical Association*, **29**, 1629

Ganong, W.F. (1989) *Review of Medical Physiology*, 14th edn, Appleton and Lange Publishers, Norwalk, p. 511

Gardiner, H. and Pembrey, M.S. (1912) Observations on the temperature of man after traumatic section of the spinal cord. *Guy's Hospital Reports*, **46**, 86–108

Glenn, W.W.L., Holcomb, W.G., Shaw, R.K., Hogan, J.F. and Holschuh, K.R. (1976) Long term ventilatory support by diaphragm pacing in quadriplegia. *Annals of Surgery*, **183**, 566–577

Gross, D., Ladd, H.W., Riley, E.J., Macklem, P.T. and Grassimo, A. (1980) The effect of training on strength and endurance of the diaphragm in quadriplegia. *American Journal of Medicine*, **68**, 27–35

Hassan, H.G. (1974) Anaesthesia in paraplegic patients. *Anaesthesia*, **29**, 629–630

Head, H. and Riddoch, G. (1917) The autonomic bladder, excessive sweating and some other reflex conditions in gross injuries of the spinal cord. *Brain*, **40**, 188–263

Howell, T., Fullerton, D.T., Harvey, R.F. and Klein, M. (1981) Depression in spinal cord injured patients. *Paraplegia*, **19**, 284–288

Johnson, B., Thomason, R., Pallares, V. and Sadove, M.S. (1975) Autonomic hyperreflexia: a review 1975. *Military Medicine*, **140**, 345–349

Johnson, R.H. (1971) Temperature regulation in paraplegia. *Paraplegia*, **9**, 137–145

Johnson, R.H., Smith, A.C. and Spalding, J.M.K. (1969) Blood pressure response to standing and to Valsalva's manoeuvre: independence of the two mechanisms in neurological diseases, including cervical cord lesions. *Clinical Science*, **36**, 77–86

Juler, G.L. and Eltorai, I.M. (1985) The acute abdomen in spinal cord injury patients. *Paraplegia*, **23**, 118–123

Kendrick, W.W., Scott, J.W., Jousse, A.T. and Botterell, E.H. (1953) Reflex sweating and hypertension in traumatic transverse myelitis. *Treatment Survey Bulletin (Ottawa)*, **8**, 437–448

Krebs, M., Ragnarrson, K.T. and Tuckman, J. (1983) Orthostatic vasomotor response in spinal man. *Paraplegia*, **21**, 72–80

Kurnick, N.B. (1956) Autonomic hyperreflexia and its control in patients with spinal cord lesions. *Annals of Internal Medicine*, **44**, 678–686

List, C.F. and Pimenta, A.D. (1944) Sweat secretion in man: spinal reflex sweating. *American Medical Association Archives of Neurology and Psychiatry*, **51**, 501–507

Mathias, C.J., Christensen, N.J., Corbett, J.L., Frankel, H.L., Goodwin, T.J. and Peart, W.S. (1975a) Plasma catecholamines, plasma renin activity and plasma aldosterone in tetraplegic man, horizontal and tilted. *Clinical Science and Molecular Medicine*, **49**, 291–299

Mathias, C.J., Christensen, N.J., Corbett, J.L., Frankel, H.L. and Spalding, J.M.K. (1976) Plasma catecholamines during paroxysmal neurogenic hypertension in quadriplegic man. *Circulation Research*, **39**, 204–208

Mathias, C.J., Christensen, N.J., Frankel, H.L. and Peart, W.S. (1980) Renin release during head-up tilt occurs independently of sympathetic nervous activity in tetraplegic man. *Clinical Science*, **59**, 251–256

Mathias, C.J., Hillier, K., Frankel, H.L. and Spalding, J.M.K. (1975b) Plasma prostaglandin E during neurogenic hypertension in tetraplegic man. *Clinical Science and Molecular Medicine*, **49**, 625–628

Mathias, C.J., Reid, J.L., Wing, L.M.H., Frankel, H.L. and Christensen, N.J. (1979) Antihypertensive effects of clonidine in tetraplegic subjects devoid of central sympathetic control. *Clinical Science*, **57**, 425–428

Naftchi, N.E., Demeny, M., Lowman, E.W. and Tuckman, J. (1978) Hypertensive crises in quadriplegic patients. *Circulation*, **57**, 336–341

Neider, R.M., O'Higgins, J.W. and Aldrete, J.A. (1970) Autonomic hyperreflexia in urological surgery. *Journal of the American Medical Association*, **213**, 867–869

Neuwirth, H., Royce, P.L. and Chaussy, C. (1986) Use of extracorporeal shock-wave lithotripsy in quadriplegic patients. *Journal of the American Medical Association*, **256**, 1295

Ohry, A., Heim, M. and Rozin, R. (1983) Peculiar septic responses in traumatic tetraplegia patients. *Paraplegia*, **21**, 318–321

Oppenheimer, W.M. (1971) Pregnancy in paraplegic patients: two case reports. *American Journal of Obstetrics and Gynaecology*, **110**, 784–786

Perkash, A. and Brown, M. (1982) Anaemia in patients with traumatic spinal cord injury. *Paraplegia*, **20**, 235–236

Quimby, C.W., Williams, R.V. and Greifenstein, F.F. (1973) Anaesthetic problems of the acute quadriplegic patient. *Anaesthesia and Analgesia*, **52**, 333–340

Rao, M.S., Barna, B.C., Vaidyanathan Gupta, C.L., Bhat, V.N., Reddy, M.J., Rao, M.K. and Singh, H. (1977) Topical or no anaesthesia for external urethral sphincterotomy in neurogenic vesical dysfunction due to spinal injury. *Paraplegia*, **15**, 226–229

Ravichandran, R.S., Cummins, D.F. and Smith, I.E. (1981) Experience with the use of nitroprusside and subsequent epidural analgesia in a pregnant quadriplegic patient. *Anesthesia and Analgesia*, **60**, 61–63

Rawal, N., Möllefors, K., Axelsson, K., Lingårdh, G. and Widman, B. (1983) An experimental study of urodynamic effects of epidural morphine and of naloxone reversal. *Anesthesia and Analgesia*, **62**, 641–647

Reid, J.L., Wing, L.M.H., Mathias, C.J., Frankel, H.L. and Neill, E. (1977) The central hypotensive effect of clonidine: studies in tetraplegic subjects 1977. *Clinical Pharmacology and Therapeutics*, **21**, 375–381

Riddoch, G. (1917) The reflex functions of the completely divided spinal cord in man compared with those associated with less severe lesions. *Brain*, **40**, 264–402

Robertson, D.N.S. (1972) Pregnancy and labour in paraplegics. *Paraplegia*, **10**, 209–212

Rocco, A.G. and Vandam, L.D. (1959) Problems in anaesthesia for paraplegics. *Anesthesiology*, **20**, 348–354

Schonwald, G., Fish, K.J. and Perkash, I. (1981) Cardiovascular complication during anesthesia in chronic spinal cord injured patients. *Anesthesiology*, **55**, 550–558

Schumacher, G.A. and Guthrie, T.C. (1951) Studies on headaches: mechanisms of headache and observations on other effects induced by distension of bladder and rectum in subjects with spinal cord injuries. *American Medical Association Archives of Neurology and Psychiatry*, **65**, 568–580

Sizemore, G.W. and Winternitz, W.W. (1970) Autonomic hyperreflexia – suppression with alpha adrenergic blocking agents. *New England Journal of Medicine*, **282**, 795

Snow, J.C., Sideropoulos, H.P., Kripke, B.J., Freed, M.M., Shah, N.K. and Schlesinger, R.M. (1977) Autonomic hyperreflexia during cystoscopy in patients with high spinal cord injuries. *Paraplegia*, **15**, 327–332

Spirnak, J.P., Bodner, D., Udayashankar, S. and Resnick, M.I. (1988) Extracorporeal shock wave lithotripsy in traumatic quadriplegic patients: can it be safely performed without anaesthesia. *Journal of Urology*, **139**, 18–19

Steinberg, F.U., Birge, S.J. and Cooke, N.E. (1978) Hypercalcaemia in adolescent tetraplegic patients: case report and review. *Paraplegia*, **16**, 60–67

Texter, J.H. Jr., Reece, R.W. and Hranowsky, N. (1976) Pentolinium in the management of autonomic hyperreflexia. *Journal of Urology*, **116**, 350–351

Thomas, D.G. (1986) The neurogenic bladder. *Surgery*, **35**, 820–827

Thompson, C.E. and Witham, A.C. (1948) Paroxysmal hypertension in spinal cord injuries. *New England Journal of Medicine*, **239**, 291–294

Thorn-Alquist, A. (1975) Prevention of hypertensive crises in patients with high spinal lesions during cystoscopy and lithotripsy. *Acta anaesthesiologica scandinavica*, suppl. 57, 79–88

Tricot, A. (1975) Annual scientific meeting discussion. *Paraplegia*, **13**, 189

Vandam, L.D. and Rossier, A.D. (1975) Circulatory, respiratory and ancillary problems in acute and chronic spinal cord injury. In *A. S. A. Refresher Courses in Anesthesiology*, Vol. 3, Lippincott, Philadelphia, pp. 171–182

Wanner, M.B., Rageth, C.J. and Zach, G.A. (1987) Pregnancy and autonomic hyperreflexia in patients with spinal cord lesions. *Paraplegia*, **25**, 482–490

Weber, W., Madler, C., Keil, B., Pollwein, B. and Laubenthal, H. (1986) Cardiovascular effects of ESWL. In *Extracorporeal Shock-Wave Lithotripsy for Renal-Stone Disease: Technical and Clinical Aspects* (eds J.S. Gravenstein and K. Peter), Butterworths, Boston, pp. 101–112

Wedley, J.R. (1976) Control of 'mass reflex' response in tetraplegia. *Anaesthesia*, **31**, 301

Welply, N.C., Mathias, C.J. and Frankel, H.L. (1975) Circulatory reflexes in tetraplegics during artificial ventilation and general anaesthesia. *Paraplegia*, **13**, 172–182

Wyndaele, J.J. (1987) Urology in spinal cord injured patients. *Paraplegia*, **25**, 267–269

Chapter 9

Nursing care of spinal cord injuries

D. Couldwell and M. Carlisle

Introduction

Spinal cord injury (SCI) used to be regarded as disastrous, with the patient's prognosis poor, but now that treatment is started very soon after injury, life expectancy can be excellent and return to a useful and active life in the community may be anticipated.

The care from admission to discharge is a team activity, with the patient and family working together with doctors, nurses, physiotherapists, occupational therapists and medical social workers. Maximum independence is the goal, with the level of physical disability and age of the patient being the limiting factors.

Prevention of complications which once caused fatality is now achievable, while pressure sores, respiratory problems, deep vein thrombosis, renal calculi and renal failure can all be minimized or ideally completely avoided.

When admitting patients with SCI, it is essential to commence treatment immediately to prevent complications. It is necessary to change the position of the patient regularly, check the condition of the skin and maintain the limbs in good alignment. A detailed care plan should be documented as soon as possible and kept updated and accurate.

Observations should include blood pressure, temperature, pulse rate and respiratory rate (vital capacity in higher lesions), fluid balance (intake and output), and bowel sounds and girth measurements. Neurological signs should be observed and recorded, including reflexes and involuntary muscle spasm, changes in the level of sensory or motor paralysis, and pain. It should be remembered that the patient will have lost sensory awareness and motor function, to a greater or lesser extent, and may not complain of any symptoms in the body below the level of injury.

Positioning the patient

Choose equipment carefully to ensure that the position of the patient can be changed, causing him or her as little discomfort as possible. The basic flat bed, with a firm mattress, is suitable, but turning-beds are available if basic staff is inadequate to turn the patient manually (Figures 9.1 and 9.2). Pillow packs may be used on a firm bed to remove pressure from any bony prominence. Whatever method of changing a patient's position is used, care must be taken to maintain the correct alignment of the spine, with all limbs supported. The turns must be timed to suit the individual patient

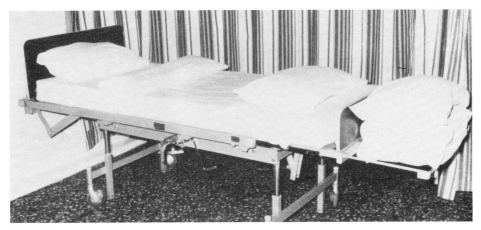

Figure 9.1 Basic flat bed with pillows, including lumbar pillow

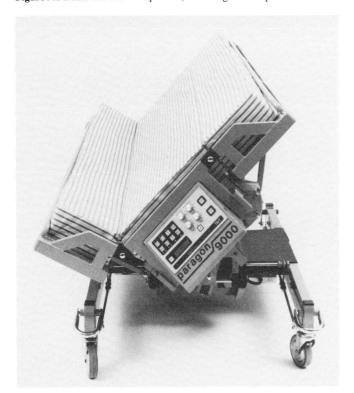

Figure 9.2 Electric turning bed. (Courtesy Egerton Hospital Equipment Ltd, Bromley, UK)

– they may be hourly in the very acute stage, but usually two-hourly turns will be tolerated. This timing must be determined by checking the state of all pressure points. When the patient has progressed to the rehabilitation stage, turns will still be necessary, but then up to 6 h may be tolerated; again this may vary and must suit the needs of the individual patient.

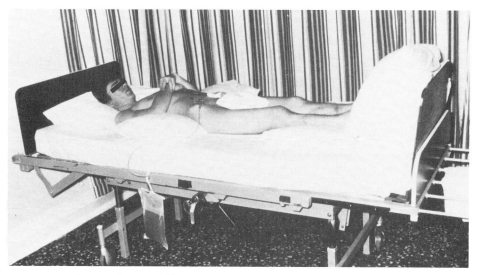

Figure 9.3 Turning the SCI patient: (i) patient supine

Dorsal and lumbar lesions

Log-rolling

Patients with these lesions can be log-rolled (see Chapter 2) by three staff, and should then be nursed in left or right lateral and supine positions two-hourly. This is an easy and quick procedure and allows inspection of all pressure points, checking of the urinary system and scrotum, observing that the legs are not swollen or discoloured due to thrombosis and that there is no abdominal distension. Since the patient may

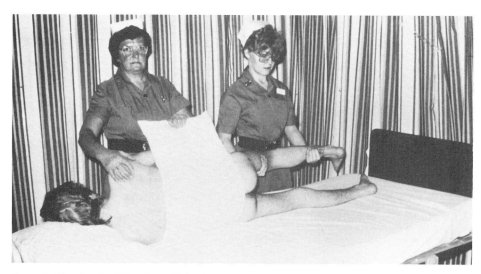

Figure 9.4 Turning the SCI patient: (ii) lumbar pillow is used to lever patient into lateral position

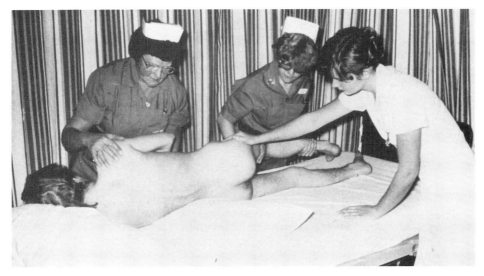

Figure 9.5 Turning the SCI patient: (iii) lumbar pillow is lowered and skin inspected, with pelvis and shoulders supported

have lost sensation below the injury level, pins and other sharp objects should not be left in the bed. The urinary catheter drainage system (if in use) should be placed clear of the patient. Nursing staff should avoid having sharp finger-nails, or sharp rings on their fingers, as the patient's skin can easily be damaged. Never drag the patient – either gently roll or, if lifting, completely clear the bed to prevent any abrasion to the skin.

Manual turning
When manually turning patients using a lumbar pillow to support the natural curve, the pillow is also used to lever the patient into a lateral position, with the shoulders being supported in line (Figures 9.3 and 9.4). Leg and foot pillows are removed and

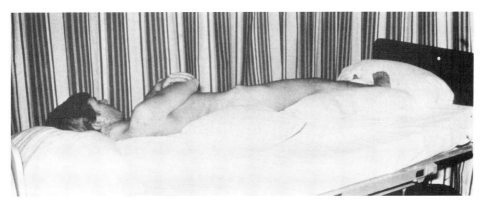

Figure 9.6 Turning the SCI patient: (iv) patient supported by pillows below spine, under upper leg and at feet

the patient is rolled onto the side using the lumbar pillow, while the upper leg is supported by another nurse. The lumbar pillow is then lowered and the skin inspected, during which the pelvis and shoulders must be supported (Figure 9.5). The patient is then supported by pillows placed behind the spine and under the upper leg, and a further pillow is used to support the feet at 90° (Figure 9.6).

Alternatively, the patient can be nursed on pillow packs and the position of these changed regularly. The patient must be lifted clear of the bed by four nurses, the packs moved to change points of pressure and the patient carefully placed back on the bed. This technique may be useful if a patient has skin problems.

If a turning-bed is used, it must be noted that the necessity for skin inspection is not eliminated.

Cervical lesions

Patients with these lesions and on traction (Figures 9.7 and 9.8) can be nursed on pillow packs, mechanical/electric turning-beds or alternatively on an ordinary bed and the pelvis turned regularly. While maintaining the alignment of the cervical spine with a nurse firmly holding the shoulders flat on the bed, the pelvis can gently be twisted (Figure 9.9), the skin inspected (Figure 9.10), and the lower trunk and pelvis and legs supported (Figures 9.11a,b). Care must be taken to inspect the occiput, and a 'halo' of sponge (shown in Figure 9.7) placed behind the head will prevent sores occurring. The elbows must be checked and the arms and hands supported on pillows in a natural line. In all cases the feet must be supported at 90°, the heels kept free from pressure and the weight of any bed covers kept off the toes.

If any pressure point becomes red (fixed erythema), the patient must *never* be placed back on that area before it has returned to *normal* appearance. Two hours in one position is usually as long as patients will tolerate initially, but by the rehabilitation stage they should progress to four- to six-hourly turns. This must be suited to the individual patient.

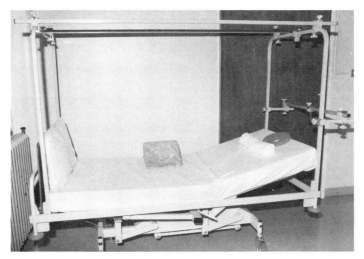

Figure 9.7 Bed suitable for cervical lesion on traction, showing neck roll occipital 'halo' and wedge to support pelvis

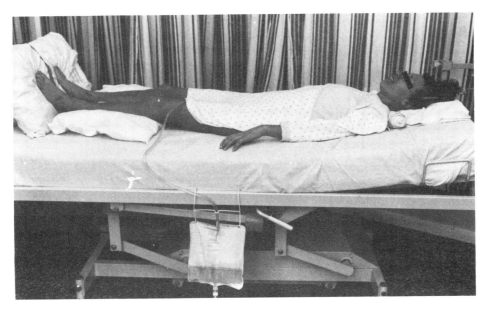

Figure 9.8 Turning the patient with cervical lesion on traction: (i) patient supine

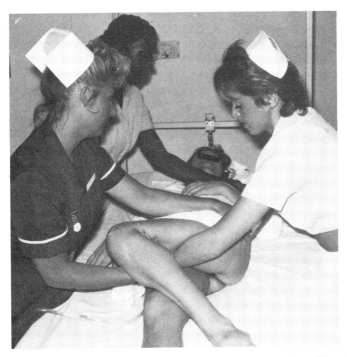

Figure 9.9 Turning the patient with cervical lesion on traction: (ii) twisting the pelvis gently, with shoulders held gently but firmly on bed

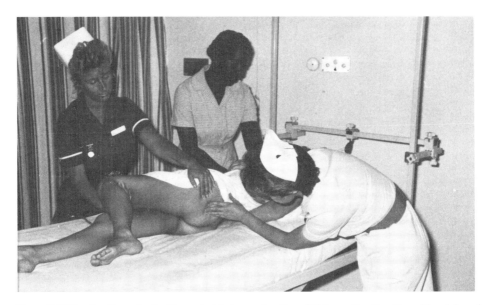

Figure 9.10 Turning the patient with cervical lesion on traction: (iii) inspecting the skin, with pelvis and shoulders still held gently in position

Hygiene

Strict hygiene must be maintained for the patients, but it should be noted that too frequent washing can destroy natural oils, while creams and sprays can be detrimental to a healthy skin. A daily bed bath is usually adequate. Clean dry bed linen is essential. Creases and darns must be avoided. Open-backed gowns should be used to avoid creases. Incontinence must be controlled by attention to bowel and bladder routines. The use of natural absorbent materials is preferable to those made of synthetic fibres.

When applying splints, care must be taken to keep the limbs in good position with adequate padding to prevent pressure.

Safety pins should not be used in areas where there is lack of sensation, as they are a potential danger.

Ensure the patient has regular oral toilet, especially when not taking oral fluids.

Maintain a clear nasal airway as far as possible, to prevent further distress to the patient. 'Drops' may be necessary.

Specific problems

Respiration
In patients with non-functional intercostal muscles and diaphragmatic breathing, it may be necessary to stabilize the rib cage to facilitate coughing or the clearing of nasal passages. Using the attendant's hands to stabilize the rib cage, a gentle push is given to expel air. This must not be done if there is injury at this level.

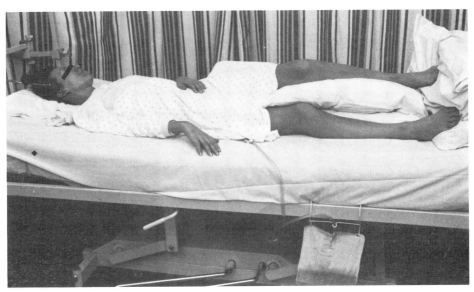

(a)

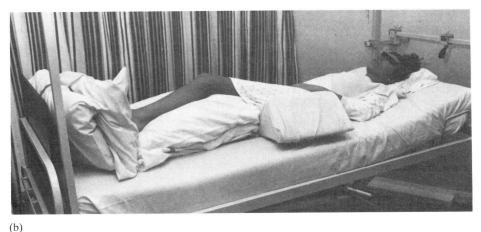

(b)

Figure 9.11 (a, b) Turning the patient with cervical lesion on traction: (iv) patient supported by pillows, with pelvis twisted and upper leg and feet supported

Paralytic ileus
This problem will occur to a greater or lesser degree. Regular measurement of girth and checking for bowel sounds is necessary. Nausea, vomiting and diminished urinary output must be regularly observed and recorded. Flatulence may have to be relieved by the passing of a flatus tube. Persistent abdominal distension can cause or increase respiratory distress. In the first few days it may be necessary to consider intravenous fluids.

Bowel function
In SCI patients, bowel function will be altered. Patients with lesions below L1, usually with lower motor neurone (atonic) lesions, will have no anal reflex and no ability to respond to suppositories or other stimuli. Gentle manual evacuation should be performed daily to prevent faecal impaction and overflow incontinence. Patients with intact anal reflex, usually upper motor neurone lesions, will respond to rectal suppositories, e.g. bisacodyl, and with good evacuation should require one to be inserted on alternate days. Toilet tissues should be placed under the buttocks only until the bowel action has been completed. They should be removed as soon as possible. Bed pans should not be used, as these may cause trauma to the skin.

Retention and/or incontinence of urine
This problem will occur in cases of SCI with paralysis. Over-distension and dyssynergia can cause long-term damage to the bladder and/or kidneys. Over-distension in upper dorsal or cervical lesions can cause respiratory problems due to pressure below the diaphragm. Autonomic disturbances needing immediate attention can also occur and if there is a rapid rise in the blood pressure and/or headache, the state of the bladder should be investigated urgently to eliminate this as a contributory cause. A strict record of fluid balance should be kept and palpation of the bladder size or an ultrasound scan to assess the residual urine volume should be carried out routinely. The patient is unaware in most cases of his or her inability to 'feel full', so this sensation must not be relied upon. Catheterization may be necessary. This can be achieved by an indwelling self-retaining catheter with a closed drainage system, or by intermittent emptying of the bladder by a small non-retaining catheter at times determined by fluid intake and physical checking of the size of the bladder. Strict asepsis must be maintained during these procedures and indwelling catheters changed regularly.

When permanent catheters are used, the bore of catheter should be the *smallest* necessary to give adequate drainage, while the balloon should be of the *smallest* volume needed to keep the catheter in position.

As an alternative to urethral catheters, suprapubic catheter drainage may be used. The medical officer's choice of method will be determined by: (a) the neurological needs of the individual patient; (b) the medical needs of the patient; and (c) the availability of trained staff.

Care must be taken to maintain strict hygiene when catheters are used. Pubic hair should be kept clean and the use of talcum powder or similar toiletries avoided. In a male, the position of the scrotum should be checked to prevent skin trauma from catheter tubing. A closed-circuit drainage system should be maintained whenever possible and a regular check made to ensure that the catheter is free-draining and output levels acceptable.

In the rehabilitation phase, the self-retaining catheters may be attached to the leg drainage bag if this is to be the permanent method of bladder control. These bags must be kept clean and replaced frequently.

Many patients will acquire a habit-controlled bladder function, in which both female and male patients maintain continence by regularly emptying their bladders by catheter after assessing the fluid intake levels. This is more a method of choice and it can be carried out quite simply in the wheelchair or on the toilet or bed after a little practice. Strict attention must again be paid to hygiene, and when disposable catheters are used, with good technique, the risk of infection is minimal.

Autonomic nervous system disturbances
These disturbances will occur in many lesions above T6 (see Chapter 8), and can easily be aggravated by many other medical conditions which may occur, e.g. blocked urinary catheter. Headache, rise in blood pressure and increased involuntary spasm should quickly be investigated, with particular attention paid to the urinary system, bowel function, and possible infection.

Deep vein thrombosis
This is an all too frequent complication in patients with paralysis. Prophylactic anticoagulation and regular movement of the limbs will lessen this risk. Care must be taken to make staff aware of the problems associated with anticoagulation therapy.

Postural hypotension
This will be a problem to overcome in patients with levels of paralysis above T5/6 when they first sit up in bed or in a chair. Mobilization must be a slow process to avoid syncope and to allow the patient to accept and feel confident in a wheelchair. If necessary, a binder may be used to support abdominal muscles, and if this is not adequate to maintain an acceptable blood pressure above 80 mmHg (10.6 kPa), the legs may be bound or elastic stockings used. These aids are not often necessary long term.

Hypothermia
This problem must be prevented in all paralysed patients, especially in the high dorsal and quadriplegic patient with impaired vasomotor control. Extremes of heat and cold must be avoided. Hot water bottles and electric blankets should not be used because of the risk of burns. Adequate room heating should be ensured and clothing must be suited to the ambient temperature.

Involuntary muscle spasm
This can be a major problem and in such cases bed cradles are a hazard to avoid, as the skin of the legs may easily be damaged. Pillows can keep the weight of the bed clothes off the feet and limbs while also supporting them.

Paramedical treatment, and counselling

Occupational therapy
Mental and physical occupational therapy should be started as soon as possible, with the patient being encouraged to do any part of the personal hygiene which is practicable. Simple aids for cleaning teeth, brushing hair, reading, writing, etc., should be made available and encouragement given to use them. Encouragement should also be given with constructive occupational therapy when the patient is well enough. Computers are now very mobile and adaptable and there is a wide choice for both academic and recreational application.

Physiotherapy
In order to minimize spasm, to encourage any return of voluntary muscle power, and to develop surviving muscle groups, physiotherapy should be given from admission. Many patients with lower lesions may walk with the aid of calipers and crutches,

sticks or walking-aids, and all patients should receive physiotherapy when the bed-rest period is over.

Involvement of the family and/or carers starts on admission of the patient. Understanding of the disability will assist in easier and quicker rehabilitation and return to the home community. These people will be taught, if necessary, to attend to all the patient's normal activities of daily living, i.e. habit-controlled bladder and bowel care, prevention of muscle contractures by physical therapy, as well as bathing and transferring from a wheelchair to bed or car, etc.

Sexual and social counselling
The social worker and community staff will be involved early in this counselling to ensure return to the community is as quick and as smooth as possible. It is necessary early in hospitalization to look, with the family, at the need for rehousing and so avoid waiting for suitable accommodation and prevent delay in final discharge. Most patients can go home for weekends as soon as the basic activities of daily living can be confidently coped with by patient or carers, provided that present housing is adequate. This is encouraged to aid social reintegration after a major accident and to ease the trauma of returning home in a wheelchair.

Sport is advised as a means of perfecting wheelchair control, building physical stamina and aiding psychological readjustment. It also helps to encourage social reintegration after becoming disabled. A high level of competitiveness is now achieved in wheelchair sport.

Regardless of age, maximum independence is aimed at in all patients. The total care, encouragement and involvement of the SCI unit team and the family will ensure a relatively fulfilled life for the wheelchair patient.

Theatre nursing of spinal cord injuries

Preoperative care

Many SCI patients have spent long periods in hospital and it is recommended that theatre staff visit the patients preoperatively in order to assess and eliminate any problems. Such a visit also gives patients the opportunity to meet the theatre staff and discuss any concerns they may have.

There are particular problems associated with SCI patients requiring surgery. Many will be unable to transfer from their beds to the theatre trolley and some who normally would be able to partially assist themselves may be too drowsy to do so if they have been premedicated with a sedative.

Patients being transferred from beds to theatre trolleys should be lifted cleanly and not dragged, as special care must be taken to protect their skin. To eliminate skin damage, it is essential that all members of the theatre team keep their finger-nails short and do not wear watches or rings, smooth wedding rings only being permissible.

The stretcher covers and sheets used on the theatre trolley must be free from creases. Patients' gowns must be untied and eased out from beneath them. Theatre staff must ensure that the patient is not laid on stretcher lifting poles.

During the transfer, care must be taken to support paralysed arms and legs. Paralysed limbs may be either flaccid or spastic, possibly fixed in a rigid position. Involuntary muscle spasm of the legs often occurs during the transfer, so it is important to secure the patient's legs firmly to prevent damage, as this spasm may be quite strong. The simplest method is for a member of the theatre staff to hold and support the legs firmly. Patients need to have confidence in the staff lifting them and made to feel secure, because many feel very vulnerable and concerned that they may fall or injure themselves. It is important to preserve their dignity at all times.

A team of three or four people may be required to support a patient with a new or an unstable fracture of the spine during transfer from bed to operating theatre trolley or to operating theatre table. It is essential to keep the patient's head, spinal column and legs in a neutral position in order to prevent further damage to the spinal cord.

If skull traction is in use, someone (preferably the surgeon) must take the responsibility of ensuring that the traction is kept steady during transfer to the theatre table.

Once the patient is on the trolley or table, pillows are used to protect bony prominences. For example, it may be necessary to place a pillow between the patient's knees or under the heels. All theatre trolleys should be fitted with padded cot sides. Cot sides with just bare, unprotected metal bars are dangerous, particularly with patients prone to muscle spasm. A sudden jerk of a leg could result in the leg being injured or trapped between the bars. Padded sides are kept in position for the duration of the journey to and from theatre.

Patients who have been paralysed for a number of years are well aware of the limitations of their own bodies. Theatre staff should never underestimate the patient's own knowledge and consideration must be given as to how they are most comfortable.

The patient's own finger-nails must be checked to ensure they are not digging into the skin. Nurses must anticipate where paralysed patients need protecting and protect them accordingly with pillows or other padding. It is often necessary for the nurse to position the fingers and arms for patients unable to do so for themselves.

Many tetraplegic patients only have feeling on their shoulders and are extra sensitive in this area, so an extra blanket tucked around the shoulders is often appreciated, particularly in cold weather or on draughty corridors.

Urinary catheters or condoms attached to drainage bags are frequently used for bladder control and care must be taken to see that they are draining freely and do not become trapped or cause pressure on the patient. If it is necessary to remove a urethral catheter, e.g. prior to transurethral surgery, then this should be done as late as possible because some patients experience headaches and sweating once their catheters have been removed. There is also the added concern of wet sheets for them to lie on.

In the anaesthetic room, the padded cot sides may be taken down provided that a designated nurse remains with the patient to care for their safety. While lifting patients across from the trolley to the theatre table, staff again must continually protect the patient, especially the limbs. Care must be taken to prevent any stretcher poles used causing abrasions when they are removed.

All arm and leg supports used should have the added protection of a layer of 'gamgee' padding. This gives extra support and also does not allow wet skin to adhere to the anti-static rubber of the table support. Pillows should also be used to protect bony prominences.

When patients are placed in the lithotomy position, it is essential to use fully adjustable, well-padded leg supports or knee crutches. As a precaution against muscle spasm, crepe bandages should be used to secure the legs in these supports.

Pillows are used to cushion the head, chest, hips and legs on the theatre table should the patient need to be in a prone position. When the patient is prone, legs should be secured, preferably by either a crepe bandage or a retaining strap over a pillow or a layer of gamgee padding.

Urinary drainage bags should be taped to the theatre table in a position where they can be seen to be draining freely; they are emptied, if necessary, during a long operation.

Corrugated drains should be stitched *in situ*, and safety pins never put through the drains in patients with SCI, as patients with limited sensation would not notice if a pin were to stick into them. Sterile surgipads are placed under any drains to prevent them from marking the patient's skin.

Similarly, gate clamps on intravenous infusions, or tubing with clamps used on bladder irrigation sets, must be kept clear of the patient because patients would be unaware of any feeling of discomfort should a clamp be pressing into them.

A pillow or other padding must be placed between a plaster of Paris cast and the patient.

Postoperative care

During and after a patient's recovery from an anaesthetic, theatre staff must continue to check that the patient's bladder is not over-distended. This is most important after transurethral surgery where bladder irrigation is being used. At this stage, patients with normal sensation would be able to say if they were experiencing any pain or discomfort, unlike patients with varying degrees of paralysis who may be unaware of any pain. It is important for the theatre staff to assess continually the level of the patient's comfort. Even small details, for example wiping a patient's eye or nose, become important for someone unable to do this for themselves.

On return to the ward, it may be necessary to lift the patient back into bed without the use of stretcher poles. Many patients are nursed on air beds or water beds with special ripple mattresses, and the use of stretcher poles could cause damage to such mattresses.

Theatre staff must ensure that the ward staff are aware of the position in which the patient has been lying in the theatre. They can then determine which position would be most suitable once the patient is back in bed. Both the theatre and the ward staff should check the condition of the skin once the patient is back in bed.

All intravenous infusions, drainage bags and/or bottles must be correctly positioned and the patient made as comfortable as possible, all relevant information being passed on to the ward staff.

Many of these guidelines for transferring patients to theatre are also applicable when a patient is being taken to another hospital department, such as radiology, for investigation or therapy.

Chapter 10

Assessment and management of the patient with spinal cord injury and pain

Chris Glynn and Peter Teddy

Introduction

The unique problem of pain following spinal cord injury (SCI) is one that has intrigued the medical profession (Tasker and Dostrovsky, 1989) for many years. Two specific questions arise:

1. What is the origin of the pain and what is the mechanism by which pain is transmitted from below the level of SCI to the brain? The investigation of the origin and transmission of this type of pain is complicated by the fact that this pain seems to be the prerogative of man, which means that there is no animal or research model for pain response/transmission (nociception) following SCI. There are obvious differences between the perception of pain by man and the response to pain by animals or the response of experimental models to noxious stimulation; this latter response to a noxious stimulus in animals or experimental models is called nociception (Merskey, 1978). There is no reliable experimental or animal model for chronic nociception. This means that at the present time all research into the pain which follows SCI must involve man.
2. How many patients with SCI suffer from this problem of chronic/intractable pain? A postal survey of over 1000 patients with SCI, conducted for a patients' spinal injury organization, revealed that 600 of these patients had a problem with pain, of whom 400 had to significantly change their life-style or their job because of the pain (Rose *et al.*, 1988). This survey also reported that only 21% of the patients who sought treatment obtained satisfactory relief of pain. It thus appears that pain following SCI is relatively common.

Why then has the problem of pain following SCI not received greater attention? One possible reason is that the results of treatment of patients with this particular pain have not been very successful and so the emphasis has been placed on rehabilitation. This is not a criticism of the therapy provided for patients with SCI, because a possible reason for the demand for pain relief by these patients may have been prompted by the dramatic improvement in their life-style as a result of their rehabilitation.

In simple terms, there are four possible sites of origin for the pain: (a) from below the level of the spinal lesion; (b) from the spinal cord of the lesion itself; (c) from above the level of the spinal lesion; (d) the pain is not related to the spinal cord lesion at all. Until there is better understanding of the mechanisms involved in the origin and transmission of this type of pain, the treatment of patients suffering such pain will remain the lottery it is now.

A frequent and concurrent problem in SCI patients is muscle spasm. This also might originate from above, at, or below the level of the spinal lesion. The possible sites of origin of muscle spasm are similar to those of pain. The relationship between the pain and the muscle spasm needs to be identified in each individual patient. It is occasionally the cause of the pain, but more commonly the muscle spasm and the pain are not related. That is, if the muscle spasm is relieved it makes no difference to the pain. The assessment and treatment of the patient with pain and muscle spasm should initially assume that the two are related because it is generally easier to abolish the muscle spasm, if only temporarily, than it is to relieve the pain. In this way, the relationship between the pain and muscle spasm should be identified and the appropriate treatment provided.

This chapter briefly discusses the present knowledge of the possible neurophysiology, pain transmission and the presumed mechanisms of muscle spasm in these patients. It then outlines a clinical assessment of the patient with pain and/or muscle spasm following SCI, and indicates possible treatment programmes.

Pain

The International Association for the Study of Pain has defined pain as an unpleasant sensory *and* emotional experience associated with tissue damage or described in terms of such damage (Merskey and Boyd, 1978). It is important to recognize that pain always has a physical and an emotional component which may or may not be significant. The art of treating patients with pain is to identify which is the principal component (Glynn, 1987). Chronic or intractable pain has been defined as pain of at least a month's duration which has not been relieved by conventional techniques (Glynn, 1988). The short duration of a month is used so as to accommodate patients with terminal cancer whose pain may only become intractable in the last months of life. Patients with SCI often have their pain for years before they are referred to a pain clinic. However, the principle is the same; the pain is unresponsive to conventional pain-relieving techniques.

It is possible that chronic or intractable pain is 'acute pain which persists' (P.D. Wall, personal communication). That is, the pain persists because the right treatment has not been given. The medical evidence for this persistence of acute pain has been available for some time, for example in the case of trigeminal neuralgia, the pain of which is not relieved by conventional analgesics but is relieved by anticonvulsants. If a patient with trigeminal neuralgia is not given anticonvulsants, then the pain persists and so becomes chronic, but if the correct drugs are prescribed, then the pain is relieved. This evidence suggests that the neurophysiological mechanisms involved in the origin of and/or the transmission of trigeminal neuralgia are different from those mechanisms involved in other types of pain which are relieved by conventional analgesics. Perhaps this analogy explains some of the pain which follows SCI, in that the pain is only chronic because the correct treatment for the acute pain is as yet unknown. Most of these patients with pain do not obtain any relief from conventional analgesics. This underlines the importance of understanding, in these patients, the possible origins and mechanisms of pain transmission which would appear to be different from normal.

The fact that animals do not suffer chronic nociception (pain) raises the question as to the possible benefits of chronic pain to man. Acute pain is generally an indication of an acute problem and will almost always resolve once the acute problem has resolved or is effectively treated. Chronic pain following SCI does not seem to serve any such useful function for the patient. It is interesting to note that these patients are often aware of differences in sensation and/or their pain when they have urinary tract infections. Once the urinary tract infection has been effectively treated, the new sensations or changes in the perception of their pain revert to 'normal' and so the relevance of their chronic pain remains a mystery. It is difficult for both patient and physician to see any benefit to be derived from, or phylogenetic reason for, chronic pain – it cannot surely serve as a warning like acute pain, and it may well be the only sensation which the patient has below the level of his or her lesion. One should learn to recognize significant change in the pain, particularly when accompanied by changes in physical signs. For example, a change in the level of normal sensation should be investigated to exclude a definitive cause such as a traumatic syrinx. Although chronic pain does not appear to serve any useful purpose, any change in the pain may equate with acute pain and should at least be an indication to re-examine the patient and reassess the situation.

Emotional component of pain

Chronic or intractable pain always has an emotional component which is made up of the unpleasant mood factors: anxiety, unhappiness (or depression) and aggression (Figure 10.1). It is normal for a patient with chronic pain to be chronically anxious because of the inability of the medical profession to provide adequate pain relief added to their inability to provide an adequate explanation for the pain. It is also normal for these patients to be angry or frustrated and unhappy for similar reasons. All these mood factors are unpleasant and, as previously defined, are therefore part of the patient's pain. It should be emphasized that the use of the word depression is as the *symptom* and not as the *syndrome* which is always abnormal. When the emotional component is the major component, then it is abnormal. The assessment

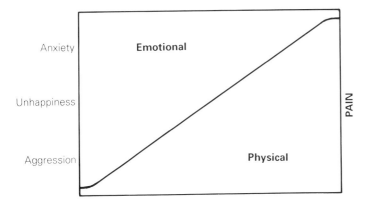

Figure 10.1 Schematic representation of the two components of chronic pain, with the three subdivisions of the emotional component – see text for explanation (After Glynn, 1988, by permission)

and treatment of this emotional component of pain will be discussed later in the chapter.

Physical component of pain

The pain that patients suffer following SCI may be broadly divided into three types: (a) deafferentation or central pain, i.e. pain in the numb area lying below the level of the lesion; (b) pain in the 'twilight zone', i.e. the area which lies between the normal sensation and the abnormal area and is usually at the level of the lesion; (c) pain that is not related to the spinal cord lesion, i.e. pain in the area of normal sensation which is above the level of the lesion.

The possible neurophysiological mechanisms for the origins and transmission of the first two types of pain will be discussed in some detail, whereas discussion of 'normal' pain is beyond the scope of this chapter.

Deafferentation pain
Deafferentation pain may be defined clinically as pain which occurs in an area of diminished or no sensation. It has been defined neurophysiologically by Zimmerman (1983):

(a) Pain is not dependent on activity in nociceptors or nocicepitive fibres.
(b) Pain involves changes in central neurones following loss of afferents due to lesions in the central or peripheral nervous system.
(c) The central changes due to loss of afferents might involve either or both excitatory and inhibitory mechanisms of the central neurones.

The three possible sites of origin of the deafferentation pain associated with SCI are: (i) the pain is originating from where the patient feels it – *peripheral*; (ii) the pain is originating from the spinal cord or the lesion itself – *spinal*; (iii) the pain is originating from above the level of the lesion – *central*. It is important to differentiate clinically these three sites because doing so should indicate possible treatment regimens (Figure 10.2).

Peripheral   There are two possible paths through which the pain may be mediated/ channelled from the periphery (i.e. where the patient feels it), and these are via the autonomic nervous system (Guttman, 1976) or via the spinal cord itself. The autonomic nervous system is extramedullary and is often not directly damaged in the patient with SCI and so is anatomically intact from the periphery to the brain. However, there is abundant evidence that the functioning of this system is altered following SCI.

Dimitrijevic (1983) tested electrophysiologically 77 patients with cervical cord injury and found that in 75% there were incomplete transections. This would allow neural conduction through the spinal cord lesion itself and it would presumably be possible for the patient to feel pain below the level of the cord lesion. However, as Dimitrijevic (1983) points out, the transmission system may be different from that in patients without SCI. This difference in transmission may be one of the reasons why the normal analgesics do not provide pain relief after SCI. Further research may indicate the relationship between incomplete spinal lesions and pain transmission.

Thus there are two possible systems available for the transmission of pain from below the level of the lesion, but there is no information available to explain why or

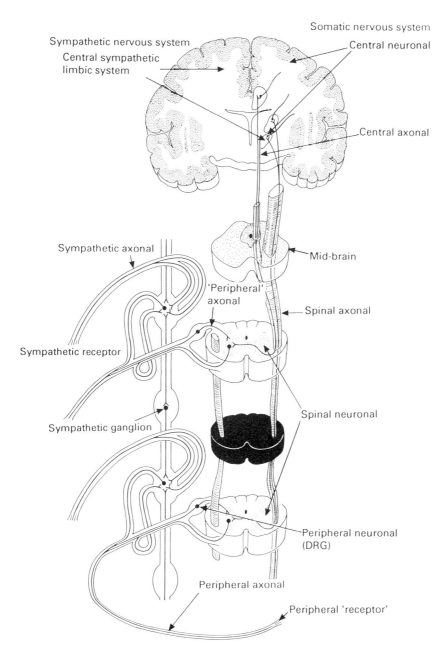

Somatic nervous system

Sympathetic nervous system

Central sympathetic
limbic system

Central neuronal

Central axonal

Sympathetic axonal

'Peripheral'
axonal

Mid-brain

Spinal axonal

Sympathetic receptor

Spinal neuronal

Sympathetic ganglion

Peripheral neuronal
(DRG)

Peripheral axonal

Peripheral 'receptor'

Figure 10.2 Possible origin of deafferentation pain in the periphery and the two methods of transmission from there to the brain

how the sensation of pain arises in the periphery. Most of the patients referred to the Oxford Regional Pain Relief Unit have other vague sensations from below the level of their lesion, as well as pain. Many of these are associated with bladder or bowel function. Some patients know when they have a urinary tract infection because of a change in sensation which, interestingly, is often not felt as pain. They seem to be able to differentiate between this sensation and their pain, although the latter may be in some way related in that it is made worse by any increase in the sensation from the bladder. The bladder sensations serve a useful clinical purpose as they indicate a need for treatment. After successful treatment, the sensation then returns to 'normal for that patient', a similar situation to acute pain in the patient without SCI; thus chronic pain in both SCI and normal patients does not seem to serve any useful function.

In summary, it is physically possible for the pain to be originating from the area where the patient feels it, although the reasons for the pain and the peripheral mechanisms initiating the pain are unknown. The transmission of this pain from the periphery to the brain is possible either via the autonomic nervous system, which is extramedullary and so not damaged, or via an incomplete lesion of the spinal cord (see Figure 10.2). Future research will hopefully identify possible peripheral mechanisms for the pain and also which of the two transmission systems is involved in the pain, because if these mechanisms are understood, then the treatment of the pain will become more effective.

Spinal   The deafferentation pain which occurs following SCI could originate from anywhere in the spinal cord, the most likely area being the site of injury. There are enormous neurophysiological changes in the spinal cord of animals following trauma to peripheral nerves (Wall and Devor, 1982). These changes are believed to be a result of the altered information from the periphery. If this is true, then the alteration in the transmission of information as a result of spinal trauma is several times greater than that which follows trauma to a peripheral nerve (Wall and Devor, 1982). The assumption is that these neurophysiological changes are in some way related to deafferentation pain. Such changes are always found after trauma to a nerve in the animal models, yet pain does not always follow nerve trauma in man. The same can be said about SCI (Brenowitz and Pubols, 1981), so that not all patients with SCI suffer deafferentation pain. The relationship between this altered neurophysiologic state and deafferentation pain remains unclear.

The mechanisms by which the pain is generated in the spinal cord are unknown, but there are numerous possibilities. The nervous system is designed to report information from the periphery; if this flow of information is interrupted, then the system tries to find another way of obtaining information. It is not a rigid system, but a plastic one; this plasticity may indeed be part of the reason why deafferentation pain seems to be the prerogative of man. It may be that man has learned the meaning of the sensations from the periphery and when some of these normal sensations are changed to unpleasant sensations, i.e. pain, he or she has not learned that this particular sensation is not serving any useful purpose. On the other hand, the return of unpleasant sensations may be a result of the phylogenetically earliest system being the most robust, that is the one that survives the trauma most effectively or the system that regenerates more effectively following trauma. The evidence in favour of these two possibilities is that deafferentation pain is (a) often poorly localized and (ii) all or any information arriving from the periphery is commonly interpreted as pain.

There are 14 possible neurotransmitters, neuro-inhibitors, neurofacilitators and

Table 10.1 Possible neurotransmitters, neuromodulators, neurofacilitators or neuro-inhibitors*

Substance P
Neurotensin
Cholecystokinin
Calcitonin gene-related peptide
Enkephalin
Vasoactive intestinal polypeptide (VIP)
Fluoride-resistant acid phosphatase (FRAP)
Glutamate
Aspartate
Glycine
Serotonin
Somatostatin
Noradrenaline (norepinephrine)
Gamma-aminobutyric acid (GABA)

* These neurotransmitters, neuromodulators, neuro-facilitators and neuro-inhibitors are found in the dorsal horn of the spinal cord and may be involved in deafferentation pain at the spinal cord level. This pain may originate from below, at, or above the site of injury; if it is below or at the site of injury, then the transmission is via the 'incomplete' lesion or via the autonomic system.

neuromodulators thought to be involved in the transmission of pain at the first synapse (Table 10.1). Thus the permutations and combinations which may result from alterations occurring at the first synapse are enormous, particularly when compared to the computer which has only one or two possibilities at the first 'synapse'. The power of the computer lies in the large numbers of 'synapses' in series and one is aware of the problems created by errors in computer programs, even more so if these errors are a result of electrical faults in the 'synapses' which give random errors.

This highlights a fundamental problem in trying to understand the mechanism of spinally originating deafferentation pain, in that it is assumed that the neuro-physiological changes that do occur in the spinal cord after trauma are logical and not random. The assumption is made that the nervous system is trying to re-establish communication with the periphery and the end result of this effort is directly related to the number and type of surviving neurones. Unfortunately, the treatment of these problems in the spinal cord is not like the computer, where an electrical error may be corrected by a new computer or board. Thus, spinal deafferentation pain may be a result of logical or random changes in any of the 14 neurotransmitters, neuro-inhibitors, neurofacilitators or neuromodulators thought to be involved in the transmission of pain at the first synapse.

There is some clinical evidence to support involvement of these spinal cord changes as the origin of the pain, in that local anaesthetics, given either epidurally or intrathecally, invariably fail to relieve the pain. These drugs exert their effect by axonal blockade and so blockade of the axons before they reach the spinal cord is generally ineffective, circumstantial evidence that the pain is arising proximal to the blockade. Thus it would seem important to examine spinal neuronal blockade to find out if this provides effective analgesia. Given the complexity of the relationships among the substances involved in the transmission of pain at the first synapse, it is difficult to know where to start. Morphine is the most effective spinal (neuronal) analgesic. However, it was effective in only 5 of the 15 patients with deafferentation pain following SCI when given either epidurally or intrathecally. Clonidine, an alpha 2 agonist, given in the same way provided a beneficial effect on pain in 10 of 15 patients studied (Glynn *et al.*, 1986). In this way, the two best known analgesic transmission systems, the opioid and the noradrenergic, were examined in the same patients. It is worth noting that 5 of these 15 patients did not obtain any analgesia from either of the drugs, suggesting that yet another transmission system was involved or that the pain was not originating from the spinal cord.

If the pain is originating from the spinal cord below the level of the lesion, then its transmission to the brain is presumably transmitted through an incomplete lesion of the cord. It is equally possible that the pain may be transmitted via the autonomic nervous system which is extramedullary and not affected by the SCI (see Figure 10.2). The deafferentation pain may also originate from above the level of the spinal cord lesion for the same reasons as described above. In summary, there are three possible sites of spinal origin for the deafferentation pain: (a) below the level of the lesion; (b) at the lesion itself; (c) above the level of the lesion (Figure 10.3).

Central   Possible sites of origin of deafferentation pain proximal to the site of injury are the most difficult to define because they are identified by a process of exclusion. If the pain is not relieved by axonal blockade of both the somatic and autonomic nervous systems (peripheral), nor by the various neuronal blocks mentioned above (spinal), then the pain is believed to be central. Given that trauma to a peripheral

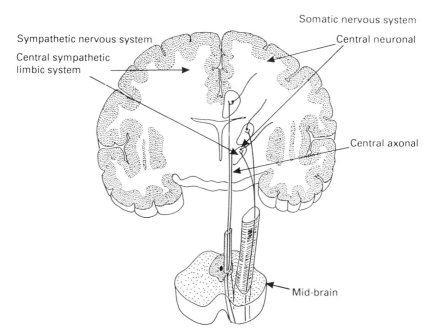

Figure 10.3 Possible areas of the brain that may be involved in central pain – both the physical and the emotional components

nerve causes changes in the spinal cord as discussed above, it is conceivable that trauma to the spinal cord may cause changes in the brain. Although these presumed changes in the brain may be a physical mechanism for the central pain, there is always a central emotional component associated with every patient's pain (see Figure 10.1). Nevertheless we assume that the pain is central because all the treatments tried have failed to provide any relief, and because the neurophysiological mechanisms for these pains are not understood, the true origin of the pain may not be central. If we do not understand the origin or the mechanism of the pain, it is difficult to know how to treat it, so from the practical point of view we treat the emotional component – the coping mechanism.

Pain in the twilight zone
Patients with SCI commonly have an area between the normal and absent sensation where there is some sensation, but this sensation is abnormal – this is the twilight zone. The pain in this border zone may be (a) deafferentation pain (see above), (b) pain peculiar to the twilight zone, or (c) chronic pain that is unrelated to the SCI – normal chronic pain. Root pain, a commonly used description of this pain in patients with SCI, has been avoided because of the confusion generated by this term, as it is often used by the medical profession to describe *all* pain below the level of the lesion.

Pain peculiar to the twilight zone   It has been suggested by Sweet (1988) that deafferentation pain is not an entity and that it should be classified by its site of origin, as above. However, pain which is peculiar to the twilight zone responds to different treatments when compared to pain found in the area of completely absent sensation. This suggests that the origins and/or mechanisms of these two pains is probably different, hence the division.

Chronic pain

The possible neurophysiological mechanisms for the transmission of chronic pain are shown in Figure 10.2 and Table 10.1. There are numerous texts devoted to this subject and further discussion is beyond the scope of this chapter.

Clinical assessment of pain

The cardinal rule of the pain clinic which is involved in the symptomatic management of pain is to be sure that there is no definitive treatment for the cause of that pain. The definition of chronic/intractable pain must be remembered and any clinically significant change in the pain must be an indication to reassess the patient. For example, in the SCI patient changes in pain perception, although vague, may be the only indication of genitourinary infection, a not uncommon problem in such patients. These changes in the perception of the pain and all new pains should be dealt with in the same way as acute pain, that is with a medical history, examination of the patient and *all* the relevant investigations indicated by the history and examination. Any change in the muscle tone below the level of the lesion is an indication to reassess the patient clinically.

These changes in the perception of pain and spasticity would appear to be the SCI patient's equivalent to acute pain or a warning that some change has occurred. It is

Table 10.2 Aims of the history, examination, investigation and treatment of the spinal cord injury patient

1. Identification of the patient's *expectations*
2. Give the patient a clear *explanation* of the special problems associated with his or her chronic pain
3. Do a full and thorough *examination*
4. Make a diagnosis and ensure that the patient's *education* is such that he or she understands the possible therapies available and their limitations
5. Decide on a treatment programme, in conjunction with the patient, designed to fulfil the *expectations* of both the patient and the physician

interesting to note that most of the causes of these involve changes in the viscera which are predominantly supplied by the autonomic nervous system. This is further observational evidence in favour of:

1. That information is transmitted past or through the spinal cord lesion.
2. The plasticity of the nervous system which is endeavouring to overcome the injury and to provide 'useful' information to the central control, i.e. the brain.
3. That the phylogenetically earlier nervous system – the autonomic – is the most robust.

The clinical assessment of a patient with an SCI and pain must involve the basic tenets of medicine, *history, examination, investigations* and, where possible, a *diagnosis* (Table 10.2 and Figure 10.4).

The second rule of the pain clinic is that all the notes, consultations and

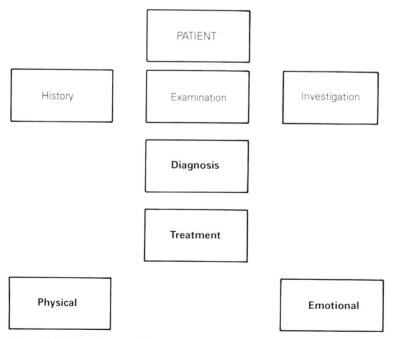

Figure 10.4 Schematic approach to the patient with spinal cord injury and pain. The most important thing to remember is that subtle changes in the perception of pain or spasticity may be clinically significant, whereas changes in the level of sensation are always significant and must be further investigated

investigations pertaining to the patient's injury and previous assessments should be available at the patient's first visit. It is obvious that it is impossible to interpret the examination of these clinically difficult patients without the baseline assessment. If there is any possible doubt in the mind of the examiner because of the examination or because of lack of information about the patient, then it is imperative that he or she consult the local expert who deals regularly with SCI patients.

History

The patient should be asked where he or she feels the pain – in the area of abnormal sensation (deafferentation pain) or in the area of normal sensation ('normal pain'). It is always helpful to have a body chart on which to record the area of the pain/pains, and the patient should be shown this at the end of the history and examination to confirm that he or she agrees with the indicated areas of pain or pains (Figure 10.5). Occasionally the patients have more than one pain and it is important to identify these different areas of pain and number them. If there is more than one area of pain or more than one pain, then each area/pain should be dealt with separately. The patient is asked when and how the pain started, and the duration of the pain is established together with any initiating, aggravating or relieving factors. All previous treatments prescribed for the pain/pains and their effect should be documented, as well as all the previous consultations with the medical and paramedical professions, together with the results of those consultations.

Classical deafferentation pain is generally not associated with any history of trauma or indeed any event; the patients most commonly say that they gradually became aware of the pain. It is often described as vague poorly localized pain in the area of abnormal sensation and it may not have any initiating, aggravating or relieving factors – it is just there all the time. If this type of pain has any association, it is with changes in genitourinary or gastrointestinal function, both normal and abnormal. For example, some of these patients' pain is aggravated by either urination or manual removal of faeces. In contrast, pain that is described in the twilight zone is commonly a variety of deafferentation pain, but it is often made worse by movement or changes in temperature or tactile stimulation. Thus there is an identifiable change associated with the pain, indeed a possible stimulus. The reasons for this division of deafferentation pain into two will become apparent when the treatment of these patients is discussed. Any pain in the area of normal sensation should be assessed as a 'normal pain' as distinct from pain associated with SCI (Wall and Melzack, 1984).

An important and alas often neglected aspect of taking a history from any patient is to identify his or her expectations of the medical profession; this is particularly important in the pain clinic. These expectations may be broadly stated as (a) having their pain relieved and (b) finding the cause of, or the meaning of, their pain.

These two expectations are related and yet are not the same. The former needs no explanation; the latter is usually a direct result of the presumed protective nature of pain which is generally true for acute pain, but probably not true for chronic pain. The patients believe that their pain is an indication that something is 'wrong' and this something needs to be put 'right'. Chronic pain does not seem to serve any useful function as far as protection of the organism is concerned. This is especially true for the deafferentation pain following SCI. The patients need to be made aware of this major difference between acute and chronic pain and it should also be made clear to them that although the actual cause of their pain cannot clearly be defined, it

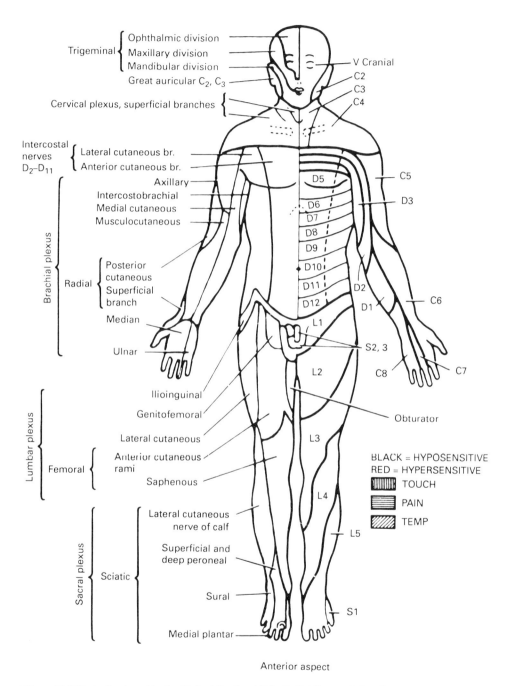

Figure 10.5 Body chart used in the Oxford Regional Pain Relief Centre. It has dermatomes on one side and peripheral nerves on the other. Because these charts vary, it is important for those working in the same unit to use the same chart so that they will be consistent among themselves

Table 10.3 Therapeutic options for the emotional component of chronic pain

1. Patients may cope with it themselves
2. Pharmacological
3. Professional counselling, both medical and paramedical

is possible to say what is *not* the cause of their pain. For these patients it is as important to state what is not the cause of the pain as to be able to say what is the cause. Chronic pain that has been present for years without identification of a definitive diagnosis despite exhaustive investigation is unlikely to have a sinister cause and patients should be made aware of this to alleviate their fears as to the possible connotations of unrelieved and undiagnosed pain.

Once the patients' expectations have been identified, then it is necessary to ensure that these are realistic, because if the patient has unrealistic expectations of what is achievable, then failure is almost certain. It is often an advantage to explain to the patient that there are two components to chronic pain – the physical and the emotional – and that these two are always present (Figure 10.1). It should clearly be explained to the patient that the unpleasant mood factors, *anxiety, unhappiness* and *aggression* (see Figure 10.1) are always present, and are part and parcel of all chronic pain. It should also be made clear that most often this emotional component requires treatment and this a reflection of the patients' ability to *cope* with the pain and all the problems that this pain creates for them. The treatment offered for the emotional component of the pain is aimed at helping the patient cope with the pain, usually a separate problem to the pain itself (Table 10.3).

Examination

The aims of physical examination are: (a) to confirm that there has been no significant neurological change since the last examination; (b) to document the clinical neurology found in the area or areas of pain; (c) to examine other systems as indicated by the symptoms and signs in order to exclude a treatable cause for the pain, such as a urinary tract infection.

There are a number of texts devoted to the SCI patient, and the reader is referred to them for a complete summary of the physical examination of such patients (Guttman, 1976; American Spinal Injury Association, 1982).

If the examination of the patient reveals a significant neurological change, then it is imperative that the patient be reassessed by someone experienced in neurological examination. One possibility is that the patient may have developed a traumatic syrinx as a cause of the pain. The cardinal rule of the pain clinic must be obeyed: pain must not be treated symptomatically if there is a treatment for the cause of the pain. Documentation of the neurological changes in the area/areas of the pain may have a bearing on the possible therapies prescribed for the patient. It is also important to have as much neurological information as possible about these patients in order to be able to understand the relationship between the neurology and the pain. The neurological changes and the pain may well, in some as yet unknown manner, be related and it is only with obsessive documentation that we shall be able to identify some or all of these relationships.

Physical examination of the other systems will be governed by their association with the patient's description of the pain; however, irrespective of the symptoms, the examination should always include the genitourinary system.

Investigations

All patients should have a urinalysis as a standard part of their examination because urinary tract infection is more common in patients with SCI than it is in the normal population. These patients are also more prone to renal and ureteric stones than the general population and so they should have regular, intravenous pyelograms. It is important to exclude any genitourinary cause for the pain. If there has been a change in the sensory level or a significant increase or decrease in motor function/spasticity, then it is imperative that a traumatic syrinx is excluded by myelography, computed tomography scan or magnetic resonance imaging. Other investigations should be undertaken as indicated.

Diagnosis

The symptomatic management of SCI patients with chronic pain generally means that we do not have a specific diagnosis for the cause of their pain, and in these circumstances we make a diagnosis based on the site of the pain in conjuction with the patient's description of their pain (Sweet, 1988). There are also circumstances where the cause of the pain is known but there is no definitive treatment and so in both situations pain is treated symptomatically. Before the patient's pain is treated symptomatically, definitive therapy for the cause of the pain must always be prescribed. It is most helpful to identify where the patient describes the pain and then to define the pain as:

1. That pain described in the area of normal sensation; in other words pain probably not related to the spinal injury.
2. Deafferentation – that pain described in the area of abnormal sensation.
3. Twilight zone – that pain described in the area between normal and abnormal sensation.

Treatment of pain

Chronic pain is generally multifactorial in origin. Broadly speaking, the problems caused by or associated with chronic pain can be divided into the two components, emotional and physical, as previously mentioned. The therapeutic options available for each of these two components are shown in Tables 10.3 and 10.4. The patient should be told that the emotional component of their pain is normal and that *all* patients with chronic pain have an emotional component. It is generally very helpful to show and explain to the patient the diagram illustrated in Figure 10.1 which indicates the mood factors which may be involved in this emotional component. The individual patient's response gives a guide to his or her insight into the problem and gives a good prognostic sign for outcome in the treatment of the emotional component of his or her pain.

After taking a history, *examining* and investigating, it should have been possible in most situations to identify that patient's *expectations*. It is probably worth while to

Table 10.4 Therapeutic options for the physical component of chronic pain

1. Physical
2. Pharmacological
3. Injections
4. Surgery

define, or to redefine, each patient's expectations of any therapeutic programme with him or her, before embarking on any treatment. It is important from the outset that each patient has realistic expectations of any therapeutic programme. The method by which a patient's expectations may be redefined is by a clear *explanation* of the physician's understanding of their pain. The end result of this explanation is that the patient understands the possible meaning of his or her pain or indeed the apparent uselessness of chronic pain and also the paucity of medical knowledge which defines the limitations of treatment. Unfortunately this may be the first time that most of these patients have been given any information about the connotations of their pain, i.e. *education*. It is important that each patient understands his or her problem as well as the limitations of the present medical knowledge and treatment of chronic pain. This definition of the lack of medical knowledge should not be nihilistic; it should be made clear to the patients that this knowledge is increasing all the time and that our understanding and therefore our treatment of their pain should improve with time.

Treatment of emotional component

As a general rule, any treatment programme should involve therapy for both components of chronic pain. The therapeutic manoeuvres available for the emotional component are shown in Table 10.3 and the decision as to which treatment is preferable should be made by the patient. If the patient decides to embark on a programme of professional counselling, then it is imperative that there is effective communication between the counsellor and the doctor who is involved with the treatment of the physical component. Chronic pain patients are past masters at playing one doctor off against another (Sternbach, 1978). Discussion of the advantages and disadvantages of the various treatment modalities for the emotional component of chronic pain is discussed elsewhere. There are very few reports of the use of these therapies in SCI patients (Grzesiak, 1977).

Treatment of physical component

The treatment of the physical component should be governed by the type of pain or pains, i.e. pain in the area of normal sensation, pain in the twilight zone or classical deafferentation pain. A discussion of the treatment of pain in the area of normal sensation is dealt with in many other texts (Wall and Melzack, 1989). Figure 10.2 shows the site of action of most of the possible treatment modalities for chronic pain.

The clinical decision as to whether the pain is deafferentation pain or not usually revolves around local anaesthetic blockade of the nerves that supply the area of the pain (Figure 10.5), and its resultant effect on the pain. If the local anaesthetic relieves the pain, then it is assumed that the source of the pain is more distal than the local anaesthetic blockade. If the converse occurs, i.e. the area of pain is made more numb without relief, then the assumption is that the pain is more central than the site of the injection. There are obvious problems with this concept in the areas of absent sensation; however, it classifies the pains that occur in the twilight zone as 'normal' or deafferentation.

It is possible that the patient has more than one type of pain in the same area, i.e. normal and deafferentation pain in the twilight zone or even in the area of absent sensation. Although the patient does not differentiate between the pains because they respond in different ways to the local anaesthetic, we infer that they are different or at least have different modes of transmission. This concept of pains being different based on their different modes of transmission is crucial to the possible understanding of mechanisms of pain and also to providing the appropriate treatment for that pain (Figures 10.3 and 10.6).

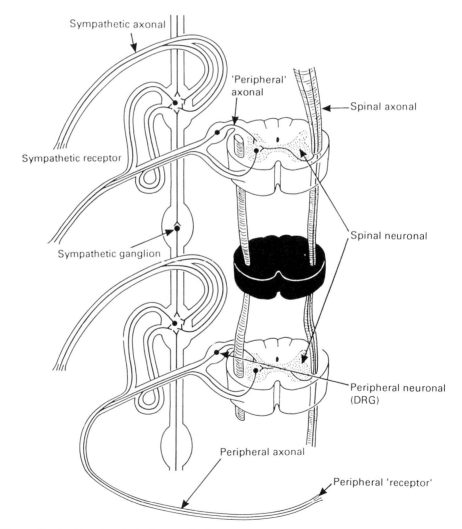

Figure 10.6 Peripheral and spinal sites of origin of the three different types of pain, highlighting the possible transmission systems

The therapeutic options available for the physical component of deafferentation pain are shown in Table 10.4. The simplest treatment is the best because it generally has the least side effects. Once again it is a good rule to discuss the merits of the various therapeutic options with the patient, because only the patient knows how much of a problem the pain creates for him or her. This is important because the occasional patient will be satisfied simply with a clear explanation of the meaning of the pain.

Physical therapies

Most patients who are referred to a pain relief unit may already have had some physical therapies, e.g. physiotherapy, but may not have had transcutaneous nerve stimulation (Banerjee, 1974; Davis and Lentini, 1975; Heilporn, 1977–78) or acupuncture. The success rate of these two modalities is not high in these patients, but they are both worth a trial because of their simplicity and lack of significant side effects.

Pharmacological treatment

The pharmacological treatment of deafferentation pain has been reviewed by McQuay (1988) and the reader is referred to that text for further information. Table 10.5 lists some of the drugs and their dosage which may be used to treat these patients. Even after using this impressive list of drugs, there are some patients who

Table 10.5 Drugs used in the management of the patient with deafferentation pain*

Antidepressants
Amitriptyline, 25–150 mg nocte
Dothiepin, 25–150 mg nocte
Mianserin, 10–100 mg nocte
Clomipramine, 10–150 mg nocte
Imipramine, 25–200 mg nocte
Lithium, in combination with amitriptyline/dothiepin†

Anticonvulsants
Phenytoin, 100 mg t.d.s.
Sodium valproate, 200 mg b.d.
Carbamazepine, 100 mg t.d.s. increasing to 400 mg t.d.s.
Clonazepam, 0.5 mg b.d. increasing to 1 mg t.d.s.

Miscellaneous
Clonidine, 25 µg t.d.s. increasing to 100 µg t.d.s.
Dexamethasone, 4 mg t.d.s.
Flecainide, 100 mg b.d. increasing to 200 mg b.d.
Mexiletine, 150 mg daily increasing to 800 mg daily
Naloxone, 0.4 mg slowly i.v.i.
Baclofen, 5 mg t.d.s. increasing to 20 mg t.d.s.
L-Tryptophan, 500 mg q.d.s. increasing to 1 g q.d.s.
Haloperidol, 1.5 mg increasing to 20 mg nocte

* The proposed mechanism of action of these drugs is discussed in McQuay (1988). This list is not complete as it mentions only those drugs that have been shown to be effective clinically and scientifically.
† The lithium should be used in conjunction with the amitriptyline/ dothiepin and the blood concentration should be measured to ensure that it is in the therapeutic range of 0.4–0.7 mg/l.

do not achieve any pain relief. There are very few controlled studies of the use of these drugs in SCI patients with deafferentation pain. One of the few reported no effect from trazadone (Davidoff *et al.*, 1987). Thus the list and dosage of drugs shown in Table 10.5 is mainly based on empirical clinical observations. There is a desperate need for controlled studies in all types of deafferentation pain.

Although controlled studies do not help the individual patient, it is only with this type of data that the rest of the medical profession will accept that these drugs do or do not have a place in the treatment of such patients. The cross the pain clinic doctors have to bear is that by educating the rest of the medical profession they make their own job more difficult, because the patients who are referred in the future will have been treated with a number if not all of these drugs. This educational role of the pain clinic for the rest of the medical profession is often not recognized.

Injections

The most commonly used injections are those involving local anaesthetics and there are two reasons for this: (a) *diagnostic* and (b) *therapeutic*. The aim is to see if the injection of local anaesthetic around the appropriate nerve(s) (Figure 10.5) results in any pain relief or if the resultant numbness is not associated with pain relief. It is possible that the patient may achieve analgesia without any numbness, e.g. some nerves do not have a cutaneous supply; this is classically the situation with most of the myofascial blocks (Schwartz, Gall and Grant, 1984). The interpretation of a positive result varies from a placebo effect at one end of the spectrum to a physiological effect at the other, and provided that the effect is repeatable and the patient achieves pain relief, then for that patient the mechanism is immaterial. On the other hand, understanding the mechanism of this pain relief would increase our knowledge of chronic pain and as a result we may be able to predict in which patients this or that particular injection would be effective.

It is one of the enigmas of chronic pain that *all* injections in some patients result in long-term pain relief, even dry needling where no drugs are injected. The best example of this is acupuncture. Again the possible reasons are similar to those proposed above: placebo, a physiological effect, or any combination of both. For the individual patient, as long as it is repeatable the mechanism does not matter. As noted above, there appears to be two nervous systems involved in the transmission of pain – the somatic and the autonomic – and the sympathetic portion of the autonomic system is generally thought to be involved (Guttman, 1976). However, it would be surprising if the parasympathetic system is not found to be involved in some patients' pain, and there is already some evidence to support this, albeit in non-SCI patients (Fitzgerald, 1989).

The history and examination will indicate the possible nerve blocks that may be appropriate for each individual patient. With deafferentation pain, the two most important questions to be answered are: (a) is the pain originating where the patient feels it, and (b) if the pain is originating where the patient feels it, then how is it being transmitted to the brain?

The quickest method of answering both of these questions is to block the somatic and sympathetic nerves that supply the area of the pain by either epidural or spinal injection. These injections do not block the parasympathetic nervous system, a fact that needs to be remembered when interpreting the results. The most common way of achieving this is to place a catheter in the epidural space and to inject local anaesthetic. Provided that the block is above L1, then it may be assumed that the lumbar sympathetic chain is blocked. In order to achieve blockade of the splanchnic nerves, the block would need to be above T6 (Figure 10.6). Both of these statements assume that the pain is not being transmitted by an extramedullary route in the sympathetic chain, as has been suggested by Guttman (1976).

If the local anaesthetic relieves the pain and the duration of that relief is short, then it may be worth while considering the use of destructive procedures to provide long-term relief. Before embarking on any destructive procedure, it is necessary to know through which nervous system the pain is transmitted – the somatic or the sympathetic. In order to find this out, one would have to block the sympathetic system independently from the somatic. The sympathetic nervous system may be blocked with local anaesthetic either at the lumbar level or higher, at the level of the coeliac plexus or splanchnic nerves. If either of these are successful, then it is possible to destroy these nerves with corrosives (phenol, alcohol) or with surgery (Figure 10.6). If the pain is somatically mediated, then it is probably better to offer the patient surgery. The arguments for and against the many different operations will be discussed later in the chapter. It is possible to inject the corrosives (phenol or alcohol) intrathecally (Turnbull, 1983), but the authors consider that it is better to be more precise with surgery.

If local anaesthetic does not relieve the pain, then it is important to examine the other possible transmission systems that may be involved in either the origin of or the transmission of the pain. These drugs have already been alluded to earlier in the chapter and they are believed to have their effect directly on the spinal cord. The pharmacokinetic basis of epidural versus intrathecal injection is discussed elsewhere (Glynn, 1988) and the reader is referred to this text. The best known of these receptor systems is the opioid receptor and it must be stressed that all deafferentation pain is not morphine insensitive (Glynn *et al.*, 1986) as suggested by Arner and Meyerson (1988). Thus if epidural morphine is effective in proving analgesia, then it is possible that a patient will obtain pain relief with oral opioid type drugs. The arguments for and against the use of opioids in patients with non-malignant pain are beyond the scope of this chapter.

Noradrenergic receptors may be blocked at the spinal cord level by epidural clonidine (Glynn *et al.*, 1986). The resultant analgesia may be prolonged by oral clonidine. GABA receptors may be blocked by midazolam (Goodchild and Noble, 1987) and if there is a positive response then it may be maintained by other benzodiazapines, e.g. clonazepam. *N*-methyl D-aspartate receptors (glutamate/aspartate) may be blocked by ketamine (Cotman and Iversen, 1987), thereby raising

Table 10.6 Diagnostic and therapeutic epidural injections*

Axonal blockade	
Local anaesthetic	Somatic and sympathetic
Neuronal blockade	
Opioid receptor	Morphine, 5 mg
Noradrenergic	Clonidine, 150 µg
Gamma-aminobutyric acid (GABA)	Midazolam, 5 mg
N-Methyl-D-aspartate	Ketamine, 10 mg
Kappa opioid	Buprenorphine, 0.3 mg

* This table shows a list of drugs and the dose which may be given epidurally to block the various receptors that are thought to be involved in the transmission of pain. There is always the possibility that if one of these injections is successful (*diagnostic*), then the duration of analgesia may be prolonged (*therapeutic*).

the possibility that other drugs with similar effects may be effective in providing analgesia, e.g. haloperidol. Buprenorphine seems to have different effect at the spinal cord level to morphine (Glynn *et al.*, 1986) and so should probably be investigated independently. The list and dose of the drugs shown in Table 10.6 is a suggested algorithm of the diagnostic/therapeutic injections for the individual patient, and as with pharmacological therapy there is a need for controlled studies.

Neurosurgery

In common with many other spheres of surgical practice, a widely held view is that neurosurgical means of treating pain should be reserved until such time as all other means of treatment have been tried and failed. This view had led, in the past, to neurosurgeons becoming involved at a very late stage in the management of chronic pain problems, sometimes at a stage when the surgical options might be restricted.

To some extent the reluctance to seek neurosurgical options in the management of chronic pain patients has been understandable. Neurosurgical procedures, even when successful, tend to be destructive in nature, they are not always totally selective and may therefore have neurological side effects. The surgical alternative to destructive operations often involves the implantation of sophisticated and expensive electrical stimulating devices or programmable drug delivery systems. Despite these drawbacks, even traditional neurosurgical treatments for pain sometimes meet with remarkable success, and newer operations and techniques are being evolved and their particular place in the overall management of pain is becoming more firmly established.

While no one could sensibly claim that neurosurgery can be dramatically or permanently effective in all, or even the majority, of chronic pain syndromes, it is sad to reflect on those patients imperfectly treated with oral or parenteral drug therapy whose pain might be better controlled by a relatively simple operation.

Neurosurgical opinion at a relatively early stage of patient management should be a useful adjunct to the assessment of any patient, not only in terms of advising whether a particular operation may be appropriate or not, but also in providing rapid and well-directed neurological history-taking and accurate neurological examination.

When planning neurosurgical intervention, one should bear in mind that the operation should aim to be as specific as possible in treating the pain, and should be localized in effect to the painful area, produce a permanent result, and carry small risk, particularly to the debilitated patient. As a general rule, one should start with the most peripheral and the simplest procedure which is likely to be effective and then progress to procedures directed more centrally within the nervous system while also giving preference to non-ablative operations.

Peripheral nerve

Nashold has described his experiences with the use of implanted stimulating devices for use on peripheral nerves in a variety of pain syndromes (Nashold, Mullen and Avery, 1979; Nashold *et al.*, 1982). Optimum pain relief was found when stimulating paraesthesia was referred to the painful zone in the affected limb.

Of 35 patients so treated, 19 had electrode systems implanted in the upper limb with relief of pain in the long term (average follow-up not given) of around 43%. The results were worse for lower limb pains. These workers stress the importance of excluding obvious lesions such as peripheral neuromas and nerve compression by adhesions or fibrous tissue at the wrist or elbow. Electrodes were placed on the nerves as far proximally as possible to allow for aberrant branches crossing from the involved nerve to adjacent nerves.

Spinal nerve roots and ganglia

The operation of dorsal rhizotomy, in which the sensory root is divided either intradurally or extradurally, has been used for some considerable time in the treatment of somatic and visceral pain. At first sight, it would seem a good operation in that it should produce an effect limited in area and should achieve a permanent result. However, dorsal rhizotomy will involve loss of all sensory modalities, so that extensive rhizotomy cannot be used in the control of limb pains. In the site where it is most appropriate, i.e. the trunk, dermatomal overlap and neural plasticity and sprouting mean that in order to derive an effect in any given dermatome, then at least two roots above and two below the affected root should be sectioned.

Before carrying out dorsal rhizotomy, an assessment as to how effective the operation might be should be carried out using nerve root blocks with local anaesthetic. The use of dorsal rhizotomy is now more or less confined to the treatment of peripheral nerve injury such as post-thoracotomy syndrome and to pain from malignant disease in the trunk in areas in which sensation is relatively well preserved. The results achieved are generally disappointing, with at least a 50% failure rate at between 5 and 10 years. Frequently, different pains from those experienced before operation appear and some patients develop a post-rhizotomy dysaesthesia which is both unpleasant and difficult to treat.

Spinal cord — open cordotomy

This operation involves a laminectomy or hemilaminectomy with opening of the dura and incision of the anterolateral quadrants of the cord to divide the ascending pain and temperature pathways. Since the introduction of this operation in the early part of this century, it has become generally recognized as an effective operation for pain relief, particularly in the treatment of malignant pain of the trunk and of the lower limbs.

Pain fibres are probably distributed widely throughout much of the anterior quadrant of the spinal cord and many workers have recommended transection of almost the entire anterior quadrant in order to cut pain afferents. The anatomy in this region is extremely variable and there are profound variations in the number of cord segments above the level of the dorsal root over which pain fibres cross to the contralateral side. In order to carry out effective cordotomy, most workers recommend that the cord incision should be within the anterolateral quadrant at around T2 or T3 for all trunk and lower limb pains.

For a while, it seemed as though open cordotomy would be supplanted by percutaneous cervical cordotomy, owing to the reportedly lower incidence of side effects and the relative ease with which this procedure should be carried out. However, it has become apparent not only that the technique of percutaneous cordotomy is not reliably replicated throughout neurosurgical clinics, but also that secondary afferent pain fibres within the cord are probably more effectively divided by open operation.

Percutaneous cordotomy

The major alternative to open cordotomy is that of percutaneous cordotomy which is invariably carried out in the cervical region. Provided the operation is performed by a skilled operator, it is associated with a low morbidity and carries the additional advantage of being performed under local anaesthetic. The indications for percutaneous cordotomy in the treatment of predominantly malignant pain of the trunk and lower limbs are much the same as for open cordotomy, but neither is particularly successful in treating pains of a dysaesthetic nature. The operative procedure essentially involves the introduction percutaneously of an insulated electrode into the anterolateral quadrant of the cord between C1 and 2. This is best carried out using a specific apparatus such as that developed by Rosomoff.

The results of both percutaneous and open cordotomy are roughly similar. Neither is particularly effective in the treatment of deafferentation pain and both may be associated with a drop in the dermatomal level of analgesia within 6 months of operation. It is partially for this reason that pains in the upper limbs are less appropriately treated by cordotomy.

Various reports suggest that around 90% of patients undergoing cordotomy will obtain immediate pain relief, but this figure would have fallen to around 50% within 1 or 2 years. This is for unilateral lesions, and bilateral cordotomy is associated with a lower success rate still. The procedure is obviously therefore most useful in those patients in whom life expectancy is short. The complications of cordotomy include motor weakness, ataxia and incoordination, hypotonia and, for the percutaneous technique, respiratory depression. Perhaps the worst side effect is that of post-cordotomy dysaesthesia, which occurs in between 5% and 10% of patients following operation.

Commissural myelotomy
This operation is based on the premise that bilateral pain relief may be obtained by division of the decussating fibres subserving pain and temperature from both sides. These cross in the mid-line commissures of the spinal cord over several segments above the entry point of the dorsal nerve roots. It has the theoretical advantage that it would be less disturbing of function than bilateral anterolateral cordotomy, but in practice there can be disruption not only of the posterior columns but risk of damage to the anterior spinal artery when the cord is divided down to the anterior median fissure.

Although a few workers have described a rather spectacular open commissural myelotomy in the cervical region, the operation is largely confined to the thoracic cord and is used in the treatment of intractable bilateral pain of malignant nature in the lower limbs, pelvis and perineum. With care, side effects (motor weakness, posterior column loss and sphincter disturbance) are mild and transient and about 60% of patients may have good pain relief for the remainder of their limited life expectancy.

Hitchcock (1970) has described a means of carrying out a stereotactic upper cervical myelotomy for treating diffuse bilateral pains in patients with tumour or central cord lesions and in a few patients with post-herpetic or causalgia. Rather bizarre and widespread deficits were noted following this operation, but with good pain relief, at least in the short-term, in many of the early and subsequent cases. It is hard to attribute the sensory losses and pain relief simply to a small lesion made in the decussation of the spinothalamic tracts.

Cordectomy
This drastic procedure must clearly be limited in its application. It has been used in the treatment of some pains following complete spinal injury or in patients who

already have effective cord transection due to malignant disease or vascular disorders. Two main series have been reported, those by Durward *et al.* (1982) and those by Jefferson (1982, 1983). It is probably more effective in treating the pains occurring at the level of the spinal injury, i.e. pain in the twilight area, rather than those occurring within the deafferented areas, particularly when of a visceral nature. Nevertheless, Jefferson reported effective pain relief in almost all his patients undergoing cordectomy for pain associated with spinal injury below the level of T11. This seemed in direct contrast to the results obtained in patients with higher lesions.

Pain in the twilight area might be better treated by cordectomy at the appropriate level, with division of one or more sensory roots above the level of the resection. The finding of most workers is that the analgesic effects following cordectomy are usually temporary and last for no more than a few months.

Dorsal root entry zone operations
In effect, there are two basic operations which attempt to produce pain relief by making lesions at the immediate point of entry of the dorsal root into the spinal cord. There is the so-called selective posterior rhizidiotomy favoured by Sindou *et al.* (1986), and that of the lesion made either by radiofrequency generator and electrode or by laser as described by Nashold and Ostdahl (1979). The dorsal root entry zone is made up of part of the dorsal nerve roots, the superficial layers of the dorsal horn and of Lissauer's tract. Lesions made in this area will interrupt nociceptive impulses generated in the spinothalamic tracts by destroying the dorsal horn neurones and the most medial part of Lissauer's tract itself.

The exact extent of the microsurgical lesions made in either operation is uncertain, particularly by virtue of possible effects on local vasculature, but the original studies of Sindou demonstrated the separation of nerve fibres within the posterior rootlets just as they entered the root entry zone. A lesion placed laterally in this area would section the small nociceptive fibres and the more medial excitatory part of Lissauer's tract. Light touch and proprioception would be preserved. This meant that unlike dorsal rhizotomy, large numbers of nerve roots in a limb could be sectioned without completely deafferenting the limb itself.

The application of the Sindou operation has been described in the treatment of a variety of limb pains and in the treatment of spasticity. The Nashold procedure was originally described for the treatment of brachial plexus avulsion injuries and then later extended to include the treatment of deafferentation (central) pain following SCI, avulsion of the lumbosacral plexus, post-herpetic neuralgia, and pains in the lower limbs following failed back surgery.

The effectiveness in treating pain following brachial plexus avulsion may be summarized by saying that effective long-term pain relief is achieved in about 80% of cases of brachial plexus injury. Nashold's figures are equally good for the lumbosacral plexus avulsions, but this has not, as yet, been substantiated by others. Although there are descriptions of only about 5% transient complications in terms of long tract, spinocerebellar and spinothalamic tract involvement together with sphincter impairment, this is by no means a universal finding and it is likely that, as the procedure is used more widely and by less experienced surgeons, the complication rate will be found to be higher. It appears to meet with variable success in the treatment of stump amputation and phantom limb pains and of the central pain in paraplegics. In the latter group it appears more successful in treating proximal, unilateral and reasonably localized pain. It appears to be of little or of no value at all in treating the intensive rectal and other visceral pains that in some cases follow SCI.

Spinal cord stimulation

Spinal (epidural) cord stimulation has been used to treat many forms of intractable pain. Its use is based on the gate control theory of Melzack and Wall (1965) in which cells within the substantia gelatinosa act as a form of barrier controlling the transmission of sensory information to the central nervous system. It was subsequently felt that stimulation of the cord (dorsal columns in particular) might activate the gate mechanism and therefore block pain transmission.

Spinal cord stimulating systems have become more refined and most nowadays comprise either a monopolar or unipolar electrode or line of electrodes which are inserted into the epidural space over the back of the spinal cord and connected to an implantable subcutaneous receiver. This is in turn activated by an external transmitting device. For a while, there was a vogue for introducing these electrodes percutaneously through a large gauge Tuohy needle. However, difficulties in wending the electrode up through the epidural space and in keeping it in position once it had reached its desired destination have now led to this technique being frequently abandoned in favour of open laminectomy and direct placement of the electrode onto the back of the dura. It may then be held in place by a small stitch.

Spinal cord stimulation has been used for a variety of intractable pain problems but, by and large, its early promise has not been fulfilled and the results are so frequently disappointing that very careful patient selection must be employed before using up valuable resources. Nevertheless, on the basis that it is better to start with non-ablative procedures before embarking upon major surgery, it is always worth considering spinal cord stimulation in cases which are refractory to drug treatment. Of some value is the test application of transcutaneous nerve stimulation. If this is either partially successful and then later is less effective or if it is entirely effective, but the patient does not wish to be encumbered with pads attached to the skin, then a trial of epidural stimulation is worth while. Complete failure of transcutaneous stimulation does not mean that epidural stimulation will not work, but it does make it less likely. One possible bar to implanting these devices is the cost, which at present exchange rates is around £3500 for the implanted system.

There has been such variability in the claims for the success of this technique that it is difficult to define precisely its indications. The authors have found it to be occasionally effective in central pain following SCI and in various deafferentation pains of the lower limbs.

Thalamotomy and deep brain stimulation

The experience needed to perform this type of stereotactic surgery, the cost involved both in terms of implanted materials and follow-up and the possibility of long-term side effects mean that these procedures are usually limited in application and are carried out in only a few major neurosurgical centres. Controversy continues as to which form of pain is most successfully treated, which targets should be used and whether lesion making or stimulation is preferable in any given case. Most of the early attempts at ameliorating intractable chronic pain of either a diffuse nature or deafferentation type were confined to centromedian thalamotomy or cingulotomy. Most often this surgery resulted in excellent temporary pain relief, but with early recurrence.

Individual results following this form of surgery might be exceptionally good, but it is probably fair to summarize the results obtained as producing a percentage of pain relief in a percentage of patients for a percentage of the time. When these three percentages are multiplied together the beneficial effects may be relatively small. This is not to say that further investigation and carefully documented work on these various techniques should not be encouraged.

Intrathecal drug administration

A possible alternative to the administration of very large doses of oral 'analgesics' in patients with intractable pain is the administration of small amounts of the drug by means of intrathecal or epidural infusion. The choice of these methods of treatment will depend very much upon individual cases, but would most commonly be applicable in cases of malignant pain with reasonable life expectancy, i.e. at least greater than 6 months. The operative procedure is very simple and relatively minor, even for severely ill patients. However, there may be multiple problems with kinking of epidural catheters and occasional pump failures. Another prohibitive factor may be the cost involved, as totally programmable systems may be as much as £4000 at current prices. The cheaper alternative, that of a manual pump which may be hand operated by the patient himself, has often been found to be unsatisfactory. This is mainly due to the extreme thinness of the subcutaneous layer overlying the pump which is necessary so that the device may be felt effectively and manipulated by the patient.

Future trends

Animals do not appear to have pain following spinal cord trauma. The best examples of this are the original experiments which described the opioid receptor μ in which a T10 spinal beagle dog was studied for the flexion response before and after morphine (Martin *et al.*, 1976). In spinal man, epidural morphine will abolish the flexion response but rarely relieves pain, reinforcing the difference between pain response (nociception) and pain perception.

The patient with SCI and pain has all the many and varied problems of the chronic pain patient added to his or her lack of mobility. Such patients offer a unique opportunity to document the different possible mechanisms of pain transmission in man.

References

American Spinal Injury Association (1982) *Standards for Neurological Classification of Spinal Injury Patients*, American Spinal Injury Association, Chicago, pp. 2–4

Arner, S. and Meyerson, B.A. (1988) Lack of analgesic effect of opioids on neuropathic and idiopathic forms of pain. *Pain*, **33**, 11–23

Banerjee, T. (1974) Transcutaneous nerve stimulation for pain after spinal injury. *New England Journal of Medicine*, **291**, 796

Brenowitz, G.L. and Pubols, L.M. (1981) Increased receptive fields size of dorsal horn neurons following chronic cord hemisection in cats. *Brain Research*, **216**, 45–49

Cotman, C.W. and Iverson, L.L. (1987) Excitatory amino acids in the brain – focus on NMDA receptors. *Trends in Neurosciences*, **7**, 263–279

Davidoff, G., Guarracini, M., Roth, E., Silwa, J. and Yarkony, G. (1987) Trazodone hydrochloride in the treatment of dysaesthetic pain in traumatic myelopathy: a randomised, double-blind, placebo-controlled study. *Pain*, **29**, 151–161

Davis, R. and Lentini, R. (1975) Transcutaneous nerve stimulation for treatment of pain in patients with spinal cord injury. *Surgical Neurology*, **4**, 100–101

Dimitrijevic, M.R. (1983) Neurophysiological evaluation and epidural stimulation in chronic spinal cord injury patients. In *Spinal Cord Reconstruction* (eds C.C. Kao, R.P. Bunge and P.J. Reier), Raven Press, New York, pp. 465–474

Durward, Q.J., Rice, G.P., Ball, M.J., Gilbert, J.J. and Kaufmann, J.C. (1982) Selective spinal cordectomy: clinicopathological correlation. *Journal of Neurosurgery*, **56**, 359–367

Fitzgerald, M. (1989) The course and termination of primary afferent fibres. In *Textbook of Pain* (eds P.D. Wall and R. Melzack), Churchill Livingstone, Edinburgh, pp. 47–62

Glynn, C.J. (1987) Intractable pain: a problem identification and solving exercise. *Update*, **13**, 44–45

Glynn, C.J., Jamous, M.A., Teddy, P.J., Moore, R.A. and Lloyd, J.W. (1986) Role of spinal noradrenergic system in transmission of pain in patients with spinal cord injury. *Lancet*, **ii**, 1249–1250

Glynn, C.J. (1988) Clinical methods in pain relief research. *Baillière's Clinical Anaesthesiology* (eds D.E.F. Newton and N.R. Webster), *Clinical Research in Anaesthesia*, **2**, 89–105

Goodchild, C.S. and Noble, J. (1987) The effects of intrathecal midazolam on sympathetic nervous system reflexes in man – a pilot study. *British Journal of Clinical Pharmacology*, **23**, 279–285

Grzesiak, R.C. (1977) Relaxation techniques in treatment of chronic pain. *Archives of Physical and Medical Rehabilitation*, **58**, 270–272

Guttman, L. (1976) *Spinal Cord Injuries*, Blackwell Scientific, Oxford, pp. 280–305

Heilporn, A. (1977–78) Two therapeutic experiments on stubborn pain in spinal cord lesions: coupling melitracen-flupenthixen and the transcutaneous nerve stimulation. *Paraplegia*, **15**, 368–372

Hitchcock, E. (1970) Stereoactic cervical myelotomy. *Journal of Neurology, Neurosurgery and Psychiatry*, **33**, 224–230

Jefferson, A. (1982) Cordectomy for the pain of paraplegics referred below the level of the lesion. Personal communication

Jefferson, A. (1983) Cordectomy for intractable pain in paraplegia. In *Persistent Pain*, Vol. 4 (eds S. Lipton and Y. Miles), Grune and Stratton, Orlando, CA, pp. 115–132

McQuay, H.J. (1988) Pharmacological treatment of neuralgic and neuropathic pain. *Cancer Surveys*, **7**, 141–159

Martin, W.R., Eades, C.G., Thompson, J.A., Huppler, R.E. and Gilbert, P.E. (1976) The effects of morphine and nalorphine like drugs in the nondependent and morphine-dependent chronic spinal dog. *Journal of Pharmacology and Experimental Therapeutics*, **187**, 517–532

Melzack, R. and Wall, P.D. (1965) Pain mechanisms: a new theory. *Science*, **150**, 971–978

Merskey, H. (1978) Emotional adjustment and chronic pain. *Pain*, **6**, 249–252

Nashold, B.S. Jr, Goldner, J.L., Mullen, J.B. and Bright, D.S. (1982) Long-term pain control by direct peripheral nerve stimulation. *Journal of Bone and Joint Surgery*, **64-A**, 1–10

Nashold, B.S. Jr, Mullen, J.B. and Avery, R. (1979) Peripheral nerve stimulation for pain relief using a multicontact electrode system. *Journal of Neurosurgery*, **51**, 872–873

Nashold, B.S. Jr and Ostdahl, R.H. (1979) Neurosurgical technique of the dorsal root entry zone lesions for pain relief. *Journal of Neurosurgery*, **51**, 59–69

Rose, M.J., Robinson, J.E., Ells, P. and Cole, J.D. (1988) Pain following spinal cord injury. Result from a postal survey. *Pain*, **34**, 101–102

Schwartz, R.G., Gall, N.G. and Grant, A.E. (1984) Abdominal pain in quadriparesis: myofascial syndrome as unsuspected cause. *Archives of Physical and Medical Rehabilitation*, **65**, 44–46

Sindou, M., Mifsud, J.J., Boission, D. and Goutelle, A. (1986) Selective posterior rhizotomy in the dorsal root entry zone for treatment of hyperspasticity and pain in the hemiplegic upper limb. *Journal of Neurosurgery*, **80**, 587–595

Sternbach, R.A. (1978) Variety of pain games. In *Advances in Neurology*, Vol. 4 (ed. J.J. Bonica), Raven Press, New York, pp. 423–430

Sweet, W.H. (1988) Deafferentation pain in man. *Applied Neurophysiology*, **51**, 117–127

Tasker, R.R. and Dostrovsky, J.O. (1989) Deafferentation and central pain. In *Textbook of Pain* (eds P.D. Wall and R. Melzack), Churchill Livingstone, Edinburgh, pp. 160–164

Turnbull, I.M. (1983) Percutaneous lumbar rhizotomy for spasms in paraplegia. *Paraplegia*, **21**, 131–136

Wall, P.D. and Devor, M. (1982) Consequence of peripheral nerve damage in the spinal cord and in neighbouring intact peripheral nerves. In *Abnormal Nerves and Muscles as Impulse Generators* (eds W.C. Culp and J. Ochoa), Oxford University Press, New York, pp. 588–603

Wall, P.D. and Melzack, R. (1989) *Textbook of Pain*, 2nd edn, Churchill Livingstone, Edinburgh
Zimmerman, M. (1983) Deafferentation pain. In *Advances in Pain Research and Therapy*, Vol. 5 (eds J.J. Bonica, U. Lindblom and A. Iggo), Raven Press, New York, pp. 661–662

Further reading

Bedbrook, G.M. (1985) Pain in paraplegia and tetraplegia. In *Lifetime Care of the Paraplegic Patient* (ed. G.M. Bedbrook), Churchill Livingstone, Edinburgh, pp. 245–256
Bors, E. (1951) Phantom limbs of patients with spinal cord injury. *Archives of Neurology and Psychiatry (Chicago)*, **66**, 610–631
Botterell, E.H., Callaghan, J.C. and Joussi, A.T. (1953) Pain in paraplegia: clinical management and surgical treatment. *Proceedings of the Royal Society of Medicine*, **47**, 281–288
Burke, D.C. (1973) Pain in paraplegia. *Paraplegia*, **10**, 297–313
Burke, D.C. and Woodward, J.M. (1976) Pain and phantom sensation in spinal paralysis. In *Handbook of Clinical Neurology*, Vol. 26 (eds P.J. Vinkin and G.W. Bruyn), Elsevier, New York, pp. 489–499
Cain, H.D. (1965) Subarachnoid phenol block in the treatment of pain and spasticity. *Paraplegia*, **3**, 152–160
Davidoff, G., Roth, R., Guarracini, M., Silwa, J. and Yarkony, G. (1987) Function-limiting dysaesthetic pain syndrome among traumatic spinal cord injury patients: a cross-sectional study. *Pain*, **29**, 39–48
Davis, L. and Martin, J. (1947) Studies upon spinal cord injuries. 2 The nature and treatment of pain. *Journal of Neurosurgery*, **4**, 483–491
Davis, R. (1975) Pain and suffering following spinal cord injury. *Clinical Orthopaedics and Related Research*, **112**, 76–80
Donovan, W.H., Dimitrijevic, M.R., Dahm, L. and Dimitrijevic, M. (1982) Neurophysiological approaches to chronic pain following spinal cord injury. *Paraplegia*, **20**, 135–146
Glynn, C.J. (1987) Intrathecal and epidural administration of opiates. *Baillière's Clinical Anaesthiology* (ed. K. Budd), *Update on Opioids*, **1**, 915–933
Laitinen, L.V., Nilsson, S. and Fugl-Meyer, A.R. (1983) *Journal of Neurosurgery*, **58**, 895–898
Michaelis, L.S. (1970) The problem of pain in paraplegia and tetraplegia. *Bulletin of the New York Academy of Medicine*, **46**, 88–96
Nashold, B.S., Jr and Bullitt, E. (1981) Dorsal root entry zone lesions to control central pain in paraplegia. *Journal of Neurosurgery*, **55**, 414–419
Nepomuceno, C., Fine, P.R., Richards, S., Gowens, H., Stover, S.L., Rantanuabol, U. and Houston, P.A. (1979) Pain in patients with spinal cord injury. *Archives of Physical and Medical Rehabilitation*, **60**, 605–609
Piepmeier, J.M. and Jenkins, N.R. (1988) Late neurological changes following traumatic spinal cord injury. *Journal of Neurosurgery*, **69**, 399–402
Pollock, L.J., Brown, M., Boshes, B., Finkleman, I., Chor, H., Arieff, A.J. and Finkle, J.R. (1951) Pain below the level of injury of the spinal cord. *Archives of Neurology and Psychiatry (Chicago)*, **65**, 319–322
Rosomoff, H.L., Carroll, F., Brown, J. and Sheptak, P. (1965) Cordotomy: technique. *Journal of Neurosurgery*, **23**, 639–644
Siegfried, J. and Lazorthes, Y. (1982) Long-term follow-up of dorsal cord stimulation for chronic pain syndrome after multiple lumbar operations. *Applied Neurophysiology*, **45**, 201–204
Sindou, M., Quoey, C. and Baleydier, C. (1974) Fiber organisation at the posterior spinal cord-rootlet junction in man. *Journal of Comparative Neurology*, **153**, 15–26
Sweet, W.H. (1984) Deafferentation pain after posterior rhizotomy, trauma to a limb and herpes zoster. *Neurosurgery*, **15**, 928–932
Tator, C.H. (1985) Pain following spinal cord injury. In *Neurosurgery* (eds R.H. Wilkins and S.R. Rengachary), McGraw-Hill, New York, pp. 2368–2371
Waisbrod, H., Hansen, D. and Gerbershagen, H.U. (1984) Chronic pain in paraplegics. *Neurosurgery*, **15**, 933–934
Wall, P.D. and Devor, M. (1978) Physiology of sensation after peripheral nerve injury, regeneration and neuroma formation. In *Physiology and Pathobiology of Axons* (ed. S.G. Wachsman) Raven Press, New York, pp. 377–388

Williams, S., Wells, C. and Hunt, S. (1988) Spinal cord neuropeptides in a case of chronic pain. *Lancet,* **ii**, 1047–1048

Woolf, C.J. (1985) Physiological, inflammatory and neuropathic pain. *Advances and Technical Standards in Neurosurgery,* **15**, 39–62

Woolsey, R.M. (1986) Chronic pain following spinal cord injury. *Journal of the American Paraplegia Society,* **9**, 39–41

Chapter 11

Anaesthesia for non-traumatic spinal disease

Peter J. Wright

Introduction

Now that100 years has passed since the first successful operation for the removal of
a spinal cord tumour, it is appropriate to review briefly some of the changes which
have occurred within the intervening period.

Sir Victor Horsley saw his first such patient at the National Hospital, London, on
9 June 1887. The symptoms were severe girdle pain radiating into the abdomen and
increasing paraplegia. The patient was in a desperate condition and readily agreed to
surgery. The operation began 2½ hours later under ether anaesthesia in the
semilateral position. A six-level thoracic laminectomy was performed for the
removal of a large intradural fibromyxoma. The early postoperative period was
stormy, marked by severe pain, muscular spasms, urinary incontinence and
decubitus ulceration. Yet within 6 weeks the patient was well enough to go to a
convalescent home, where he improved to the extent that he could walk with the aid
of two sticks, and a year later the patient was back at work (Gowers and Horsley,
1888).

Horsley's success encouraged other surgeons to take on such patients at a time
when surgery for the spinal cord was generally thought to be too dangerous. By 1920
Sir Percy Sargent had sufficient experience to report on 27 cases with favourable
results. Working in close cooperation with the anaesthetist, Sargent commented that
he was much in favour of intratracheal ether as it aided positioning of the patient in
the prone position. He also stated that in his practice 'the amount of blood lost
depends more on the surgeon's technique and resource than upon the anaesthetist'
(Sargent, 1920).

Both of the above reports represent landmarks in the history of the development
of surgical and anaesthetic techniques for spinal surgery. Within 13 years the method
of intratracheal anaesthesia for maintenance of a clear airway and ensuring the
adequacy of ventilation had been incorporated together with observations of pulse,
blood pressure and peripheral oxygenation (Challis, 1933). The importance of
posture and airway management, with emphasis on low resistance breathing circuits,
was established shortly (Gillespie, 1935; Ayre, 1937). These are the solid
foundations upon which we have built today's anaesthetic management of spinal
cord surgery.

Preoperative assessment

Anaesthesia for the patient with non-traumatic spinal disease is a routine procedure for the majority of cases, with little chance of anaesthetic-related morbidity. A normal preoperative history and physical examination relevant to anaesthesia, supported by appropriate x-rays, laboratory tests and electrocardiogram (ECG) will prove adequate for uncomplicated procedures. However, anaesthetic literature indicates that, in retrospect, underlying pathology may be associated with apparently uncomplicated orthopaedic surgery and that these abnormalities are usually detected either in the anaesthetic room, or perioperatively.

In order to avoid some of the more common pitfalls, when presented with a long elective spinal surgical session, a few minutes' enquiry into the patient's past anaesthetic experience and family history is worth while, combined with simple tests to try to anticipate a difficult intubation. Examination of the lower limbs may reveal signs of muscle wasting, decubitus ulceration or deep venous thrombosis. All of the above have implications for future anaesthetic management, but are unlikely to be elicited during a routine anaesthetic enquiry.

Patients with neuromuscular disorders and skeletal deformities require thorough assessment of respiratory function in order to determine whether or not the patient is likely to require postoperative respiratory support (see below). Arterial blood gas analysis may reveal unexpected hypoxaemia in the early stages of lung volume restriction due to thoracic deformity, as seen in scoliosis, but not in cases of ankylosing spondylitis where lung function is surprisingly normal (Zorab, 1962). Only rarely do such patients exhibit upper lobe fibrosis and cyst formation and as a result are prone to developing pneumonia (Leading Article, 1971).

When vital capacity is significantly below predicted values, as for example with cervical cord compression, it is likely that the patient will suffer from postoperative respiratory insufficiency, and risks developing pulmonary atelectasis, lobar collapse and respiratory infection. These conditions are encouraged if patient mobility is restricted by traction or inadequate pain relief. Severe cases, with a vital capacity of 50% or less than predicted, should be considered as candidates for elective postoperative respiratory support (Hall, Levine and Sudhir, 1978). It is wise to discuss the matter fully with the patient and relatives in advance of the operation, in order to diminish the demoralizing effect of such treatment. Regrettably some patients will present in such an advanced condition that they cannot be expected to benefit from surgery. The management of such cases, including home ventilatory care, is discussed in detail elsewhere (Bjure and Nachemsona, 1973; Spencer, 1977).

Patients with chronic pain and disability will usually be taking regular analgesic medication, often in combination with sedative drugs. The salicylates and non-steroidal anti-inflammatory agents (NSAIDs) interfere with blood clotting and may cause gastric irritation and contribute to iron deficiency anaemia. More potent analgesics used in the long term may produce habituation and relative resistance to opiates used for postoperative analgesia.

The use of steroid therapy is generally restricted to severe cases. These patients must have perioperative steroid therapy designed to maintain a therapeutic blood level. Such patients are more likely to develop chest infections and are at high risk for decubitus ulceration. Other 'Cushingoid' stigmata may be present, so that it is mandatory regularly to check serum electrolytes and blood sugar levels. If the patient is already in traction, or severe deformity has resulted in a lack of mobility, there is a higher risk of deep vein thrombosis and prophylaxis should be considered (see below).

Preoperative medication should include analgesia if the patient is in pain; if not, anxiolytic agents such as the benzodiazepines are appropriate to allay anxiety. In general, patients with chronic pain and disability will be less apprehensive than the patient presenting with an acute neurological deficit. Opiate medication is best avoided when tests show significant reduction in respiratory function, and is contraindicated in patients with evidence of hypercarbia. Such patients respond well to mild anxiolytics and reassurance.

General anaesthesia for spinal surgery

All personnel involved in the operative process should be made aware of the degree of neurological deficit where it is present, in order to emphasize the need to protect the affected areas from damage during transport and positioning. The patient should not be required to position himself after medication, as the degree of weakness may become unexpectedly pronounced after sedation. This is distressing for the patient and may lead to an inappropriate diagnosis of acute neurological deterioration. All movements should be passive and adequate numbers of assistants must be present to enable safe lifting and manipulation. The latter is particularly important for those patients in splints or traction.

It is not uncommon to find that the patient has adopted an unusual posture in bed, often with the aid of numerous pillows. If possible this position should be maintained until the patient is asleep. A note should be made of this preference for future use, as there is often a good reason for the adopted position. It is probably the one that causes the least pain or respiratory effort and this knowledge may be helpful in the postoperative period.

After reassurance that surgery will not begin before the patient is asleep, ECG leads and a blood pressure cuff can be attached and a wide-bore intravenous infusion established using local anaesthesia. If a difficult intubation is anticipated, then full precautions to deal with the situation should be taken (see later under Difficult Intubation).

The pathophysiology of spinal cord damage and blood flow has been dealt with in earlier chapters. The same principles apply to non-traumatic disease where the aim of the operating team is not to contribute to any existing neurological deficit. The method chosen to anaesthetize the patient should reflect the need to maintain spinal cord blood flow (SCBF) by avoiding unnecessary hypotension, and being aware of the effect of Pa_{CO_2} on SCBF. Free communication of the paravertebral and epidural veins with the abdominal and thoracic vessels is well known, and the importance of positioning the patient in order to minimalize venous pressure cannot be over-stressed.

Children may prefer an inhalational induction, otherwise it is usual to induce anaesthesia with intravenous thiopentone (or other short-acting agent) and give a muscle relaxant to facilitate endotracheal intubation. Unless there is a specific indication, suxamethonium should be avoided, as potassium efflux from denervated muscle may cause hyperkalaemia (Gronert and Theye, 1975), and should only be used with extreme caution in patients with neuromuscular disease (Ellis, 1980). Pancuronium can be recommended in this context as tried and tested over many years, with the knowledge that it will not contribute to postural hypotension when positioning the patient in the prone or sitting positions. Good relaxation aids intubation, which should be smooth to avoid raised thoracic venous pressure. It is also essential to allow efficient mechanical ventilation in a variety of postures. A low-pressure cuffed polyvinyl chloride endotracheal tube is sufficient for the majority of cases, and is to be preferred to latex armoured tubes (Wright, 1986a; Wright and Mundy, 1987; Wright, Mundy and Mansfield, 1988). If the surgical field is to encroach upon the airway, a wire-reinforced tube may be required to prevent obstruction.

When positioning the patient, utmost care is required to ensure that the neck is not placed in an unnatural position, as this inhibits venous drainage as well as compromising the airway. The endotracheal tube and its connections should be visible and accessible at all times, and monitoring should include a disconnection alarm. Other monitoring should include airway pressure, inspired oxygen concentration, end tidal CO_2 concentration and peripheral oxygen saturation. If humidified gases are not available, an exchange humidifier and bacterial filter incorporated in the circuit provides necessary humidification and isolates the patient from any bacterial flora in the anaesthetic apparatus (Shelley, Bethune and Latimer, 1986).

If heavy blood loss can be anticipated, additional intravenous lines can be set up, including central venous pressure monitoring. Direct arterial pressure recording is advisable when deliberate hypotension is to be induced. Temperature probes, peripheral nerve stimulator and an oesophageal stethoscope can be inserted at this stage, together with a urinary catheter for long procedures. Respiration is controlled using an inspiratory waveform which produces the lowest mean intrathoracic pressure.

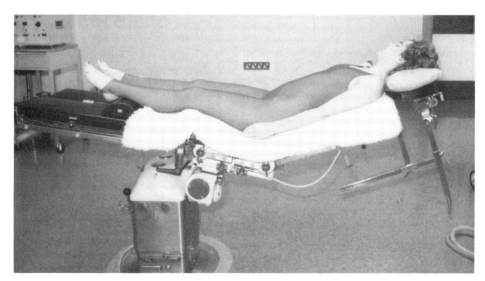

Figure 11.1 Supine position. Posterior cervical spine is well supported, with a head-up tilt to encourage venous drainage

Patient positions for anaesthesia

Positioning the patient has a profound effect on anaesthetic management and is dealt with in greater detail in other texts (Gilbert, Brindle and Galindo, 1966; Martin, 1978). General measures should include eye protection and padding of pressure points, especially where peripheral nerves are vulnerable or where there is potential for acceleration of decubitus ulceration. In patients with skeletal abnormalities, joint laxity and metastatic disease, the risk of joint dislocation and pathological fracture should be remembered. When turning patients, the technique of 'log-rolling' (see Chapter 2) is the safest, particularly when traction is in place. When limbs are manipulated, the rule of 'both together' places least stress on the rest of the body.

Supine position
This position poses little challenge to the anaesthetist and least risk to the patient. Unfortunately it only provides access to the anterior cervical spine. It is easy to establish and maintain traction in this position without complicated equipment (Figure 11.1). In the context of anterior cervical fusion (Cloward's procedure), it is worth mentioning that the practice of placing a sandbag under the shoulders to extend the neck is inherently dangerous, as it leaves the cervical spine unsupported. The intended position for the sandbag is directly underneath the cervical spine, where it affords stability to the spine during surgical instrumentation.

Prone position
Familiarity with the operating table is essential if this manoeuvre is to be carried out safely. Blood pressure monitoring is required frequently to detect hypotension associated with sudden pronation. The development of a natural posture is desirable in order to avoid compression of the abdomen and thoracic cage. Early workers favoured the 'Mohammedan prayer' position (Lipton, 1950), but unfortunately it puts enormous strain on the knee joints, can compress the contents of the popliteal fossa (Martin, 1978), and has been associated with postoperative renal failure (Keim and Weinstein, 1970). In addition, once the position has been set up, it is virtually impossible to modify. Some centres rely on pillows, towels and bolsters to provide support for the hips and shoulders with great success; indeed, when dealing with children and severely deformed adults, this may be the only satisfactory solution.

   In general, however, a purpose-built frame for the operating table is more reliable and has the advantage of allowing intraoperative changes in posture. The Relton–Hall frame (Relton and Hall, 1967; Callan and Brown, 1981) was designed in North America for the operative correction of scoliosis. In the UK the Wilson frame is a popular device for the prone position (Figures 11.2 and 11.3). Both can be modified for lumbar or thoracic work, and may be used to create the prone cerebellar position. When operating on the lumbar spine the arms are brought forward to rest on a foam mattress, and the frame is covered loosely in lambswool. Note the use of leg supports to prevent venous pooling, in conjunction with calf compression garments to provide prophylaxis against deep venous thrombosis (Allemby et al., 1973; McKenna et al., 1980). During thoracic operations it may be necessary to strap the arms down by the side of the patient, making access difficult. Under these circumstances it is desirable to establish a second intravenous infusion and an arterial line at the onset, in case they become necessary later on.

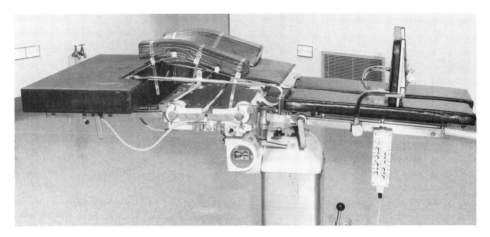

Figure 11.2 Wilson frame on operating table, for use in prone position

Prone cerebellar position
The equipment described above can easily be modified for this position by the addition of a horseshoe head rest or head clamp (Figure 11.4). This position is used for high thoracic and cervical lesions, and also provides access to the atlanto-axial joint. A reverse Trendelenburg tilt on the table reduces venous pressure at the operative site and helps to prevent the patient from slipping toward the surgeon during instrumentation. A simple head rest is satisfactory for most procedures, and encourages a natural anatomical position. When using clamp fixation it is possible to over-flex the neck and cause both venous and airway obstruction.

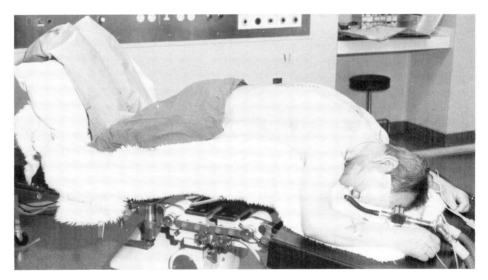

Figure 11.3 Prone position for dorsal laminectomy. Frame and leg supports are well padded, and calf compression garments are applied

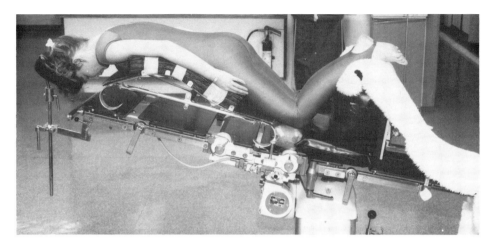

Figure 11.4 Prone cerebellar position using Wilson frame and horseshoe head rest

Park bench position
The best description of this position is to be found in Gilbert's text from Montreal (Gilbert, Brindle and Galindo, 1966), which also deals with other positions in some detail. Unfortunately this book is no longer in print. We have found this modified lateral position extremely versatile, useful for exploration of the cerellar-pontine angle, the atlanto-axial joint, and a transthoracic approach to the anterior thoracic spine is facilitated. Solid hip and chest supports are replaced by a large evacuation mattress which provide all-round contoured support for the patient. The surgical approach is made through a right costotransverse incision, necessitating deflation of the right lung. All the usual precautions and monitoring associated with one-lung anaesthesia and thoracic surgery must be observed.

Sitting position
This position represents the greatest challenge to the anaesthetist because of the risk of postural hypotension and air embolism. However, the excellent operating conditions obtained for cervical decompression justify its continued use. Provided that rigorous precautions are taken to prevent and detect air embolism, and the patient is physically able to withstand being sat up under anaesthesia, the risk need be no greater than for other positions. In order to avoid hypotension, the patient should be sat up in slow graded movements, beginning from a Trendelenburg position, so that when the table has been broken into a chair, the patient is in fact still reclining. The whole table is then tipped forward with the head coming to rest naturally on a horseshoe head rest (Figure 11.5). If the manoeuvre is carried out with care and attention to detail there will be very little change in blood pressure, and there is no need for any kind of fixation as the patient is literally sitting. Head clamps may be used with caution, as extreme flexion of the neck may result in complete venous obstruction and macroglossia (McAllister, 1974; Ellis, Bryan-Brown and Hyderally, 1975). A precordial ultrasound air embolus detector is placed over the right atrium and its position verified by the injection of saline through a central venous catheter. When air is detected, the neck veins are compressed and the

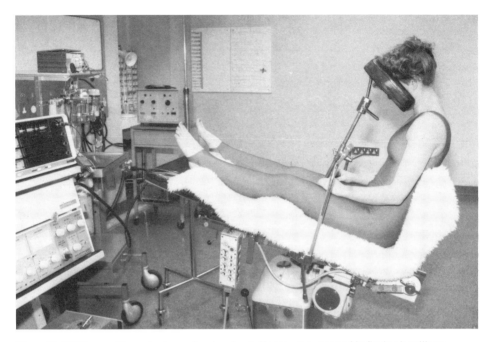

Figure 11.5 Sitting position using horseshoe head rest. Knees are supported in flexion by pillows

operator uses diathermy, bone wax and saline packs to block the ingress of air. Because of the poor physical condition of some of these patients, particularly those with quadriplegia, a nasal endotracheal tube may be preferred which facilitates early postoperative respiratory support (Wright, 1986b).

Maintenance of anaesthesia

Most anaesthetic techniques used for spinal surgery are based on controlled respiration using nitrous oxide as the carrier gas. It is a matter of personal preference and choice of spinal cord monitoring devices (if any) which are likely to determine how this is supplemented. SCBF behaves in much the same way as cerebral blood flow in its response to anaesthetic agents (Griffiths, 1973a, 1973b; Kobrine, Doyle and Martins, 1975; Marcus *et al.*, 1977; Scremin and Decima, 1983; Messick *et al.*, 1985), so that their effects ought to be predictable. In the absence of monitoring devices one should remember that, although volatile agents should increase SCBF, it will be counteracted by hypotension or direct mechanical pressure. Most anaesthetic agents reduce cerebral metabolism, and the same probably applies to the human spinal cord, although the ratio of grey : white matter is not comparable. Opiates and neuroleptic agents probably have little or no effect on either spinal cord blood flow or metabolism.

With this knowledge, it would be prudent to avoid hypotension before the spinal cord is decompressed and if hypotension is required later, then a volatile agent will reduce metabolism but not blood flow. Monitoring spinal cord pathway function is always desirable when the cord is compressed or hypotension is to be used. The neuroleptic agents are preferred by some workers for the relative lack of effect on evoked potentials, but others find that they can obtain satisfactory results using the volatile agents. The final choice will depend very much on the past experience and degree of expertise of the whole operating team. Provided that the principles of careful positioning, good airway management and adequate relaxation are observed, the actual anaesthetic agents used are unlikely materially to affect the results of surgery.

Intradural and extradural anaesthesia

It is interesting that the preparation of this work almost coincides with the 100th anniversary of the publication of *Local Anaesthesia in General Medicine and Surgery* (New York, 1886) by Corning. In that same year, Corning accidentally injected cocaine into the extradural space producing spinal anaesthesia, giving rise to the frequently quoted misconception that he was the founding father of spinal anaesthesia (Lee and Atkinson, 1978). In fact, the first two papers describing intradural anaesthesia as we practice it today were published by different authors within a few months of each other in 1899 (Beir, 1899; Tuffier, 1899). The relative merits of spinal and general anaesthesia have been in constant debate ever since.

The subject causes much controversy in the context of orthopaedic surgery, particularly when the hip joint is involved, and is discussed in detail elsewhere (Loach, 1973). So far as spinal surgery is concerned, there are very few specific contraindications to intradural or extradural anaesthesia. Complete blockage of the intradural space at myelography is one such example (Bonica *et al.*, 1957; Silver, Dunsmore and Dickson, 1976). The majority of studies of intradural anaesthesia have shown consistently good results. Two large series of lumbar laminectomies using intradural anaesthesia found no evidence of neurological defect attributable to the technique (Ditzler *et al.*, 1959; Rosenburg and Berner, 1965), and one series evaluating the method for surgery in the presence of severe neurological disease including adhesive arachnoiditis was equally in favour (Ditzler *et al.*, 1959). A review of 9000 intradural anaesthetics for lumbar disc surgery reported one perioperative death, due to myocardial infarction, giving an apparent mortality rate of 0.01% (Silver, Dunsmore and Dickson, 1976). The statistical analysis used would not be accepted today, and this figure cannot be regarded as representative of the true perioperative mortality rate.

Extradural anaesthesia was enthusiastically recommended for surgery of the lumbar spine, after considerable personal experience, by Bromage (1954) and other favourable reports were soon to follow (Bonica *et al.*, 1957; Tice, 1957; Lucca Escobar and Castillo, 1958; Matheson, 1966). Experiences of surgical lesions at higher levels are mostly anecdotal and therefore difficult to evaluate.

Experienced practitioners have used both the lateral and prone positions for injection and subsequent operation. The site of injection in all reports was one or two spaces above the lesion. Over the years, different drugs and methods of administration have evolved, with extradural anaesthesia gaining in popularity. Bromage commented in 1954 that he thought that there was a decrease in surgical blood loss as a result of adrenaline in the extradural space. Others attribute the same effect to a combination of muscle relaxation and a degree of hypotension. Recently there have been investigations of the effects of vasoconstrictors administered by both intradural and extradural routes. These studies appear to demonstrate that intradural adrenaline (epinephrine) does not affect SCBF, nor does the application of local anaesthetic agents. Spinal cord reactivity to Pa_{CO_2} is also maintained during intradural anaesthesia, but there is some evidence to suggest that autoregulation is impaired after blood loss (Dohl, Takeshima and Naito, 1987).

The neurological side effects of both intradural and extradural anaesthesia have also been more recently reviewed (Kane, 1981). The overall incidence was not equated, but the author concluded that neurological sequelae were rare and that the pathophysiological mechanism remains unknown. Many of the cases reported subsequently revealed pre-existing neurological disease, and other cases were inadequately documented. In conclusion, there is no evidence in man to suggest that properly administered intradural or extradural anaesthesia has any adverse effect on outcome after spinal surgery. Neither is there yet any evidence to unequivocally support its use in favour of a carefully administered general anaesthetic.

Postoperative care

Fluid balance, oxygenation and analgesia are the most important factors in the postoperative care of spinal patients. In uncomplicated decompression, blood loss should be minimal and maintenance fluids are sufficient. When blood loss has been partially replaced intraoperatively, and when bleeding continues into the postoperative period (e.g. scoliosis, metastatic disease), blood transfusion and haematocrit measurement are mandatory in the recovery period. All patients should receive oxygen therapy, with special attention given to the adequacy of ventilation in patients with restrictive respiratory disease, immobilizing casts and traction devices.

Spinal surgery causes severe pain, and adequate pain relief should be achieved with intravenous narcotics initially, supplemented by the intramuscular route on the ward. Where available, patient-controlled administration of intravenous narcotics can provide excellent analgesia without respiratory depression (Keeri-Szanto and Heamans, 1972; Evans et al., 1976; Tamsen et al., 1979; White, Pearce and Norman, 1979). Sublingual buprenorphine may be introduced early on, bypassing the need for complicated apparatus, and avoids the usual delays associated with the issue of controlled drugs on the ward (Rolly and Versichedlen, 1976, Edge, Cooper and Morgan, 1979; Fry, 1979). Recently there has been a great deal of interest in the applications of intradural (Wang, Nauss and Thomas, 1979) and extradural opiates (Bahar et al., 1979), for the relief of postoperative pain, and these are reviewed in detail elsewhere (Loach, 1983). To summarize, lyophilic opiates are faster in onset of action, and the intradural route of administration requires smaller amounts of the drug which exerts a long-lasting effect. The extradural route may be more appropriate for thoracic lesions, where respiratory depression is more likely to occur with intradural administration (Glynn et al., 1979; Liolios and Anderson, 1979; Gjessing and Tomlin, 1981; Sidi et al., 1981). Given in moderate doses, extradural opiates are unlikely to give rise to respiratory problems (Torda, 1980; Rutter, Skewes and Morgan, 1981; Gustafsson, Schildt and Jacobsen, 1982).

The objective of postoperative care, regardless of the methods used, is to keep the patient safe and comfortable. Simple measures, such as constructing a supportive cradle of pillows and allowing the patient to determine the most comfortable position for different therapies, will recruit confidence and gain cooperation with the team delivering postoperative care. Compliance with painful physiotherapy and ambulation should be rewarded with equally important periods of mental recreation and sleep.

Spinal haematomas

A chapter on anaesthesia for spinal disease would not be complete without reference to spinal anaesthesia and spinal haematomas and abscess formation. The reader should, however, be reassured by the relative rarity of such sequelae. Spinal haematomas are classified anatomically as intraspinal (Clarke, 1954; Kreyenbuhl, Yasargil and McClintock, 1969; Ommaya, Di Chiro and Doppman, 1969), subarachnoid (Douglas-Wilson, Miller and Watson, 1973; Slavin, 1937; Henson and Croft, 1956; Plotkin, Ronthal and Froman, 1966), subdural (SSH) and epidural (SEH). The latter two have received considerable reporting and may be classified further as acute, arising over hours or days, and chronic, taking weeks or even years to give rise to symptoms (Edelson, 1976). For academic reasons they should be regarded as separate entities, but in practice their presentation and treatment are the same.

The presenting complaint is usually radicular pain followed by weakness and, later, bowel and bladder malfunction (Guthikonda *et al.*, 1979). Chronic haematomas are more common in the elderly, and are probably related to atherosclerosis and hypertension (Rader, 1955; Stewart and Watkins, 1969; Guy and Zahra, 1979; Brandt, 1980). The thoracic spine is more frequently involved than lumbar or cervical.

The diagnosis depends on successful interpretation of myelography, which may be technically difficult due to obliteration of the relevant space by blood clot. Spinal tomography and computed tomography scanning may be necessary to distinguish between SSH and SEH (Zilka and Nicolletti, 1947; Edelson, 1976; Tomarken, 1985). It is important to avoid excessive delay in making the diagnosis, as the prognosis for useful recovery is directly related to the degree of preoperative deficit and the time taken to achieve decompression of the cord (Jellinger, 1976; Mattle *et al.*, 1987).

Spinal subdural haematoma

This is a rare but well-documented phenomenon, occurring spontaneously in the majority of cases. Although there is an association with major spinal trauma it is not a common finding (Russell and Benoit, 1983), and is even less likely to be associated with minor degrees of trauma (Edelson, 1976; Black, Zervas and Caplan, 1978).

The aetiology of non-traumatic SSH remains unclear and the relative lack of blood vessels in the subdural space makes explanation of the pathophysiological process difficult (Edelson, 1976; Black, Zervas and Caplan, 1978). The subarachnoid and radicular vessels are very small and run longitudinally along the lateral margins of the cord. The only vessels of significant calibre are the artery and vein of Adamkiewicz. A full list of factors previously associated with this condition is given in Table 11.1.

Examination of case reports and review of the authors' comments leave no doubt that anticoagulant therapy, particularly in excess of the normal therapeutic range, is the most important risk factor.

Spinal epidural haematoma

Haemorrhage into the epidural space is also well documented, yet despite the comparatively rich blood supply in the form of venous complexes, it remains an

Table 11.1 Factors associated with spinal subdural haematoma

Factor	References
Anticoagulant therapy	Sclang, Carmichael and Freund (1962); Tricot, Nogrette and Ragot (1964); Edelson (1976); Hurt, Shaw and Russell (1977); Reynolds and Turner (1978); Dunn, Phopesh and Mobini (1979); Guthikonda *et al.* (1979); Tomarken (1985)
Lumbar puncture	Schiller, Neligan and Brudtz-Olsen (1948); Carrea, Girado and Eurnekian (1954); King and Glass (1960); Wolcott, Grunnet and Lahey (1970); De Angelis (1972); Edelson, Chernick and Posner (1974); Kohli, Palmer and Gray (1974); Kirkpatrick and Goodman (1975); Gutterman (1977); Hurt, Shaw and Russell (1977); Dunn, Phopesh and Mobini (1979)
Blood dyscrasias	Schiller, Neligan and Brudtz-Olsen (1948); Alajouanine, Castaigne and Lhermitte (1949); King and Glass (1960); Wolcott, Grunnet and Lahey (1970); Hurt, Shaw and Russell (1977); Dunn, Phopesh and Mobini (1979)
Epidural anaesthesia	Lombarbi and Passerini (1964); Greensite and Katz (1980); Roscoe and Barrington (1984)
Arteriovenous malformation	Harris (1911); Schaake and Schafer (1970); Guy, Zahra and Sengupta (1979)
Idiopathic	Harris (1911); Ainslie (1956); Sanchez-Juan and Lopez-Escobar (1964); Schaake and Schafer (1970); Sakata and Kurihara (1984)
Neoplasm	Toledo, Shalit and Segal (1981); Roscoe and Barrington (1984); Smith (1985)
Spinal surgery	Lombardi (1970)

uncommon entity. Analysis of case reports and reviews reveals many factors in common with SSH. Approximately 20% are associated with anticoagulant therapy (Alderman, 1956; Spurry, Robin and Wolf, 1964; Piotrowski, Kroger and Tornow, 1979; Oldenkott, Preger and Todorow, 1981), and 10% bleed from vascular abnormalities (Solero, Forani and Savoirardo, 1980; Koyama *et al..*, 1982; Muller *et al.*, 1982). Most of the rest may be classified as idiopathic (Hehman and Norrell, 1964; Cooper, 1967; Markham, Lynge and Stahlman, 1967; Harris, 1969; Boyd and Pear, 1972; Horne and Muller, 1977; Mracek, 1980; Phillips, Kling and McGillicudy, 1981), since no definite cause was found. Uncommon associations include epidural anaesthesia (Gingrich, 1968; Janis, 1972; Selwyn Crawford, 1975; Sollman, Gaab and Panning, 1987), lumbar puncture (Lenerer, Gutterman and Jenkins, 1973), blood dyscrasias (Jackson, 1869) and vascular malformation of the vertebra (Kosary *et al.*, 1977).

Not unexpectedly, the combination of anticoagulant therapy, alcoholism or antirheumatic drug therapy has been found to be dangerous. As with SSH the lesions are more commonly found in the thoracic spine than cervical or lumbar. The anatomical position may be significant in terms of outcome, as there is some evidence to show that lumbar lesions respond more favourably to surgical intervention (Foo and Rossier, 1981; Klossek and Huller, 1984). One recent advance in the treatment of SEH is percutaneous aspiration under local anaesthesia at the time of myelography, using a radiographic technique similar to discography (Solymosi and Wappenscmidt, 1985).

Spinal epidural abscess

Spinal epidural abscesses (SEA) are thought to occur mainly as a result of haematogenous spread of bacteria, usually from the skin, but also from the respiratory and urinary tracts (Hulme and Dott, 1954; Danner and Hartman, 1987). The most common infective agent is *Staphylococcus aureus*, but in children more unusual bacteria such as Pneumococcus may be cultured (Marks and Bodensteiner, 1988).

Anaesthetists should be aware that there have been cases associated with epidural anaesthesia (Selwyn Crawford, 1975; Saady, 1976; Abouliesh, Amortegui and Taylor, 1977; Nerubay, Volpin and Katznelson, 1978; North and Brophy, 1979; Konig, Schleep and Krahling, 1985; Wanscher, Riishede and Krogh, 1985; Sollman, Gaab and Panning, 1987), multiple lumbar punctures, spinal anaesthesia (Bergman *et al.*, 1983; Beaudoin and Klein, 1984), and local anaesthetic injections into the sacrum (Rustin, Flynn and Coomes, 1983). More rarely, there are reports following spondolysis (Yu and Emans, 1988), vertebral osteomyelitis (Gardner, 1985), bacterial endocarditis (Elian *et al.*, 1984) and aspergillosis (Chee and Poh, 1983; Wagner *et al.*, 1985).

The presentation of infective lesions is similar to SSH and SEH, except that localized tenderness may be prominent. Speed in diagnosis and treatment is equally important, as is the degree of preoperative deficit. Treatment is usually surgical decompression combined with the appropriate anti-infective agent.

Anaesthetic management

The anaesthetic management of spinal haematoma or abscess is, in general, according to the principles outlined for non-traumatic spinal disease. Patients receiving anticoagulant therapy will require preoperative reversal with fresh frozen plasma and phytomenadione, with due regard for the consequences in the postoperative period. The advice of a haematologist should be sought whenever possible, and is mandatory when dealing with patients with blood dyscrasias.

The choice between local and general anaesthesia is somewhat limited, since it is likely that the disease process will contraindicate spinal subarachnoid or epidural anaesthesia. There is also some evidence that obliteration of the relevant space by the lesion itself might limit effective spread of local anaesthetic agents (Rainbird and Pfitzner, 1983). General anaesthesia would appear to be most appropriate for these cases, with emphasis on preparing the debilitated patient for prolonged and often bloody surgery.

Scoliosis

Scoliosis is the result of progressive degeneration of the spine. The multiple disease processes associated with the resulting kyphoscoliosis were largely the province of the paediatrician, until the pioneering work of Harrington (1962) and Dwyer *et al.* (1969) made surgical correction a possibility. The challenge of surgical correction has led to advances in the understanding of the mechanisms of spinal cord neurological damage, and has highlighted the need for close cooperation between all members of the operating team. The present classification of scoliosis (Table 11.2) helps to underline the collective nature of complex pathologies which may present together with an apparently simple orthopaedic deformity.

Preoperative assessment is primarily directed toward the respiratory and cardiovascular status of the patient, which in many cases will show little, if any, change from predicted values (Relton, 1977). However, patients with curvature greater than 50%, long-standing kyphoscoliosis and associated congenital defects

**Table 11.2 Classification of scoliosis
(After Kafer, 1980)**

Idiopathic
  Infantile   <4 years old
  Juvenile   4–9 years old
  Adolescent   >9 years old

Congenital
  Spinal deformity
  Abnormal cord development
  Congenital rib fusion

Neuromuscular
  Neuropathic
  Lower motor neurone, e.g. poliomyelitis
  Upper motor neurone, e.g. cerebral palsy
  Others, e.g. syringomyelia

Myopathic
  Progressive, e.g. muscular dystrophy
  Static, e.g. amyotonia
  Others, e.g. Friedreich's ataxia

Mesenchymal disorders
  Congenital, e.g. Marfan's syndrome
  Acquired, e.g. rheumatoid
  Others, e.g. juvenile apophysis

Trauma
Associated with neurofibromatosis
Secondary to spinal lesion, e.g. tumour

will require more in-depth investigation (Shannon *et al.*, 1970). Spirometry and blood gas analysis show that the early decrease in lung volume results in ventilation : perfusion inequality and hypoxaemia (Shannon *et al.*, 1970; Secker-Walker, Ho and Gill, 1979). As the thoracic deformity progresses, vital capacity is reduced as a restrictive pattern of lung function develops (Kafer, 1975; Zorab, Prime and Harrison, 1979; Kafer, 1980). Hypercarbia is a rare and late finding in advanced disease, indicative of impending respiratory failure (Spencer, 1977). The subject of disorders of the thorax and respiratory function is detailed elsewhere (Berkovsky, 1979). Put in its simplest form, many experienced workers have found that a decrease in vital capacity of 50% or less than predicted indicates that postoperative respiratory support may be necessary (Dyer, Newton and Sherwood, 1969; Westgate and Johnson, 1971; Hall, Levine and Sudhir, 1978).

In addition to respiratory problems, the incidence of congenital myocardial defects and pulmonary hypertension is considerable (Moe, 1967; Kafer, 1975). Other conditions associated with kyphoscoliosis are Marfan's syndrome, Friedreich's ataxia, neurofibromatosis and syringomyelia. Among the younger patients there is a distinct subgroup with congenital muscular disorders including muscular dystrophy and the myotonias. A review of such patients (Ellis, 1980) found that these children respond abnormally to depolarizing muscle relaxants and anticholinesterases. Dystrophic patients may exhibit hyperkalaemia and benign hyperthermia in response to suxamethonium, and myotonic patients may develop abnormal reactions resulting in muscular spasm.

The incidence of cardiac defects is high in myopathic children, and there is also the risk of aspiration pneumonia if the cough and swallow reflexes are inhibited. Because of this and other associated factors, there is high risk of preoperative respiratory infections. Other workers have drawn attention to the unusually high incidence of non-neurological manifestations in scoliotic patients undergoing general anaesthesia. These include malignant hyperthermia (Britt and Kalow, 1970), myoglobinuria (Moore, Watson and Summery, 1976) and cardiac instability, particularly in association with suxamethonium and halothane (Richards, 1972; Miller, Sanders and Rowlingson, 1978; Seay, Ziter and Thompson, 1978).

General anaesthesia and monitoring

Anaesthetic technique for scoliosis patients should conform to that outlined earlier in this chapter. Induced hypotension is frequently requested by the surgical team in order to reduce blood loss during bone decortication (Mallory, 1973; Bennett and Abbot, 1977; Mandel et al., 1981). Intra-arterial blood pressure monitoring is mandatory and central venous pressure catheterization is advisable, since blood loss can be rapid and considerable. In patients with myocardial defects and right heart failure, Swan-Ganz catherization is indicated (Zorab, Prime and Harrison, 1979).

A wide variety of drugs have been successfully used to induce hypotension, including trimetaphan (Dyer, Newton and Sherwood, 1969), sodium nitroprusside (Bennett and Abbot, 1977) and labetalol (Schofield, 1973). Preoperative haemodilution and autologous transfusion have also been recommended as methods of dealing with excessive blood loss (Messmer, 1975; Mandel et al., 1981). Whichever method is used it is essential to restore blood pressure to normal levels before instrumentation of the spine. Hypotension *per se* is unlikely to lead to spinal cord ischaemia, but the combination of direct mechanical pressure and hypotension is thought to be the major cause of intraoperative neurological damage in scoliosis surgery (Brodkey et al., 1972; Hardy, Naser and Brodkey, 1973; Pontes, 1974; Spielholz et al., 1979; Grundy, Nash and Brown, 1981; Grundy, Nelson and Doyle, 1982).

Monitoring spinal cord function during scoliosis surgery takes two basic forms. The wake-up test first performed by Vauzelle, Stagnara and Jouvinroux (1973) has since been confirmed as a useful test by others (Sudhir et al., 1976; Hall, Levine and Sudhir, 1978; Abbot and Bentley, 1980). It involves lightening of anaesthesia after spinal distraction in order to test lower limb movements. It has the major advantage of testing motor function at the time of greatest risk. The anaesthetic technique is relatively simple. Opiates are discontinued while distraction is in progress and nitrous oxide is replaced with 100% oxygen, and the patient allowed to wake up. Reversal of narcotics or neuromuscular blockade should be avoided if possible. After testing, the patient is put back to sleep and a benzodiazxepine is often administered to reduce the incidence of recall. With experience, painful recall is rare (Hall, Levine and Sudhir, 1978). Occasional complications include disconnection of the endotracheal tube, distraction of the rods and air embolus (Engler et al., 1978; Hall, Levine and Sudhir, 1978). False-positive results are possible (Diaz and Lockhardt, 1987). The method is unsuitable for children, uncooperative adults and patients with existing paralysis of the legs.

Alternatively somatosensory evoked potential (SSEP) monitoring may be used to monitor spinal cord function continuously. First described by Dawson (1974), cortical evoked potentials showed distinct limitations. Major refinements in technique have been made since then to eliminate interference from outside sources, and to standardize the computed signal (Clark and Rosner, 1973; Donchin, Calaway and Cooper, 1977; Nash *et al.*, 1977; Engler *et al.*, 1978; Brown and Nash, 1979; Grundy *et al.*, 1982; Grundy, 1983; Jones *et al.*, 1983; Thornton *et al.*, 1984). The greatest advantage of this method is that it provides continuous information about changes in spinal cord function. Unfortunately, expensive equipment is required and an experienced specialist is usually needed to interpret signals that are frequently ambiguous. Changes in waveform may be caused by all anaesthetic agents (Grundy, 1983; Thornton *et al.*, 1984; Baines *et al.*, 1985; Diaz and Lockhardt, 1987), and movement of instruments or recording electrodes (Grundy *et al.*, 1982; Grundy, 1983; Jones *et al.*, 1983; Lamont *et al.*, 1983; Whittle, Johnson and Besser, 1984). However, during steady-state anaesthesia, useful SSEP monitoring is possible with most anaesthetic drugs (Grundy, 1983; Thornton *et al.*, 1984; Peterson, Drummond and Todd, 1986; Sebel *et al.*, 1986). Because sensory pathways are being monitored, it is possible to create motor tract lesions without affecting dorsal column activity (Halliday and Wakefield, 1963), and this may partly explain the occurrence of false-positive results (McCallum and Bennett, 1975; Ginsberg, Shetter and Radzens, 1985).

Postoperatively these patients are best managed in an intensive care unit so that adequate nursing care can be provided. Attention must be given to adequate blood replacement, analgesia, chest drains and respiratory function. The major cause of morbidity is respiratory failure, and this is most common in patients with pre-existing reduction in vital capacity, and those with inherited neuromuscular disorders. Correction of spinal curvature may fail to improve lung volumes (Prime, 1977; Zorab, Prime and Harrison, 1979) and some may be temporarily reduced. Respiratory therapy should therefore be directed toward the prevention of atelectasis and sputum retention. Some patients may benefit from elective overnight ventilation, when hypoxaemia and hypercarbia are most likely to develop (Spencer, 1977). Others may require mandatory ventilation for a period of days or even weeks, with a planned weaning programme in order to establish independence.

Syringomyelia

Syringomyelia may present as pain in the head, neck or upper limbs, typically with dissociated sensory loss. There may be progressive weakness of the limbs depending on the level of the lesion (Williams, 1979). There might also be a history of birth injury or spinal trauma (Oakley, Ojemann and Alvord, 1981). More than half will have an associated scoliotic deformity of the spine. Less common associations include Arnold–Chiari malformation, basilar impression, Klippel–Fiel syndrome, cervical rib and spina bifida (Huebert and MacKinnon, 1969).

Uncomplicated cases are treated with cerebrospinal fluid drainage procedures, usually into the pleural or peritoneal cavities. The Arnold–Chiari malformation requires a more extensive decompression, often involving the base of the skull and the cervical spine. The sitting position may have advantages in relatively fit patients, but experience has shown that in patients with pronounced scoliosis the prone cerebellar position is to be preferred. Intraoperative cardiac instability may occur as a result of autonomic dysfunction (Thornton, 1980), and unexpected cardiac arrest has been observed following apparently uncomplicated decompression. The mechanism behind this phenomenon is not clear.

Neurofibromatosis

Spinal cord compression may result from an extradural fibroma or because of associated kyphoscoliosis (Moe, 1967). Patients may exhibit other manifestations of the disease which include hydrocephalus, mental retardation, spina bifida and honeycomb lung cysts. Intubation can be made difficult by laryngeal tumour or stenosis (Fisher, 1975). There are also reports of patients showing unusual sensitivity to both depolarizing and non-depolarizing muscle relaxants (Magbagbeola, 1970; Manser, 1970; Yamashita and Matsuki, 1975), although these are rare. Preoperative screening for hypertension is important because of the well-recognized association with phaeochromocytoma (13%) and renal artery stenosis.

Rheumatoid arthritis

The incidence of rheumatoid arthritis in the general population has been estimated to be 1–2%, is more likely to occur in females, and its incidence appears to be accelerating (Hughes, 1979). The disease process is widely acknowledged to be an autoimmune process affecting extravascular connective tissue. Joints and tendons are primarily affected, but immune complex deposition in other systems results in nodule formation, peripheral neuropathy and pulmonary involvement (Holborow, 1979). The pulmonary manifestations include pleurisy, with or without effusion, Caplan's syndrome, pulmonary fibrosis, arteritis and Sjögren's syndrome. The above are, of course, relatively rare and when a solitary shadow is detected on the chest x-ray it is most likely to be carcinoma. Rheumatoid nodules tend to be multiple and located at the periphery (Hughes, 1979).

Anaemia with low serum iron is a common feature, frequently aggravated by gastrointestinal blood loss as a result of medication (Table 11.3). A full blood coagulation screen is recommended in order to detect the effects of treatment with salicylates or non-steroidal anti-inflammatory drugs (NSAIDs). The platelet count is often high and severe neutrophilia suggests the rare possibility of Felty's syndrome.

Pulmonary function tests should be requested for any patients with pulmonary

Table 11.3 Drugs commonly used in rheumatoid arthritis

Aspirin and salicylates

Non-steroidal anti-inflammatory drugs
  Naproxen, propionic acid derivative
  Diflunisal, salicylate derivative
  Ibuprofen, fenoprofen and ketoprofen
  Azapropazone, phenylbutazone derivative
  Mefenamic acid
  Indomethacin
  Phenylbutazone

Corticosteroids

Gold

Penicillamine

Immunosuppressants
  Azathioprine
  Cyclophosphamide

involvement to give a valuable baseline to refer to in the postoperative period. There is an increased tendency towards atelectasis and pulmonary infection, which may be further aggravated by concurrent steroid or immunosuppressant therapy.

The cervical spine is frequently involved, causing synovitis and laxity of the transverse ligament of the atlas and resulting in antlanto-axial instability. Subluxation of the lower cervical joints is also seen. The overall incidence of cervical spine degeneration is approximately 30% (Boyle, 1971). Fortunately the incidence of spinal cord compression is low by comparison (Mathews, 1974). The risk of further injury to the neck must be constantly kept in mind, particularly during myelography and endotracheal intubation.

Unfortunately the progressive deformities and pain associated with the disease may mask underlying spinal cord compression. When constriction does occur it is most often at the atlanto-axial level, but lower cervical subluxation can also occur and is equally dangerous (Figure 11.6). The resulting anatomical deviations and deformity of the airway itself make intubation difficult and hazardous for the patient.

Conservative management using collars and traction are preferred to surgery unless there is severe pain or evidence of progressive neurological damage (Editorial, 1985; Fehring and Brooks, 1987). Traction devices such as halo frames or skull tongs may reduce access to the airway even further. Before attempting intubation, the degree of involvement of the temporal-mandibular joint should be assessed by asking the patient to open the mouth (Eisele, 1981). Crico-arytenoid arthritis with resulting fixation of the vocal cords and narrowing of the airway should be anticipated in advanced cases (Funk and Raymond, 1975).

Positioning the patient for surgery presents many difficulties, since in addition to

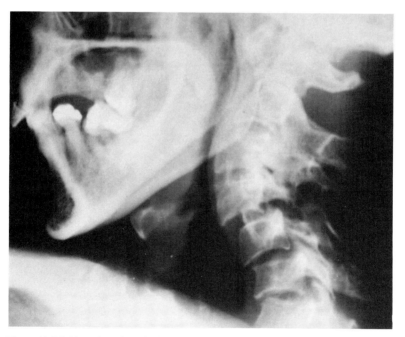

Figure 11.6 Subluxation of cervical spine in rheumatoid arthritis. Note degree of bony degeneration and deformity of neck, making endotracheal intubation extremely difficult

general frailty and deformity it may be necessary to maintain traction on the neck while turning the patient. Long-term steroid therapy produces thin parchment-like skin, and great care is necessary in order to prevent decubitus ulceration. In those patients where restrictive pulmonary disease has developed, the use of prophylactic antibiotic therapy and aggressive respiratory therapy is advised. Postoperative mandatory ventilation should only be considered where indicated by a high level of neurological deficit, as these patients respond poorly to prolonged periods of immobility.

Spinal cord compression by tumour, disc and arteriovenous malformation

Although distinctly different pathological processes, these three lesions share common trends in presentation, investigation and treatment. Disc prolapse is usually associated with spondylitis and is by nature associated with progressive pain and limitation of movement. Non-aggressive spinal cord tumours may also present subacutely with pain or anaesthesia pre-empting paralysis. Intramedullary tumours are an exception and present with more acute symptoms including rapidly increasing neurological deficit and autonomic dysfunction. Arteriovenous malformations (AVMs) are present at birth and can be found throughout the central nervous system. Symptoms similar to disc lesions are produced by the slowly advancing space-occupying effect in the spinal canal.

Between periods of normality there may be repeated exacerbation of pain, paraesthesia or weakness affecting the limbs. For a variety of reasons at present, the majority of patients are deferred from neurosurgical assessment until there is complete spinal occlusion with resulting paresis. There is frequently a history of recent mild trauma or physical exertion, which is taken to be the precipitating factor. Patients also present after manipulation under general anaesthesia, after myelography and spinal anaesthesia (Warner, Danielson and Restall, 1987). The threshold for tolerance of mechanical pressure is obviously different for each patient. This is aptly demonstrated in one patient with an AVM whose symptoms were precipitated by eating a large meal (Whitcomb, 1975).

The anaesthetic management of such cases is affected by the level of the lesion, which will determine the likelihood of respiratory insufficiency and sympathetic blockade. The majority of cases will present for elective surgical exploration, although precipitate changes in neurological status do occasionally give rise to more urgent action. Such patients must be treated as for any other acute surgical emergency, with a rapid sequence induction and the appropriate measures to prevent aspiration of gastric contents. Gastric emptying is frequently delayed in higher lesions and the anaesthetist would be well advised to pass a nasogastric tube and aspirate stomach contents before induction. The use of suxamethonium in these circumstances is fully justified and has been proven safe in experienced hands (Zorab, Prime and Harrison, 1979; Deacock, 1980).

Decompression is usually performed in the prone position, with little blood loss or cardiovascular disturbance. Heavy blood loss may be anticipated with AVMs, vascular tumours and metastatic disease. Unexpected hypertension and cardiac arrhythmias may be observed as a direct result of spinal cord compression (Evans, Kobrine and Rizzoli, 1980), often inappropriate to the degree of surgical stimulation. Symptomatic treatment for persistent arrhythmias is necessary, but no attempt should be made to induce hypotension until the spinal cord has been decompressed. If time permits and the equipment is available, SSEP monitoring can be most valuable in determining the effect of anaesthetic manipulations and surgical intervention.

Down's syndrome

Generalized laxity of ligaments and hypotonia make these patients liable to suffer from joint laxity and hyperextension (Rabe, 1964), and this is particularly important when the cervical joints are involved. The incidence of atlanto-axial instability in young Down's patients is 14–22% (Rabe, 1964; Semine et al., 1978; Hreidarsson, Magram and Singer, 1982), but rather like rheumatoid disease the majority of patients remain asymptomatic for many years. Gradual onset of paraplegia is the most common presentation of atlanto-axial subluxation, which may be idiopathic (Dzenitis, 1966), associated with physical exertion (Committee on Sports Medicine, 1984) or manipulation under general anaesthesia (Moore, McNicholas and Warran, 1987). In addition to C1–2 instability, there is an increased tendency toward cervical and lumbar disc lesions (Tishler and Martel, 1965; Martel and Tishler, 1966).

Preoperative assessment of the patient should include examination of the cardiovascular system for congenital defects and chronic respiratory disease (Kobel, Creighton and Steward, 1982). Intubation may be made difficult by macroglossia, and obese hypotonic individuals may suffer from sleep apnoea. The latter group require constant supervision throughout the postoperative period. When positioning patients on the operating table, the limbs should be supported in such a way as to avoid hyperextension of any joints. Where there is no long-standing neurological defect and atlanto-axial subluxation is treated electively, the outcome from surgery is usually good.

Metastatic disease

Preoperative evaluation should include evaluation of the effects of any radiation or chemotherapy. General cachexia may be aggravated by dehydration or electrolyte imbalance induced by such therapy (Desmond, 1970). Radiation to the thorax may induce pneumonitis, progressing to fibrosis with a restrictive pattern of lung function (Dvorak, 1982). Immunosuppressive therapy may predispose the patient towards anaemia and thrombocytopenia, and pulmonary lesions such as pleural effusion and pneumonia may coexist. Gentle positioning of the patient on the operating table is required in cases with bone metastasis. Provision should be made for rapid blood transfusion, as blood loss is frequently in excess of that associated with routine spinal decompression (Kitihana, 1971).

Acromegaly

As the disease progresses, adults are at increasing risk of spinal stenosis requiring decompression. The anaesthetist should be forewarned of the difficulty presented by macroglossia, and the symptom of hoarseness of the voice may be the result of thickening of the vocal cords and restricted laryngeal aperture. Subglottic stenosis can also occur, making intubation difficult with a normal sized endotracheal tube (Kitihana, 1971; Hassan et al., 1976; Dvorak, 1982; Tindal, 1987).

Difficult intubation

Information about specific spinal disorders should clarify the need to be prepared for difficult intubation. Limitation of jaw movement, restriction of the cervical joints (Brechner, 1968) and problems associated with specific conditions such as neurofibromatosis and Down's syndrome may all present the anaesthetist with airway problems. Moreover, traction devices designed to limit the progression of neurological damage may further inhibit visualization of the larynx. The subject of difficult intubation is dealt with comprehensively in other texts (Latto, 1985).

When treating patients with spinal disease, the anaesthetist becomes accustomed to difficult intubations and will ensure that there is a wide range of laryngoscopes, endotracheal tubes and introducers readily available. An unexpected difficult intubation in an anaesthetized patient may first be approached using the oldest established method of blind nasal intubation (Magill and Robotham, 1921). This is by no means the ideal method, however, and it is hoped that preoperative evaluation of the patient supplemented by lateral cervical x-rays and indirect laryngoscopy will allow adequate preparation. The retrograde cannulation technique (Butler and Cirillo, 1960; Waters, 1963) has much to recommend it, as it can be used safely in the awake patient, using local anaesthesia. Alternatively, fibre optic methods have been more recently demonstrated (Murphy, 1967; Taylor and Towey, 1972) which are particularly suitable for patients with cervical instability, and which with practice can achieve consistently good results (Prithvi et al., 1974; Messeter and Petterson, 1980; Ovassapian, 1983).

Prevention of deep venous thrombosis

It is not appropriate to review this subject in great detail, although certain observations can be made which may help the operating team reach a satisfactory solution to this problem. One of the greatest difficulties is in first assessing the incidence of pulmonary embolism and whether the clotting process is initiated in the calf or the iliofemoral veins. The incidence of fatal pulmonary embolism is highest in elderly patients with femoral fractures (10%), and falls to 2% for elective hip replacement. The incidence is lowest in general surgery, where the rate approximates to 1% of all patients (Morris and Mitchell, 1977; Morris, 1980). The rate of embolism for elective spinal surgery is unknown, but can be presumed to lie within 1–2%. It may be higher in specific groups of patients, for example elderly patients, patients in prolonged traction and so on.

Orthopaedic surgeons have established in several trials that oral anticoagulants given in sufficient dosage to significantly prolong the bleeding time are effective in high-risk groups (Johnson, Green and Charnley, 1976; Morris, 1980; Hirsch, 1981; Evarts, 1987). Direct trauma to veins is less likely in the lower risk groups and the incidence of thrombosis is related to the duration of immobilization. For these patients, subcutaneous heparin has been found to be effective in preventing deep vein thrombosis in the lower limbs (Kakkar et al., 1972). Low molecular weight dextran infusions given perioperatively have also been found useful during general surgery and orthopaedic procedures (Johnson, Green and Charnley, 1976). It is important to recognize the danger of concurrent heparin and dextran therapy which may result in excessive bleeding (Charnley, 1972). Early mobilization is widely advocated as prophylactic, despite the lack of evidence to support this theory. The benefit to the patient may not be related to the circulatory system at all.

If the cause of venous thrombosis is vein damage, venous stasis and increased blood viscosity secondary to inadequate fluid replacement, then certain preventative measures would seem obvious. Protection of the lower limbs during surgery and measures to actively increase limb blood flow are to be encouraged (Knight and Dawson, 1976; McKenna *et al.*, 1980; Hirsch, 1981), and early mobilization and adequate fluid replacement therapy seem to be established practice in most centres. Elasticized stockings have also been shown to reduce thrombosis, but only if they are fitted correctly (Lawrence and Kakkar, 1980). If access to the limbs is required, for example to apply an electrical ground plate, the garment should be completely removed, and not partly rolled down the leg.

The decision to use anticoagulants depends upon the level of risk incurred by the nature and duration of surgery, the patient's age, and degree of immobility of the patient. Since minor degrees of haematoma formation in the extradural space can result in significant neurological deficit, many surgeons prefer to avoid the use of anticoagulants entirely.

Malignant hyperthermia

This specific myopathy is an inherited condition characterized by hyperthermia and triggered by volatile anaesthetic agents and depolarizing muscle relaxants. The pattern of inheritance is autosomal dominance with partial expression. Therefore it does not skip generations and it is important to investigate the whole family when a case is identified (Ellis and Halsall, 1980; Gronert, 1980). Since its discovery in 1960 (Denborough and Lovell, 1960), the incidence of the disease has been estimated to be between 1 : 14 000 and 1 : 200 000 (Britt and Kalow, 1970; Ellis and Halsall, 1980). It is a rare condition, but one with which all anaesthetists should be familiar, particularly because early detection of symptoms and treatment seem to be leading to a decrease in mortality. Patients with spinal deformities, particularly kyphoscoliosis, have been identified as a high-risk group, males are more frequently affected and the incidence is higher in young patients (Ellis and Halsall, 1980).

The diagnosis is made by recognition of one or more of the following symptoms: rise in temperature at the rate of 2–6 °C/h, muscle rigidity, inappropriate tachycardia, tachypnoea and rising Fe_{CO_2}. Cyanosis, disseminated intravascular coagulation and heart failure are late, often terminal symptoms. A patient may experience very mild symptoms with one anaesthetic and then go on to exhibit a fulminant episode with a later anaesthetic. This is in part due to the nature of partially expressed genetic susceptibility. All of the volatile anaesthetics, including nitrous oxide, have been implicated, and there is a high incidence of reports of triggering malignant hyperthermia using the combination of suxamethonium and halothane (Harrison, 1975; Ellis, 1980).

Treatment must begin by discontinuation of the provocative agents. If surgery cannot be postponed, anaesthesia may be continued using barbiturates, neuroleptanalgesia and pancuronium (Ellis and Halsall, 1980; Gronert, 1980). Dantrolene is the only effective treatment (Harrison, 1975), giving 1 mg/kg initially, which may be repeated up to a maximum of 10 mg/kg. Symptomatic treatment should follow and includes active cooling, intravenous fluid replacement and electrolyte therapy. Serum potassium is likely to rise and may be treated with a glucose and insulin infusion. Acidosis is corrected using bicarbonate solution, and mannitol is given to protect the renal tubules from myoglobinuria. Large doses of steroids are still recommended by some authorities, but the evidence of any beneficial effect is lacking. Once the patient is out of theatre, treatment is best given in an intensive care environment. Continuous monitoring (ECG) of arterial and central venous pressures, blood gas and pH measurement, urinary output and serum electrolytes is essential.

When a known malignant hyperthermia patient presents for surgery which cannot be performed under local anaesthesia, diazepam or morphine may be given for premedication. The phenothiazines and atropine should be avoided. A vapour-free anaesthetic machine should be used. Anaesthesia is induced, with thiopentone and pancuronium used to facilitate endotracheal intubation. Maintaining anaesthesia with a continuous infusion of a short-acting synthetic opiate such as alfentanil, or more traditional neuroleptic analgesic agents combined with oxygen-enriched air, is recommended. Reversal of neuromuscular blockade with neostigmine should be avoided (Ellis, 1980). The use of nitrous oxide, and prophylactic treatment of malignant hyperthermia patients with preoperative dantrolene, remains controversial (Gronert, 1980). The recommended dose of dantrolene is 5 mg/kg orally in divided doses, starting on the day before surgery.

References

Abbot, T.R. and Bentley, G. (1980) Intraoperative awakening during scoliosis surgery. *Anaesthesia*, **35**, 298–302

Abouliesh, E., Amortegui, A.J. and Taylor, F. (1977) Are bacterial filters needed in continuous epidural analgesia for obstetrics. *Anaesthesiology*, **46**, 351–354

Ainslie, J. (1956) Paraplegia due to spontaneous extradural or subdural haemorrhage. *British Journal of Surgery*, **45**, 565–567

Alajouanine, T., Castaigne, P. and Lhermitte, F. (1949) L'hématoma sous dural intrarachidienne á évolution fatal, complication rare de l'hémophilie. *Centenaire Soc. Med. Hosp., Paris*, **22**, 194–201

Alderman, D.B. (1956) Extradural spinal cord hematoma. Report of a case due to dicoumarol and a review of the literature. *New England Journal of Medicine*, **225**, 839–842

Allemby, F., Boardman, L., Pflug, J.J. and Calnan, J.S. (1973) Effects of external pneumatic intermittent compression on fibrinolysis in man. *Lancet*, **1**, 1412–1414

Ayre, P. (1937) Anaesthesia for intracranial operation. *Lancet*, **1**, 561–563

Bahar, M., Olshwand, D., Magora, F. and Davidson, J.T. (1979) Epidural morphine treatment of pain. *Lancet*, **1**, 527–529

Baines, D.B., Whittle, I.R., Chaseling, R.W., Overton, J.H. and Johnson, I.H. (1985) Effect of halothane on spinal somatosensory evoked potentials in sheep. *British Journal of Anaesthesia*, **57**, 896–899

Beaudoin, M.G. and Klein, L. (1984) Epidural abscess following multiple spinal anaesthetics. *Anaesthesia in Intensive Care*, **12**, 163–164

Beir, A. (1899) Ver über Cocainisierung des Ruckenmark. *Deutsche Zeitschrift Chirurg*, **51**, 361–364

Bennett, N.R. and Abbot, T.R. (1977) Use of sodium nitroprusside in children. *Anaesthesia*, **32**, 456–463

Bergman, I., Wald, E.R., Meyer, J.D. and Painter, M.J. (1983) Epidural abscess and vertebral osteomyelitis following multiple lumbar punctures. *Pediatrics*, **72**, 476–480

Bergofsky, E.H. (1979) Respiratory failure in disorders of the thoracic cage. *American Review of Respiratory Diseases*, **119**, 643–669

Bjure, J. (1973) Nachemsona. Non treated scoliosis. *Clinical Orthopaedics*, **93**, 44–52

Black, P.M., Zervas, N.T. and Caplan, L.R. (1978) Subdural hygroma of the spinal meninges: a case report. *Neurosurgery*, **2**, 52–54

Bonica, J.J., Backup, P.H., Anderson, C.E., Hadfield, D., Crepps, W.F. and Monk, B.F. (1957) Peridural block: analysis of 3,637 cases and a review. *Anaesthesiology*, **18**, 723–784

Boyd, H.R. and Pear, B.L. (1972) Chronic spontaneous spinal epidural hematoma. Report of two cases. *Journal of Neurosurgery*, **36**, 234–242

Boyle, A.C. (1971) The rheumatoid neck. *Proceedings of the Royal Society of Medicine*, **64**, 1161–1165

Brandt, R.A. (1980) Chronic spinal subdural haematoma. *Surgery and Neurology*, **13**, 121–123

Brechner, V.L. (1968) Unusual problems in the management of airways I. Flexion-extension mobility of the cervical vertebrae. *Anesthetics and Analgesia*, **47**, 362–373

Britt, B.A. and Kalow, W. (1970) Malignant hyperthermia. A statistical review. *Canadian Anaesthetists Society Journal*, **17**, 293–315

Brodkey, J.S., Richards, D.E., Blasingame, J.P. and Nulsen, F.E. (1972) Reversible spinal cord trauma in cats. Additive effects of direct pressure and ischaemia. *Journal of Neurosurgery*, **37**, 591–593

Bromage, P.R. (1954) *Spinal Epidural Analgesia*, Livingstone, London

Brown, R.H. and Nash, C.L. (1979) Current status of spinal cord monitoring. *Spine*, **4**, 466–470

Butler, F.S. and Cirillo, A.A. (1960) Retrograde tracheal intubation. *Anesthetics and Analgesia*, **39**, 333–338

Callan, R.A. and Brown, M.D. (1981) Positioning techniques in spinal surgery. *Clinical Orthopaedics*, **154**, 22–26

Carrea, R., Girado, M. and Eurnekian, A. (1954) Hematoma cronico epidural y subdural espinal. Relato de tres casos y analisis de la literatura sobre el tema. *Medicina (Buenos Aires)*, **14**, 179–197

Challis, J.H.T. (1933) Discussion on anaesthesia in intracranial surgery. *Proceedings of the Royal Society of Medicine*, **26**, 957–958

Chapman, R.C., Kemp, E.V. and Taliaferro, I. (1959) Phaeochromocytoma associated with multiple neurofibromatosis and intracranial hemangioma. *American Journal of Medicine*, **26**, 883–890

Charnley, J. (1972) Prophylaxis of post operative thromboembolism. *Lancet*, **2**, 134–135

Chee, Y.C. and Poh, S.C. Aspergillus epidural abscess in a patient with obstructive airways disease. *Postgraduate Medical Journal*, **59**, 43–45

Clark, D.L. and Rosner, B.S. (1973) Neurophysiologic effects of general anesthetics I. The electroencephalogram and sensory evoked responses in man. *Anesthesiology*, **38**, 564–582

Clarke, J.M.P. (1954) Traumatic haematomyelia from rupture of intramedullary angioma. Report of a case. *Journal of Bone and Joint Surgery*, **36-B**, 419–422

Cloward, R.B. and Yuhl, E.T. (1955) Spontaneous intraspinal hemorrhage and paraplegia complicating dicoumarol therapy. *Neurology*, **5**, 600–602

Committee on Sports Medicine (1984) Atlantoaxial instability in Down's syndrome. *Pediatrics*, **74**, 152–154

Cooper, D.W. (1967) Spontaneous spinal epidural hematoma. Case Report. *Journal of Neurosurgery*, **26**, 343–345

Danner, R.L. and Hartman, B.J. (1987) Update on spinal epidural abscess: 35 cases and a review of the literature. *Review of Infectious Diseases*, **9**, 265–274

Dawson, G.D. (1974) Cerebral responses to electrical stimulation of peripheral nerve in man. *Journal of Neurology, Neurosurgery and Psychiatry*, **10**, 137–140

De Angelis, J. (1972) Hazards of subdural and epidural anesthesia during anticoagulant therapy, a case report and review. *Anesthesia and Analgesia*, **51**, 676–679

Deacock, A.R. DeC. (1980) Anaesthesia for orthopaedic surgery. In *General Anaesthesia* (eds T.C. Gray, J.F. Nunn and J.E. Utting), Butterworths, London

Denborough, M.A. and Lovell, R.R.H. (1960) Anaesthetic deaths in a family. *Lancet*, **2**, 45

Desmond, J. (1970) Paraplegia: problems confronting the anesthesiologist. *Canadian Anaesthesia Society Journal*, **17**, 435–451

Diaz, J.H. and Lockhardt, C.H. (1987) Post operative quadriplegia after spinal fusion for scoliosis with intraoperative awakening. *Anesthetics and Analgesia*, **66**, 1039–1042

Ditzler, J.W., Dumke, P.R., Harrington, J.J. and DeWitt Fox, J. (1959) Should spinal anesthesia be used for herniated intravertebral disc. *Anesthetics and Analgesia*, **38**, 118–124

Dohl, S., Takeshima, R. and Naito, H. (1987) Spinal cord blood flow during spinal anesthesia in dogs. The effects of tetracaine, epinephrine, acute blood loss and hypercarbia. *Anesthetics and Analgesia*, **66**, 599–606

Donchin, E., Calaway, E. and Cooper, E. (1977) Publication criteria for studies of evoked potentials in man. Attention, voluntary contraction and event-related cerebral potentials. In *Progress in Clinical Neurophysiology*, Vol. 5 (ed. J.E. Desmej), Karger, Basel

Douglas-Wilson, J., Miller, S. and Watson, G.W. (1933) Spontaneous subarachnoid haemorrhage of intraspinal origin. *British Medical Journal*, **1**, 554–555

Dunn, D., Phopesh, V. and Mobini, J. (1979) Spinal subdural hematoma, a possible hazard of lumbar puncture in an alcoholic. *Journal of the American Medical Association*, **241**, 1712–1713

Dvorak, E. (1982) Peracute radiation pneumonitis. *Strahlentherapie*, **158**, 23–29

Dyer, A.F., Newton, N.C. and Sherwood, A.A. (1969) An anterior approach to scoliosis. A preliminary report. *Clinical Orthopaedics*, **62**, 192–203

Dzenitis, A.J. (1966) Spontaneous atlantoaxial dislocation in a mongoloid child with spinal cord compression. *Journal of Neurosurgery*, **25**, 458–460

Edelson, R.N. (1976) Spinal subdural hematoma. In *Handbook of Clinical Neurology*, Vol. 26 (eds P.J. Vinken and G.W. Bruyn), Elsevier, New York

Edelson, R.N., Chernick, N.L. and Posner, J.B. (1974) Spinal subdural hematomas complicating lumbar puncture. Occurrence in thrombocytopenic patients. *Archives of Neurology*, **31**, 134–137

Edge, W.G., Cooper, G.M. and Morgan, M. (1979) Analgesic effects of sublingual buprenorphine. *Anaesthesia*, **34**, 463–467

Editorial (1985) Rheumatoid subluxation of the cervical spine. *Annals of Rheumatic Diseases*, **44**, 807–808

Eisele, J.H. Jr. (1981) Connective tissue diseases. In *Anesthesia and Uncommon Diseases* (eds J. Katz, J. Benumof and L.B. Kadis), Saunders, Philadelphia

Elian, D., Hassin, D., Tomer, A., Bank, H. and Eisenstein, Z. (1984) Spinal epidural abscess: an unusual complication of bacterial endocarditis. *Infection*, **12**, 258–259

Ellis, F.R. (1980) Inherited muscle disease. *British Journal of Anaesthesia*, **52**, 153–164

Ellis, F.R. and Halsall, R.J. (1980) Malignant hyperpyrexia. *British Journal of Hospital Medicine*, **24**, 318–327

Ellis, S.C., Bryan-Brown, C.W. and Hyderally, H. (1975) Massive swelling of the head and neck. *Anesthesiology*, **42**, 102–103

Engler, G.L., Spielholz, N.I., Bernard, W.N., Danziger, F., Merkin, H. and Wolff, T. (1978) Somatosensory evoked potentials during Harrington instrumentation for scoliosis. *Journal of Bone and Joint Surgery*, **60-A**, 528–532

Evans, D.E., Kobrine, A.I. and Rizzoli, H.V. (1980) Cardiac arrhythmias accompanying acute compression of the spinal cord. *Journal of Neurosurgery*, **52**, 52–59

Evans, J.M., David, H., Rosen, M., Revill, S., Robinson, J., McCarthy, J. and Hogg, M.I.J. (1976) Patient activated intravenous narcotic. *Anaesthesia*, **31**, 847–848

Evarts, C. (1987) Prevention of venous thromboembolism. *Clinical Orthopaedics*, **222**, 98–104

Fee, J.H.P., McDonald, J.R., Dundee, J.W. and Clarke, R.S.J. (1978) Frequency of previous anaesthesia in an anaesthetic population. *British Journal of Anaesthesia*, **50**, 917–920

Fehring, T.K. and Brooks, A.L. (1987) Upper cervical instability in rheumatoid arthritis. *Clinical Orthopaedics*, **221**, 137–148

Fisher, M.D. (1975) Anaesthetic difficulties in neurofibromatosis. *Anaesthesia*, **30**, 648–650

Foo, D. and Rossier, A.B. (1981) Preoperative neurological status in predicting surgical outcome of spinal epidural hematomas. *Surgery and Neurology*, **15**, 389–401

Fry, E.N.S. (1979) Relief of pain after surgery. A comparison of sublingual buprenorphine with intramuscular papaveretum. *Anaesthesia*, **34**, 549–551

Funk, D. and Raymond, F. (1975) Rheumatoid arthritis of the cricoarytenoid joints. An airway hazard. *Anesthetics and Analgesia*, **54**, 724–725

Gardner, R.V. (1985) Salmonella vertebral osteomyelitis and epidural abscess in a child with sickle cell anemia. *Pediatric Emergency Care*, **1**, 87–89

Gilbert, R.G.B., Brindle, G.F. and Galindo, A. (1966) *Anaesthesia for Neurosurgery*, Churchill, London

Gillespie, N.A. (1935) Endotracheal nitrous oxide oxygen ether anaesthesia in neurological surgery. *Anesthetics and Analgesia*, **14**, 225–229

Gingrich, T.F. (1968) Spinal epidural hematoma following continuous epidural anesthesia. *Anesthesiology*, **29**, 162–163

Ginsberg, H.H., Shetter, A.G. and Radzens, P.A. (1985) Post operative paraplegia with preserved intraoperative somatosensory evoked potentials. *Journal of Neurosurgery*, **63**, 296–300

Gjessing, J. and Tomlin, P.J. (1981) Post operative pain control with intrathecal morphine. *Anaesthesia*, **36**, 268–276

Glynn, C.J., Mather, L.E., Cousins, M.J., Wilson, P.R. and Graham, J.R. (1979) Spinal narcotics and respiratory depression. *Lancet*, **2**, 356–357

Gowers, W.R. and Horsley, V. (1888) A case of tumour of the spinal cord. Removal, recovery. *Proceedings of the Medical and Chirurgical Society*, **lxxxi**, 377–428

Greensite, F.S. and Katz, J. (1980) Spinal subdural hematoma associated with attempted epidural anesthesia and subsequent continuous spinal anesthesia. *Anesthetics and Analgesia*, **59**, 72–73

Griffiths, I.R. (1973a) Spinal cord blood flow in dogs 2. The effect of blood gases. *Journal of Neurology, Neurosurgery and Psychiatry*, **36**, 42–49

Griffiths, I.R. (1973b) Spinal cord blood flow in dogs. The effect of blood pressure. *Journal of Neurology, Neurosurgery and Psychiatry*, **36**, 914–920

Gronert, G.A. (1980) Malignant hyperthermia. *Anesthesiology*, **53**, 395–423

Gronert, G.A. and Theye, R.A. (1975) Pathophysiology of hyperkalaemia induced by succinylcholine. *Anesthesiology*, **43**, 88–99

Grundy, B.L. (1983) Intraoperative monitoring of somatosensory evoked potentials. *Anesthesiology*, **58**, 72–82

Grundy, B.L., Luna, A., Doyle, E. and Procopio, P. (1982) Somatosensory cortical evoked potential monitoring during neurosurgical operations. *Anesthetics and Analgesia*, **61**, 186–187

Grundy, B.L., Nash, C.L. and Brown, R.H. (1981) Arterial pressure manipulation alters spinal cord function during correction of scoliosis. *Anesthesiology*, **54**, 249–253

Grundy, B.L., Nelson, P.B. and Doyle, E.P. (1982) Intraoperative loss of somatosensory evoked potentials predicts loss of spinal cord function. *Anesthesiology*, **57**, 321–322

Gustafsson, L.L., Schildt, B. and Jacobsen, K. (1982) Adverse effects of extradural and intradural opiates. *British Journal of Anaesthesia*, **54**, 479–486

Guthikonda, M., Schmideck, H.M., Wallman, L.J. and Snyder, T.M. (1979) Spinal subdural hematoma. Case report and review of the literature. *Neurosurgery*, **5**, 614–616

Gutterman, P. (1977) Acute spinal subdural hematoma following lumbar puncture. *Surgery and Neurology*, **7**, 355–356

Guy, M.J., Zahra, M. and Sengupta, R.P. (1979) Spontaneous spinal subdural hematoma during general anaesthesia. *Surgery and Neurology*, **11**, 199–200

Hall, J.E., Levine, C.R. and Sudhir, K.G. (1978) Intraoperative awakening to monitor spinal cord function during Harrington rod instrumentation and spine fusion. *Journal of Bone and Joint Surgery*, **60-A**, 533–536

Halliday, A.M. and Wakefield, G.S. (1963) Cerebral evoked potentials in patients with dissociated sensory loss. *Journal of Neurology, Neurosurgery and Psychiatry*, **26**, 211–219

Hardy, R.W., Naser, C.L. and Brodkey, J.S. (1973) Experience and clinical studies in spinal cord monitoring. The effects of pressure, anoxia and ischaemia on spinal cord function. *Journal of Bone and Joint Surgery*, **55-A**, 435

Harrington, P.R. (1962) Treatment of scoliosis. *Journal of Bone and Joint Surgery*, **44-A**, 591–595

Harris, M.E. (1969) Spontaneous epidural spinal hemorrhage. *American Journal of Roentgenology*, **105**, 383–385

Harris, W. (1911) Two cases of spontaneous haematorrhachis or intrameningeal spinal haemorrhage, one cured by laminectomy. *Proceedings of the Royal Society of Medicine*, **5**, 115, 122

Harrison, G.G. (1975) Control of the malignant hyperpyrexic syndrome in MHS swine by dantrolene sodium. *British Journal of Anaesthesia*, **47**, 62–65

Hassan, S.Z., Matz, G.J., Lawrence, A.M. and Collins, P.A. (1976) Laryngeal stenosis in acromegaly. A possible cause of airway difficulties associated with anesthesia. *Anesthetics and Analgesia*, **55**, 57–60

Hehman, K. and Norrell, H. (1964) Massive chronic spinal epidural hematoma in a child. *American Journal of Diseases in Childhood*, **116**, 308–310

Henson, R.A. and Croft, P.B. (1956) Spontaneous spinal subarachnoid haemorrhage. *Quarterly Journal of Medicine*, **125**, 53–66

Hirsch, J. (1981) Prevention of deep venous thrombosis. *British Journal of Hospital Medicine*, **26**, 143–147

Holborow, J. (1979) Current concepts in corrective tissue disorders. *British Journal of Hospital Medicine*, **21**, 8–14

Horne, J.G. and Muller, P. (1977) Spontaneous spinal extradural hematoma. *Canadian Journal of Surgery*, **20**, 379–384

Hreidarsson, S., Magram, G. and Singer, H. (1982) Symptomatic atlantoaxial dislocation in Down's syndrome. *Pediatrics*, **69**, 568–571

Huebert, H.T. and MacKinnon, W.B. (1969) Syringomyelia and scoliosis. *Journal of Bone and Joint Surgery*, **51-B**, 338–343

Hughes, G.R.V. (1979) Rheumatoid arthritis. *British Journal of Hospital Medicine*, **21**, 584–592

Hulme, A. and Dott, N.M. (1954) Spinal epidural abscess. *British Medical Journal*, **1**, 64–68

Hurt, R.W., Shaw, M.D. and Russell, J.A. (1977) Spinal subdural hematoma: an unusual complication of lumbar puncture. *Surgery and Neurology*, **8**, 296–297

Jackson, R. (1869) Case of spinal apoplexy. *Lancet*, **2**, 5–6

Janis, K.M. (1972) Epidural hematoma following postoperative epidural analgesia. *Anesthetics and Analgesia*, **51**, 689–692

Jellinger, K. (1976) Traumatic vascular disease of the spinal cord. In *Handbook of Clinical Neurology*, Vol. 26 (eds P.J. Vinken and G.W. Bruyn), Elsevier, New York

Johnson, R., Green, J.R. and Charnley, J. (1976) Pulmonary embolism and its prophylaxis following Charnley total hip replacement. *Clinical Orthopaedics*, **127**, 123–132

Jones, S.J., Edgar, M.A., Rasford, O. and Thomas, N.P. (1983) A system for the electrophysiological monitoring of the spinal cord during operations for scoliosis. *Journal of Bone and Joint Surgery*, **65-B**, 134–139

Kafer, E.R. (1975) Idiopathic scoliosis. Mechanical properties of the respiratory system and ventilatory response to carbon dioxide. *Journal of Clinical Investigation*, **55**, 1153–1163

Kafer, E.R. (1980) Respiratory and cardiovascular functions in scoliosis and the principles of anaesthetic management. *Anesthesiology*, **52**, 339–351

Kakkar, V.V., Spindler, J., Flute, P.T., Corrigan, T., Fossard, D.P. and Crellin, R.Q. (1972) Efficacy of low doses of heparin in the prevention of deep vein thrombosis after major surgery. *Lancet*, **2**, 101–106

Kane, R.E. (1981) Neurologic deficits following epidural or spinal anesthesia. *Anesthetics and Analgesia*, **60**, 150–161

Kavan, E.M. and Julien, R.M. (1974) Central nervous system effects of isoflurane. *Canadian Anaesthetists Society Journal*, **21**, 390–402

Keeri-Szanto, M. and Heamans, S. (1972) Post operative demand analgesia. *Surgery, Gynecology and Obstetrics*, **134**, 647–651

Keim, H.A. and Weinstein, J.D. (1970) Acute renal failure. A complication of spine fusion in the tuck position. *Journal of Bone and Joint Surgery*, **52-A**, 1248–1250

King, O.J. and Glass, W.W. (1960) Spinal subarachnoid haemorrhage following lumbar puncture. *Archives of Surgery*, **80**, 574–577

Kirkpatrick, D. and Goodman, S.J. (1975) Combined subarachnoid and spinal subdural hematoma following spinal puncture. *Surgery and Neurology*, **3**, 109–111

Kitihana, L.M. (1971) Airway difficulties associated with anaesthesia in acromegaly. *British Journal of Anaesthesia*, **43**, 1187–1190

Klossek, H. and Huller, E. (1984) Zur Problematik de spotanen spinale Epiduralhamatome. *Zentralblatt für Neurochirurgie*, **45**, 116–123

Knight, M.Y.N. and Dawson, R. (1976) Effect of intermittent compression of the arms on deep venous thrombosis in the legs. *Lancet*, **2**, 1265–1267

Kobel, M., Creighton, R.E. and Steward, D.J. (1982) Anaesthetic considerations in Down's syndrome. Experience with 100 patients and a review of the literature. *Canadian Anaesthetists Society Journal*, **29**, 593–599

Kobrine, A.I., Doyle, T.F. and Martins, A.N. (1975) Autoregulation of spinal cord blood flow. *Clinical Neurosurgery*, **22**, 573–581

Kohli, C.M., Palmer, A.H. and Gray, G.H. (1974) Spontaneous intraspinal haemorrhage causing paraplegia. A complication of heparin therapy. *Annals of Surgery*, **179**, 197–199

Konig, H.J., Schleep, J. and Krahling, K.H. (1985) A case of transverse spinal cord syndrome following contamination of a peridural catheter. *Regional Anaesthesia*, **8**, 60–62

Kosary, I.Z., Braham, J., Shacked, I. and Shacked, R. (1977) Spinal epidural hematoma due to hemangioma of vertebra. *Surgery and Neurology*, **7**, 61–62

Koyama, T., Igarashi, S., Hanakita, J. and Handa, J. (1982) Das spinale epidurale Hamatome. *Neurochirurgia*, **25**, 11–13

Kreyenbuhl, H., Yasargil, M.G. and McClintock, H.G. (1969) Treatment of spinal cord vascular malformations by surgical excision. *Journal of Neurosurgery*, **30**, 472–485

Krishna, G. (1975) Neurofibromatosis, renal hypertension and cardiac dysrhythmias. *Anesthetics and Analgesia*, **54**, 542–545

Lamont, R.L., Watson, S.L. and Green, M.A. (1983) Spinal cord monitoring during spinal surgery using somatosensory spinal evoked potentials. *Journal of Pediatric Orthopedics*, **3**, 31–36

Latto, I.P. (1985) Management of difficult intubation. In *Difficulties in Tracheal Intubation* (eds I.P. Latto and M. Rosen), Baillière Tindall, Sussex, UK

Lawrence, D. and Kakkar, V.V. (1980) Graduated static external compression of the lower limbs: a physiological assessment. *British Journal of Surgery*, **67**, 119–121

Leading Article (1971) The lungs in ankylosing spondylitis. *British Medical Journal*, **3**, 492–493

Lee, J.A. and Atkinson, R.S. (1978) *Lumbar Puncture and Spinal Anaesthesia*, Churchill Livingstone, London

Lenerer, M.L., Gutterman, P. and Jenkins, F. (1973) Epidural hematoma and paraplegia after numerous lumbar punctures. *Anesthesiology*, **39**, 550–551

Liolios, A. and Anderson, F.H. (1979) Selective spinal analgesia. *Lancet*, **2**, 357

Lipton, S. (1950) Anaesthesia in the surgery of retropulsed vertebral discs. *Anaesthesia*, **5**, 208–212

Loach, A. (1973) *Anaesthesia for Orthopaedic Patients*, Edward Arnold, London

Lombarbi, G. and Passerini, A. (1964) *Spinal Cord Disease. A Radiographic and Myelographic Analysis*, Williams and Wilkins, Baltimore

Lombardi, V. (1970) Postoperative subdural haematoma with associated extradural arachnoid cyst of the spine. Case report. *Acta neurologica*, **25**, 123–125

Lucca Escobar, R.J. and Castillo, R. (1958) Continuous epidural anesthesia for laminectomy. *Anesthetics and Analgesia*, **37**, 328–331

McAllister, R. (1974) Macroglossia, a positional complication. *Anesthesiology*, **40**, 199–200

McCallum, J.E. and Bennett, M.H. (1975) Electrophysiological monitoring of spinal cord function during intraspinal surgery. *Surgical Forum*, **26**, 469–471

McKenna, R., Galante, J., Wallace, D.L., Kaushal, S.P. and Meredith, P. (1980) Prevention of venous thromboembolism after total knee replacement by high dose aspirin or intermittent calf and thigh compression. *British Medical Journal*, **1**, 514–517

Magbagbeola, J.A.O. (1970) Abnormal responses to muscle relaxants in patients with Von Recklinghausen's disease (multiple neurofibromatosis). *British Journal of Anaesthesia*, **42**, 710

Magill, I.W. and Robotham, I.S. (1921) Anaesthetics in the plastic surgery of the face and jaws. *Proceedings of the Royal Society of Medicine*, **14**, 17–27

Mallory, T.M. (1973) Use of hypotensive anesthesia in total hip replacement. *Journal of the American Medical Association*, **24**, 248–253

Mandel, R.J., Brown, M.D., McCollough, N.C., Pallares, V. and Varlotta, R. (1981) Hypotensive anaesthesia and autotransfusion in spinal surgery. *Clinical Orthopaedics*, **154**, 27–33

Manser, J. (1970) Abnormal responses in Von Recklinghausen's disease. *British Journal of Anaesthesia*, **42**, 183–184

Marcus, M.L., Heistad, D.D., Ehrhardt, J.C. and Abboud, F.M. (1977) Regulation of total and regional spinal cord blood flow. *Circulation Research*, **41**, 128–134

Markham, J.W., Lynge, H.W. and Stahlman, E.B.S. (1967) The syndrome of spontaneous epidural haematoma, report of 3 cases. *Journal of Neurosurgery*, **26**, 334–339

Marks, W.A. and Bodensteiner, J.B. (1988) Anterior cervical epidural abscess with pneumococcus in an infant. *Journal of Childhood Neurology*, **3**, 25–29

Martel, W. and Tishler, J.M. (1966) Observations on the spine in mongolism. *American Journal of Roentgenology*, **97**, 630–638

Markham, J.W., Lynge, H.W. and Stahlman, E.B.S. (1967) The syndrome of spontaneous epidural haematoma, report of 3 cases. *Journal of Neurosurgery*, **26**, 334–339

Martin, J.T. (1978) *Positioning in Anaesthesia and Surgery*, Saunders, Philadelphia

Masdue, J.C., Breuer, M.D. and Schoene, W.C. (1979) Spinal subarachnoid hematomas: clue to a source of bleeding in traumatic lumbar puncture. *Neurology (Minneapolis)*, **29**, 872–876

Matheson, D. (1966) Epidural anaesthesia for lumbar laminectomy and spinal fusion. *Canadian Anaesthesia Society Journal*, **7**, 149–157

Mathews, J.A. (1974) Atlantoaxial subluxation. *Annals of Rheumatic Diseases*, **33**, 526–531

Mattle, H., Seib, J.P., Rohner, M. and Menenthaler, M. (1987) Nontraumatic spinal epidural and subdural hematomas. *Neurology*, **37**, 1351–1356

Messeter, K.H. and Petterson, K.I. (1980) Endotracheal intubation with the fibreoptic bronchoscope. *Anaesthesia*, **35**, 294–298

Messick, J.M., Newberg, L.A., Nugent, M. and Faust, R.J. (1985) Principles of neuroanaesthesia for the non neurosurgical patient with CNS pathology. *Anesthetics and Analgesia*, **64**, 143–174

Messmer, K. (1975) Hemodilution. *Surgical Clinics of North America*, **55**, 659–678

Miller, E.D., Sanders, D.B. and Rowlingson, J.C. (1978) Anesthesia induced rhabdomyolysis in a patient with Duchenne's muscular dystrophy. *Anesthesiology*, **48**, 146–148

Moe, J.H. (1967) Complications of scoliosis treatment. *Clinical Orthopaedics*, **53**, 21–30

Moore, R.A., McNicholas, K.W. and Warran, S.P. (1987) Atlantoaxial subluxation with symptomatic spinal cord compression in a child with Down's syndrome. *Anesthetics and Analgesia*, **66**, 89–90

Moore, W.E., Watson, R.L. and Summery, J.J. (1976) Massive myoglobinuria precipitated by halothane and succinylcholine in a member of a family with elevation of serum creatine phosphokinase. *Anaesthetics and Analgesia*, **55**, 680–682

Morris, G.K. (1980) Prevention of venous thromboembolism. A survey of methods by orthopaedic and general surgeons. *Lancet*, **2**, 572–574

Morris, G.K. and Mitchell, J.R.A. (1977) The aetiology of acute pulmonary embolism and the identification of high risk groups. *British Journal of Hospital Medicine*, **18**, 6–12

Mracek, Z. (1980) Spontaneous spinal extradural haematoma. Experiences with four patients and a review of the literature. *Zentralblatt für Neurochirurgie*, **41**, 12–30

Muller, H., Schramm, J., Roggendorf, W. and Brock, M. (1982) Vascular malformations as a cause of spontaneous spinal epidural haematoma. *Acta neurochirurgica*, **62**, 297–305

Murphy, P. (1967) A fibreoptic endoscope used for nasal intubation. *Anaesthesia*, **22**, 489–491

Nash, C.L., Lorig, R.A., Schatzinger, L.A. and Brown, R.H. (1977) Spinal cord monitoring during operative treatment of the spine. *Clinical Orthopaedics*, **126**, 100–105

Nerubay, J., Volpin, G. and Katznelson, A. (1978) Spinal epidural abscess following epidural anaesthesia. *Harefuah*, **95**, 341–342

North, J.B. and Brophy, B.P. (1979) Epidural abscess: a hazard of spinal epidural anaesthesia. *Australian and New Zealand Journal of Surgery*, **49**, 484–489

Oakley, J.C., Ojemann, G.A. and Alvord, E.C. (1981) Post traumatic syringomyelia. *Journal of Neurosurgery*, **55**, 276–281

Oldenkott, P., Preger, R. and Todorow, S. (1981) Spinale epidurale Hamatome und Antikoagulantienbenhandlung. *Medizinische Welt*, **32**, 46–49

Ommaya, A.K., Di Chiro, G. and Doppman, J.L. (1969) Ligation of arterial supply in the treatment of spinal cord arteriovenous malformations. *Journal of Neurosurgery*, **30**, 679–692

Ovassapian, A., Yelich, S.J., Dykes, M.H.M. and Brunner, E.E. (1983) Fiberoptic nasotracheal intubation. Incidence and causes of failure. *Anesthetics and Analgesia*, **62**, 692–695

Peterson, D.O., Drummond, J.C. and Todd, M.M. (1986) Effects of halothane, enflurane, isoflurane and nitrous oxide on somatosensory evoked potentials in humans. *Anesthesiology*, **65**, 35–40

Phillips, T.W., Kling, T.H.F. and McGillicudy, J.E. (1981) Spontaneous ventral spinal epidural haematoma with anterior cord syndrome. Report of a case. *Neurosurgery*, **9**, 440–443

Piotrowski, W., Kroger, M. and Tornow, K. (1979) Das spinale epidurale Hamatome. *Nervenarzt*, **50**, 426–431

Plotkin, R., Ronthal, M. and Froman, C. (1966) Spontaneous spinal subarachnoid haemorrhage. Report of three cases. *Journal of Neurosurgery*, **25**, 443–446

Ponte, A. (1974) Post operative paraplegia due to hypercorrection of scoliosis and drop of blood pressure. *Journal of Bone and Joint Surgery*, **56-A**, 444–456

Potts, C.S. (1910) Intradural cyst of the spinal meninges removed by operation. Remarks on the location of the spinal centres for testicular sensibility. *Journal of Nervous and Mental Diseases*, **37**, 621–625

Prime, F.J. (1977) A review of lung function in scoliotic patients. In *Scoliosis* (ed. P.A. Zorab), Academic Press, London

Prithvi Raj, P., Forestner, J., Watson, T.D., Morris, R.E. and Jenkins, M.T. (1974) Technics for fiberoptic laryngoscopy in anesthesia. *Anesthetics and Analgesia*, **53**, 708–713

Pueschel, S.M., Herndon, J.H., Gelch, M.M., Senft, K.E., Scola, F.H. and Golberg, M.J. (1984) Symptomatic atlantoaxial subluxation in persons with Down's syndrome. *Journal of Pediatric Orthopaedics*, **4**, 682–688

Rabe, E.F. (1964) The hypotonic infant. *Journal of Pediatrics*, **64**, 422–440

Rader, J.P. (1955) Chronic subdural hematoma of the spinal cord. Review of a case. *New England Journal of Medicine*, **253**, 374–376

Rainbird, A. and Pfitzner, J. (1983) Restricted spread of analgesia following epidural blood patch. *Anaesthesia*, **38**, 481–484

Relton, J.E.S. (1977) Anaesthesia in scoliosis. In *Scoliosis* (ed. P.A. Zorab), Academic Press, London

Relton, J.E.S. and Hall, J.E. (1967) An operation frame for spinal fusion. A new apparatus designed to reduce haemorrhage during operation. *Journal of Bone and Joint Surgery*, **49-B**, 327–330

Reynolds, A.F. and Turner, P.T. (1978) Spinal subdural hematoma. *Rocky Mountains Medical Journal*, **75**, 199–200

Richards, W.C. (1972) Anaesthesia and serum creatinine phosphokinase levels in patients with Duchenne's pseudohypertrophic muscular dystrophy. *Anaesthesia in Intensive Care*, **1**, 150–153

Rolly, G. and Versicheclen, L. (1976) Buprenorphine as post operative analgesic. *Acta anaesthesiologica belgica*, **27**, 183

Roscoe, M.W.A. and Barrington, T.W. (1984) Acute spinal subdural hematoma. *Spine*, **9**, 672–675

Rosenburg, M.K. and Berner, G. (1965) Spinal anesthesia in lumbar disc surgery: review of 200 cases with a case history. *Anesthetics and Analgesia*, **44**, 419–423

Russell, N.A. and Benoit, B.G. (1983) Spinal subdural hematoma. A review. *Surgery and Neurology*, **20**, 133–137

Russell, N., Maroun, F.B. and Jacob, J.C. (1981) Spinal subdural hematoma in association with anticoagulant therapy. *Canadian Journal of Neurological Science*, **8**, 87–89

Rustin, M.H., Flynn, M.D. and Coomes, E.N. (1983) Acute sacral epidural abscess following local anaesthetic injection. *Postgraduate Medical Journal*, **58**, 399–400

Rutter, D.V., Skewes, D.G. and Morgan, M. (1981) Extradural opiates for post operative analgesia. *British Journal of Anaesthesia*, **53**, 915–919

Saady, A. (1976) Epidural abscess complicating thoracic epidural analgesia. *Anesthesiology*, **44**, 244–246

Sakata, T. and Kurihara, A. (1984) Spontaneous spinal subdural hematoma. *Spine*, **9**, 324–326

Sanchez-Juan, J. and Lopez-Escobar, F. (1964) Hematoma subdural raquideo. *Revista española de oto-neuro-oftalmologia y neurocirugia*, **23**, 248–252

Sargent, P. (1920) A clinical lecture on the surgical aspect of spinal tumours. *British Medical Journal*, **1**, 37–40

Schaake, T. and Schafer, E.R. (1970) Spontaneous hemorrhage in the spinal canal (Abstract). *Journal of Neurology, Neurosurgery and Psychiatry*, **3**, 715–716

Schiller, F., Neligan, B. and Brudtz-Olsen, O. (1948) Surgery in haemophilia: a case of spinal subdural haematoma producing paraplegia. *Lancet*, **2**, 842–845

Schofield, N.McC. (1973) Anaesthesia for spinal disorders. In *Anaesthesia for Orthopaedic Patients* (ed. A. Loach), Edward Arnold, London

Sclang, H.A., Carmichael, A.H. and Freund, C.J. (1962) Spontaneous subdural hematoma in anticoagulant therapy. *American Practitioner*, **13**, 247–250

Scremin, O.U. and Decima, E.E. (1983) Control of blood flow in the cat spinal cord. *Journal of Neurosurgery*, **58**, 742–748

Seay, A.R., Ziter, F.A. and Thompson, J.A. (1978) Cardiac arrest during induction of anaesthesia in Duchenne muscular dystrophy. *Journal of Paediatrics*, **93**, 88–90

Sebel, P.S., Ingram, D.A., Flynn, P.J., Rutherford, C.F. and Rogers, H. (1986) Evoked potentials during isoflurane anaesthesia. *British Journal of Anaesthesia*, **58**, 580–585

Secker-Walker, R.H., Ho, J.E. and Gill, I.S. (1979) Observations on regional ventilation and perfusion in kyphoscoliosis. *Respiration*, **38**, 194–203

Selwyn Crawford, J.S. (1975) Pathology in the extradural space. *British Journal of Anaesthesia*, **47**, 412–415

Semine, A.A., Ertel, A.N., Goldberg, M.J. and Bull, M.J. (1978) Cervical spine instability in children with Down's syndrome (trisomy 21). *Journal of Bone and Joint Surgery*, **60-A**, 649–652

Shannon, D.C., Riseborough, E.J., Valenca, L.M. and Kazemi, H. (1970) The distribution of abnormal lung function in kyphoscoliosis. *Journal of Bone and Joint Surgery*, **52-A**, 131–144

Shelley, M., Bethune, D.W. and Latimer, R.D. (1986) A comparison of five heat and moisture exchangers. *Anaesthesia*, **41**, 527–532

Shimoji, K., Kano, T., Nakashima, H. and Shimizu, H. (1974) The effects of thiamyl sodium on electrical activity of the central and peripheral nervous system in man. *Anesthesiology*, **40**, 234–240

Sidi, A., Davidson, J.T., Bahar, M. and Oldshwang, D. (1981) Spinal narcotics and central nervous system depression. *Anaesthesia*, **36**, 1044–1047

Silver, D.J., Dunsmore, R.H. and Dickson, C.M. (1976) Spinal anesthesia for lumbar disc surgery. Review of 576 operations. *Anesthetics and Analgesia*, **55**, 550–554

Slavin, H.B. (1937) Spontaneous intraspinal subarachnoid haemorrhage. Report of a case. *Journal of Nervous and Mental Diseases*, **86**, 425–427

Smith, R.A. (1985) Spinal subdural hematoma, neurilemmoma and acute transverse myelopathy. *Surgery and Neurology*, **23**, 367–370

Solero, C.L., Forani, M. and Savoirardo, M. (1980) Spontaneous spinal epidural haematoma arising from ruptured vascular malformation. *Acta neurochirurgica*, **53**, 169–174

Sollman, W.P., Gaab, M.R. and Panning, B. (1987) Lumbar epidural hematoma and spinal abscess following peridural anesthesia. *Regional Anaesthesie*, **10**, 121–124

Solymosi, L. and Wappenscmidt, J. (1985) A new radiological method for therapy of spinal epidural hematomas. *Neuroradiology*, **27**, 67–69

Spencer, G. (1977) Respiratory insufficiency in scoliosis. Clinical management and home care. In *Scoliosis* (ed. P.A. Zorab), Academic Press, London

Spielholz, N.I., Benjamin, M.V., Engler, G.L. and Ransohof, J. (1979) Somatosensory evoked potentials during compression and stabilization of the spine. *Spine*, **4**, 500–505

Spurry, O.M., Rubin, S. and Wolf, J.W. (1964) Spinal epidural hematoma during anticoagulant therapy. *Archives of Internal Medicine*, **114**, 103–107

Stewart, D.H. and Watkins, E.S. (1969) Spinal cord compression by chronic subdural hematoma. Case report. *Journal of Neurosurgery*, **31**, 80–82

Sudhir, K.G., Smith, R.M., Hall, J.E. and Hansen, D.D. (1976) Intraoperative awakening for early recognition of possible neurological sequelae during Harrington rod spinal fusion. *Anaesthetics and Analgesia*, **55**, 526–528

Tamsen, A., Hartvig, P., Dahlstrom, B., Lindstrom, B. and Holmdahl, H. (1979) Patient controlled analgesic therapy in the early post operative period. *Acta anaesthesiologica scandinavica*, **26**, 462–470

Taylor, P.A. and Towey, R.M. (1972) The bronchoscope as an aid to endotracheal intubation. *Anaesthesia*, **44**, 611–612

Thornton, C., Heneghan, C.P.H., James, M.F.M. and Jones, J.G. (1984) Effects of halothane or enflurane with controlled ventilation on auditory evoked potentials. *British Journal of Anaesthesia*, **56**, 315–323

Thornton, J.A. (1980) Neurological and muscular disorders. In *General Anaesthesia* (eds T.C. Gray, J.F. Nunn and J.E. Utting), Butterworths, London

Tice, W.P. (1957) The use of epidural anesthesia for excision of the lumbar disc. *Journal of Neurosurgery*, **14**, 1–4

Tindal, S. (1987) Anesthesia for spinal decompression for metastatic disease. *Anesthetics and Analgesia*, **66**, 894–898

Tishler, J.M. and Martel, W. (1965) Dislocation of the atlas in mongolism. *Radiology*, **84**, 904–906

Toledo, E., Shalit, M.N. and Segal, R. (1981) Spinal subdural hematoma associated with anticoagulant therapy in a patient with spinal meningioma. *Neurosurgery*, **8**, 600–603

Tomarken, J.L. (1985) Spinal subdural hematoma. *Annals of Emergency Medicine*, **14**, 261–263

Torda, T.A. (1980) Epidural morphine. *Anaesthesia in Intensive Care*, **8**, 218–219

Tricot, R., Nogrette, P. and Ragot, M. (1964) Hemorragie sous durale, interrachidienne hemorragie et ramollisement medullaires au cours d'un traitement anticoagulant chez un mitrale. *Bulletin de la Société de médecine de Paris*, **115**, 627–637

Tuffier, T. (1899) Analgesic Chirurgicale per l'injection sous arachnoidienne lombaire de cocaine. *Compte rendu des séances de la Société de biologie*, **51**, 882–884

Uhl, R.R., Squires, K.C., Bruce, D.L. and Starr, A. (1980) Effect of halothane anesthesia on the human cortical visual evoked response. *Anesthesiology*, **53**, 273–276

Vauzelle, C., Stagnara, P. and Jouvinroux, P. (1973) Functional monitoring of spinal cord activity during spinal cord surgery. *Clinical Orthopaedics*, **93**, 173–178

Wagner, D.K., Varkey, B., Sheth, N.K. and Da Mert, G.J. (1985) Epidural abscess, vertebral destruction and paraplegia caused by an extending infection from an aspergilloma. *American Journal of Medicine*, **78**, 518–522

Wang, J.K., Nauss, L.A. and Thomas, J.E. (1979) Pain relief by intrathecally applied morphine in man. *Anesthesiology*, **50**, 149–151

Wanscher, M., Riishede, L. and Krogh, B. (1985) Fistula formation following epidural catheter. *Acta anaesthesiologica scandinavica*, **29**, 552–553

Warner, D.O., Danielson, D.R. and Restall, C.J. (1987) Temporary paraplegia following spinal anesthesia in a patient with spinal cord arteriovenous malformation. *Anesthesiology*, **66**, 236–237

Waters, D.J. (1963) Guided blind endotracheal intubation for patients with deformities of the upper airway. *Anaesthesia*, **18**, 158–162

Westgate, H.D. and Johnson, B.E. (1971) Preoperative pulmonary evaluation and postoperative respiratory management of patients with severe thoracic scoliosis. *Journal of Bone and Joint Surgery*, **53-A**, 195–204

Whitcomb, B.B. (1975) Complications from surgery on a vulnerable spinal cord. *Advances in Neurosurgery*, **3**, 331–333

White, W.D., Pearce, D.J. and Norman, J. (1979) Postoperative analgesia. A comparison of intravenous on demand fentanyl with epidural bupivicaine. *British Medical Journal*, **2**, 166–167

Whittle, I.R., Johnston, I.H. and Besser, M. (1984) Spinal cord monitoring during surgery by direct recording of somatosensory evoked potentials. *Journal of Neurosurgery*, **60**, 440–443

Williams, B. (1979) Orthopaedic features in the presentation of syringomyelia. *Journal of Bone and Joint Surgery*, **61-B**, 314–323

Wolcott, G.J., Grunnet, M.L. and Lahey, M.E. (1970) Spinal subdural hematoma in a leukemic child. *Journal of Pediatrics*, **77**, 1060–1062

Wright, P.J. (1986a) Are armoured tracheal tubes really necessary for neuroanaesthesia. *Anaesthesia*, **41**, 213

Wright, P.J. (1986b) Nasotracheal intubation, another approach. *Anaesthesia*, **41**, 1057–1058

Wright, P.J. and Mundy, J.V.B. (1987) Tracheal tubes in neuroanaesthesia. Nylon reinforced latex rubber tracheal tubes. *Anaesthesia*, **42**, 1012–1014

Wright, P.J., Mundy, J.V.B. and Mansfield, C.J. (1988) Obstruction of armoured tracheal tubes. Case report and discussion. *Canadian Journal of Anaesthesia*, **35**, 195–197

Yamashita, M. and Matsuki, A. (1975) Muscle relaxant requirements in patients with Von Recklinghausen's disease. *British Journal of Anaesthesia*, **47**, 1032

Yu, I. and Emans, J.B. (1988) Epidural abscess associated with spondylolysis. A case report. *Journal of Bone and Joint Surgery*, **70-A**, 444–447

Zilka, A. and Nicolletti, J.M. (1947) Acute spinal subdural haematoma. Case report. *Journal of Neurosurgery*, **4**, 627–630

Zorab, P.A. (1962) The lungs in ankylosing spondylitis. *Quarterly Journal of Medicine*, **31**, 267–277

Zorab, P.A., Prime, F.J. and Harrison, A. (1979) Lung function in young persons after spinal fusion for scoliosis. *Spine*, **4**, 22–28

Chapter 12

Trends in spinal cord injury research

Alan Hirschfeld and Wise Young

Introduction

The search for an effective treatment to prevent or reverse the neurological sequelae of spinal cord injury (SCI) has proved to be an arduous pursuit of an elusive goal. Despite extensive research into the mechanisms of secondary tissue damage in SCI, our understanding of these mechanisms remains incomplete. Even with the understanding that has been achieved, the surgical, physiological and pharmacological strategies devised to treat SCI based on these theories still leave much room for improvement when applied in clinical situations (Hansebout, 1982; Janssen and Hansebout, 1989). Although there has been a significant decrease in mortality in the last half-century (Hartwell, 1917), the neurological outcome, especially in complete lesions (when there is loss of all sensorimotor function below the level of injury), remains unchanged by aggressive therapy. One problem of assessing the relative merits of different therapeutic approaches has been the inherent difficulties of performing randomized, controlled clinical trials (Maynard *et al.*, 1979; Bracken and Collins, 1985).

The principal concept which continues to give hope that an effective treatment will eventually be developed is that of 'secondary injury'. According to this concept, the effects produced by trauma to the cord may be divided into 'primary' injury effects, such as axonal shearing and vascular disruption, which are largely non-reversible, and progressive or 'secondary' effects, such as tissue edema, ischemia, ionic fluxes, and free-radical damage, which may contribute to neurological dysfunction, and which may also be preventable or reversible (Young, 1985; Janssen and Hansebout, 1989). The period over which these secondary effects develop may be minutes, hours or days. In some SCI models, progressive pathological changes were observed beyond 24 hours after the injury (Balentine, 1978a). Time-dependent pathophysiological changes have been described in many of the articles to be discussed in this chapter.

Our understanding of the mechanisms of secondary SCI is based on groundwork laid over 70 years ago, when Allen (1914) developed the first reproducible animal model for SCI. This and subsequent models will be the main topic of the first section. Subsequent sections will deal with the pathological, physiological, biochemical and therapeutic observations made in these models. We will also briefly discuss the findings of some researchers concerning the possibility of re-establishing central nervous system (CNS) integrity, or CNS regeneration.

Models of spinal cord injury

Basic medical researchers develop and study animal models of human disease. Such models allow a more detailed investigation of the disease process on the cellular level and under controlled conditions. The effectiveness of experimental treatments can be measured and compared with the natural course of the disease. Because the spinal cords of humans are only rarely available for study and almost never during the very early phases of injury, much of what we know about SCI stems from the investigation of animal models.

A potential animal model of SCI should fulfill several criteria. First, it should approximate the physical events which occur in human SCI. Second, the pathological results should be similar to those seen in human SCI. Third, reproducible injuries and results should be obtainable within a given laboratory and between laboratories. Fourth, the results of injury and treatment should be quantifiable. Fifth, the model must be humane. Other desirable features of an ideal model are that it not be prohibitively expensive, and that the degree of injury and neurological deficit can be reproducibly varied.

Many of these criteria are inconsistent or incompatible with one another. For example, most humane animal models require the use of anesthetic agents, which adds a controllable but nevertheless confounding factor to the models, because these agents have profound effects on neural function, metabolism, and blood flow. The response to injury in experimental SCI models can therefore be expected to differ from that in clinical SCI in unanesthetized humans. Another problem derives from the concepts of 'standardization' and 'reproducibility'. Experimental conditions, including physiological parameters such as blood pressure, blood gases and temperature, have to be strictly controlled. The mechanical parameters of the injury also have to be standardized in order to achieve reproducible tissue damage. In the clinical situation, the magnitude, duration, and direction of force differs considerably from case to case. Concurrent systemic insult, especially in motor vehicle accidents, may influence outcome considerably. Finally, in order to demonstrate the degree of effectiveness of various treatments aimed at reducing secondary tissue damage, experimental SCI models must be designed to allow a certain proportion of the damage to be primary and a certain known proportion to be due to secondary injury mechanisms. In the clinical situation, the proportion of primary and secondary tissue damage is likely to vary considerably from case to case.

The model of SCI developed by Allen (1914) has remained, with some variations, the most commonly used model by researchers in this field. The Allen model involves the dropping of a known weight from a known height onto a posteriorly exposed segment of spinal cord. The force imparted to the cord is both quantifiable and transient, creating a cord 'contusion'. The energy of the contusion can be expressed as the product of the weight and height. For example, a 20 g weight dropped from a height of 20 cm produces a 400 g-cm lesion. This nomenclature is misleading, since the primary tissue damage is related to the displacement velocity of the spinal cord which is nonlinearly related to the height from which the weight is dropped. For example, the tissue damage from a 20 g mass dropped 20 cm differs from that of a 10 g mass dropped 40 cm or a 4 g mass dropped 100 cm (Windle, 1980). Therefore, unless all parameters including weight, height, and area of the contusing surface are duplicated, it is inappropriate to compare different models with the same g-cm energy of contusion (Koozekanani, Vise and McGhee, 1976). Many of the experiments using the weight-drop technique have been performed on cats, but

Wrathall and her co-workers, among others, have reported gradable and reproducible results using rats, a more cost-effective animal (Gale, Kerasidis and Wrathall, 1985; Noble and Wrathall, 1985). Dog (Griffiths, 1975), sheep (Yeo, Payne and Hinwood, 1975) and ferret (Eidelberg et al., 1976) models have also been developed. A sophisticated, feedback-controlled electromechanical impactor has been developed by Noyes (1987a) and has been reported to give reproducible and graded anatomic and behavioral changes in rats (Bresnahan et al., 1987; Noyes, 1987b).

These concussive, or 'dynamic load', techniques are analogous to the clinical situation in which the spinal cord, during a hyperextension injury, is transiently pinched between a bulging disc or osteophytes anteriorly and a buckling of the ligamentum flavum posteriorly. Many cases of SCI, however, involve a more prolonged compression of the spinal cord, due to anterior subluxation of one cervical vertebra on top of another. These clinical situations have been mimicked in the laboratory by several 'static load' models. These include the use of a finger (McVeigh, 1923), scalpel handle (Thompson, 1923), Kocher clamp (Fontaine, Mandel and Dany, 1954), aneurysm clip (Dolan and Tator, 1979), or an inflatable balloon or cuff placed in the epidural space (Ayer, 1919; Tarlov, Klinger and Vitale, 1953; Tator, 1973). With the last technique, the balloon may be left deflated for a few hours, and then inflated to produce injury in the awake animal, thereby eliminating anesthetic-associated artefacts. In the static load models, the application of compressive forces may last from minutes to hours, thereby blurring the distinction between primary and secondary injury and adding a component of directly-induced local ischemia due to vascular compression (Holtz, Nystrom and Gerdin, 1989). A study by Khan and Griebel (1983), comparing the weight drop, aneurysm clip and inflatable cuff techniques in rats, favored the latter approach, but Black et al. (1988a) felt that a dynamic load model produced lesions which approximated the pathologic findings in human SCI better than those seen in their previously-described static load model (Black et al., 1986a; Kushner et al., 1986).

Some models of SCI create a complete physical discontinuity in the cord, either by crush or severance of the cord, followed sometimes by removal of the necrotic segment after the injury (de la Torre, 1984; Benes and Rokyta, 1988). In these models, secondary events are of importance only in so far as they may affect axonal regeneration across the physical gap. These models have therefore been utilized primarily for the study of spinal cord regeneration (Guth et al., 1980a, 1980b). Since complete transection of the spinal cord is very rare clinically, such models have little basis in reality. Furthermore, transections allow the invasion of external cellular elements into the spinal cord and produce gaps across which axons may not cross readily.

Changes seen in spinal cord injury

Studies of pathological changes seen after experimental SCI have established a surprisingly similar reaction of the spinal cord to injuries, regardless of the type or cause of injury. Contusion, compression, ischemia, or even toxic substances produce similar pathological, physiological and biochemical changes in the spinal cords, leading to central hemorrhagic necrosis. These findings have provided the basis for several current hypotheses of secondary injury mechanisms.

Pathological changes

The earliest gross pathological changes seen in both clinical and experimental SCI are petechial hemorrhages, primarily within the central gray matter of the cord (Balentine, 1978). The small veins at the site of impact may be the most sensitive to injury (Dohrman, Wagner and Bucy, 1971). In the first 15 min there may be relatively little else, even upon microscopic examination, to indicate that a devastating neurological lesion has been created. The majority of cells and nerve fibers may appear intact at the lesion site, even though the conduction of impulses through the injury site may be lost and the animal may be rendered paraplegic. The paucity of morphologic changes in individual tissue sections may be misleading, however. Focal axonal damage may be scattered so that no single cross-section of the spinal cord will reveal all the axonal disruption. With time, however, as degenerative processes take place, more axonal damage will appear.

Within the first hour, edema will develop, even in areas where the vessels appear intact (Beggs and Waggener, 1976). This may manifest itself as an increase in the extracellular space in both white and gray matter and tends to spread centrifugally from the gray to the white matter, and longitudinally along the axis of the spinal cord (Griffiths and Miller, 1974; Nemecek et al., 1977). Within a certain range of injury forces, there appears to be a dose dependence of the extent of edema formation (Wagner and Stewart, 1981), although a recent study suggests that edema is independent of injury severity when examined within 6 h after weight-drop contusions in rats (Kwo, Young and De Crescito, 1989). Although the same dose-dependence is seen in neurological function in some animal models (Rivlin and Tator, 1977; Khan and Griebel, 1983; Gale, Kerasidis and Wrathall, 1985), the exact role played by edema in the production or perpetuation of these deficits has not been determined. Spinal cord edema starts to develop within minutes, peaks at 2–3 days post-injury, and starts to resolve by 4–7 days (Yashon et al., 1973; Beggs and Waggener, 1976; Janssen and Hansebout, 1989). This 'vasogenic' edema may be due to 'loosening' of the tight junctions between capillary endothelial cells and to increased pinocytotic activity, as well as to physical disruption of the capillaries (Brightman et al., 1970; Beggs and Waggener, 1976; Kapadia, 1984).

Early morphological changes seen within the axons include fragmentation of the axolemma and tubovesicular invagination of axonal membranes into the axoplasm (Balentine, 1978b). Loss of neurofilament can be observed within minutes. In addition, gross myelin changes can be seen, associated with loss of myelin basic protein. Neuronal loss occurs early in the gray matter at the injury site. Progressive degeneration of white matter takes place in the long tract fibers (Means, Anderson and Gutierrez, 1976; Pallini, Fernandez and Sbriccoli, 1988). Axonal degeneration in the lumbosacral cord was quantified by Iizuka et al. (1986), and correlated well with the loss of neurological function at 7 days after injury. Benoist et al. (1979) showed that axoplasmic transport in short-range spinal interneurons neither improved nor deteriorated with time after the initial impact. Both ultrastructural (Banik et al., 1982) and electrophoretic (Iizuka et al., 1987) analyses have demonstrated degradation of neuronal cytoskeletal protein within the first few hours following injury.

Time-dependent morphological changes in the myelin sheaths have been described in the 2–7-day post-injury period (Blight, 1985). These are associated with a local infiltration by inflammatory cells (Means and Anderson, 1983; Blight, 1985). It is uncertain whether these inflammatory cells play an important role in secondary damage to surviving axons or merely scavenge tissue debris. The release of chemotactic and pro-inflammatory factors, and of histolytic and proteolytic enzymes, by these cells may further enhance tissue necrosis. Macrophages probably play a role in the formation of the central cavity which develops within the cord as early as 9 days post-injury and remains as a chronic gross pathological reminder of the injury. This central cavity may enlarge with time and is sometimes called post-traumatic syringomyelia, although the mechanisms of its formation probably are not the same as those responsible for congenital syringomyelia.

The existence of potentially reversible secondary injury processes provides the rationale for early treatments of acute SCI. Although attractive, this rationale may not be applicable to all types of SCI. Secondary effects may be overshadowed by primary injury in most clinical cases of SCI. After all, only a relatively small percentage of patients undergo clinically recognizable deterioration over time (Phillippi *et al.*, 1980). However, such deterioration may be subclinical. The challenge of the future will be to detect, using *in situ* measurement techniques, subgroups of patients who may benefit from treatment devised to minimize secondary injury processes.

Neurological changes

Most experimental models of SCI traumatize the spinal cord at thoracic or lumbar levels, rather than at the cervical level, where most human SCI occurs. Thoracic and lumbar injuries do not impair respiration, so respiratory complications do not have to be factored into the experimental design or conclusions of such models. Also damage to gray matter in thoracic SCI will have minimal consequences, whereas gray matter loss in the cervical segments will have major motor and sensory consequences.

Contusions, whether mild, moderate, or severe, produce very rapid losses of axonal conduction across the lesion site, even though pathological changes evolve over a matter of hours. The initial loss of conduction can be explained by a very large rise in extracellular potassium activity (Young *et al.*, 1982) and other ionic derangements that occur within seconds after contusion.

Three variables should be considered in the loss of neurological function after SCI. First, injury causes ionic and metabolic derangements in the spinal cord which can result in prolonged blockade of axonal conduction and even segmental reflexes far from the injury site. Second, primary or secondary tissue damage causes loss of axons. Third, loss of supporting structures such as oligodendroglia can cause long-term axonal dysfunction. These factors contribute to the complex and variable time course of neurological loss and recovery after injury.

In chronic SCI, the number of variables contributing to neurological changes increases. These include the remyelination of axons at the lesion site, the presence and quality of spasticity, and other adaptations of the animal or person to the injury. A clear example of how much influence these variables have on recovery of function comes from animal studies showing recovery of near-normal locomotory and sensory function with < 10% of the spinal cord white matter (Blight and Young, 1989a, 1989b). The number and types of axons surviving injury are not the only determinants of functional recovery. The measurement of neurological function or losses in spinal injured animals continues to be a central problem in SCI research. Most researchers use a crude scoring system modified from one described by Tarlow

(1957). Others have developed more objective approaches, such as the length of time that animals can cling to a serrated board inclined at different angles, the number of hindpaw licks that a rat will do when the hindpaw is placed on a hot plate, the number of misses by an animal walking on a wiremesh, etc. The problem with all these methods is that neither the linearity nor the quantitative relationships between behavior and axon number at the lesion site have been established.

Neurophysiological changes

To circumvent the limitations of behavioral tests, many researchers have turned to neurophysiological tests of function, based on electrical stimulation and recording of neural responses. The most commonly utilized monitoring approach is the somatosensory evoked potential (SSEP or SEP). This directly measures the conduction of electrical impulses by the dorsal columns (the long tracts which subserve proprioception). The assumption is usually made that sensory function may be generalized to all long tract functions in the spinal cord. The motor evoked potential (MEP), as a means of directly monitoring the corticospinal pathways, has also been described, but has not been utilized to the same extent as the SEP (Fehlings et al., 1987).

Severe injury of the spinal cord will cause a rapid disappearance of the SEP (Martin and Bloedel, 1973; Fehlings et al., 1987). This is accompanied by the clinical findings of paraplegia, as has been described in a number of animal and clinical studies (Deecke and Tator, 1973; Griffiths, Trench and Crawford, 1979; de la Torre and Boggan, 1980; Young, 1982; Schramm et al., 1983). The converse is not always true, for SEPs may be present, though diminished in amplitude, in the presence of clinical paraplegia (Young, 1982). If the SEPs are present, however attenuated, there may be some chance of neurological recovery (Young, 1982). Animals with moderate contusions may show a transient return of evoked potentials at 1–3 h after contusion, only to lose these evoked potentials with the onset of progressive central hemorrhagic necrosis. Animals with mild contusions recover evoked potentials with no delayed loss.

The degree of abnormality of the waveform correlates well with the degree of neurological dysfunction in acute SCI studies (Blight and Young, 1989b). Raines et al. (1988) have shown in rats that the amplitude and the integrated areas of SEPs predict behavioral outcome at 4 weeks after injury, but that the response latency does not.

Somatosensory evoked potentials may recover transiently, only to be lost hours, or even days, later (Cusick et al., 1979; Young et al., 1980; Flamm et al., 1982). This secondary loss of neurophysiological responses does not occur in injuries which do not produce long-term paraplegia (Young et al., 1980). The primary loss of SEPs is probably due to mechanical disruption of axonal membranes and to rapid changes in the intracellular and extracellar ionic concentrations. The secondary loss of SEPs may be caused by more gradually evolving processes, including white matter ischemia.

In chronic SCI, SEPs do not correlate well with the neurological status of animals or patients except for gross differentiation of complete and incomplete spinal injuries (Young, 1982). While patients with no sensory function below the lesion level almost never have normal SEPs, and patients with sensation almost never have absent SEPs, the amplitudes and latencies of SEPs at 6 weeks after SCI are not good general predictors of the quality or usefulness of sensation. Completely paralyzed patients may show robust SEPs. Alternatively, some patients with useful motor function may show little or no SEPs. Several studies have reported that SEPs obtained within 4 h after injury are most predictive of eventual outcome, but the correlation diminishes with time after injury (Rowed, 1982; Young, 1982).

Physiological changes and spinal cord ischemia

Trauma to the brain (Evans et al., 1976) or to the spinal cord (Evans, Kobrine and Rizzoli, 1980) produces disturbances in the autonomic nervous system leading to cardiac arrhythmias and to profound changes in blood pressure. An initial hypertensive response is followed by prolonged hypotension (Young et al., 1982). Such hypotension is frequently seen in human victims of SCI (Lehman et al., 1987). Guha and Tator (1988), in a clip compression rat model, showed an immediate post-injury increase in mean arterial pressure from $105 + 8$ mmHg ($13.9 + 1.0$ kPa) to $178 + 11$ mmHg ($23.7 + 1.5$ kPa), followed by a hypotensive phase, to $46 + 15$ mmHg ($6.1 + 2.0$ kPa), which lasted at least 135 min. There was a parallel decrease in cardiac output (CO). In the absence of changes in total peripheral resistance, central venous pressure or heart rate, they concluded that the decline in CO was due to myocardial changes, rather than to a loss of sympathetic tone. Young et al. (1980) have implicated the sympathetic nervous system in the initial hypertensive response in cats.

The spinal cord vasculature, like that of the brain, normally compensates for changes in systemic blood pressure (autoregulation), to ensure that spinal cord blood flow (SCBF) remains relatively constant. Since SCBF is a major determinant of spinal cord oxygenation, the measurement of SCBF and the ability of the cord to autoregulate have been extensively studied (Sandler and Tator, 1976). The results have been conflicting. This may be due to differences either in experimental protocols, methods of producing injury, or SCBF measurement techniques. The two most frequently used methods are the hydrogen clearance technique, which measures the rate of hydrogen washout from different regions of the cord using platinum electrodes, and the autoradiography technique, which uses local concentrations of radiolabeled tracers like ^{14}C-antipyrine to infer local blood flow (Cawthon, Senter and Stewart, 1980). Each technique has its advantages and disadvantages. The hydrogen clearance technique permits serial measurements in living animals but, because of the diffusibility of hydrogen, does not permit fine spatial resolution. Autoradiographic techniques have good spatial resolution, but only permit a single measurement in time.

Most studies of SCBF have found a rapid fall in blood flow in the central gray matter (Sandler and Tator, 1976; Rivlin and Tator, 1978; Cawthon, Senter and Stewart, 1980) which may be attributable to the direct vascular damage seen in pathological studies (Balentine, 1978). In severe contusion injuries, blood flow in lateral column white matter tends to vary in the first 2–3 h after injury, but then falls to about 50% of pre-injury values (Sandler and Tator, 1976; Senter and Venes, 1978; Hayashi, de la Torre and Green, 1980) after 3 h. Some workers, however, have reported hyperemia in less severe injuries (Kobrine and Doyle, 1976). Many factors influence SCBF, including impaired autoregulation to systemic blood flow (Kobrine, Doyle and Martins, 1975; Sandler and Tator, 1976; Senter and Venes, 1978; Smith et al., 1978), effects of anesthetic agents (e.g. pentobarbital will depress SCBF), injury severity (milder injuries have been associated with hyperemia in some studies – Lohse et al., 1980), focal areas of hemorrhage (Goodman, Bingham and Hunt, 1978; Wallace, Tator and Frazee, 1986) or edema (Stewart, 1985), or the release of vasoconstricting neurotransmitters such as norepinephrine (noradrenaline) (Osterholm, 1974) by damaged neurons.

The catecholamine hypothesis is based on initial reports of catecholamine accumulation at the injury site. However, these findings could not be replicated (Schoultz, DeLucca and Reding, 1976; Alderman et al., 1980). Nevertheless, the potential role of released neurotransmitters, including the opiates, excitatory amino acids, substance P, and other vasoactive substances, has attracted much attention and continues to stimulate therapeutic studies (Anden et al., 1964; Misra, Singh and Bhargava, 1967; Naftchi et al., 1974; Brodner and Dohrmann, 1977; Naftchi et al., 1978; Faden et al., 1981a; Kuruvilla, Theodore and Abraham, 1985). Likewise, the release of prostaglandins and leukotrienes has been noted in several recent studies (see below). Monoamines and other vasoactive substances are likely to alter blood flow, but may also affect spinal cord cells directly by inducing lipid peroxidation (Kurihara, 1985) or interacting with raphe–spinal nerve terminals (Salzman et al., 1987a). The sum total of the vasoactive effects determines spinal cord blood flow. However, the precise role of post-traumatic ischemia still remains a matter of speculation.

Metabolic changes

Whether or not decreased blood flow and spinal cord ischemia cause secondary injury, significant metabolic and ionic derangements do occur in spinal cords after injury. These derangements may play a major role in, but also may simply be consequences of, cell death.

The most significant metabolic change is the rapid reduction in high-energy phosphate bond substrates and other energy stores at the injury site. Adenosine triphosphate (ATP) and phosphocreatine levels are reduced by over 70% within the first 15 min, and remain reduced for at least 24 h (Walker, Yates and Yashon, 1979; Anderson et al., 1980). Increased levels of adenosine monophosphate (AMP) have also been noted. In addition, decreased tissue levels of pyruvate (Braughler and Hall, 1983), a marked increase in tissue lactate levels (Anderson et al., 1980; Braughler and Hall, 1983; Goldman, Elowitz and Flamm, 1983), and oxidative shifts of NAD–NADH ratios (Rosenthal et al., 1979) have been reported, all of which suggests an uncoupling of oxidative metabolism with a shift to anaerobic glycolysis (Ito, Allen and Yashon, 1978). The rapidity and magnitude of these changes are difficult to explain purely on the basis of ischemia, edema or hypoxia, since these take longer to evolve. The loss of high-energy substrates denotes the failure of all energy-dependent cellular functions at the injury site, including sodium/potassium-dependent ATPase (Clendenon et al., 1978; Hall and Braughler, 1982a).

Ionic changes

There has been considerable interest in measuring ionic fluxes in the injured spinal cord, particularly those of potassium, sodium, and calcium, because of the effects these would have on axonal conduction, neurotransmitter release and, in the case of calcium, on cellular viability. Eidelberg, Sullivan and Brigham (1975) described a release of K^+ into the superfusants of compressed spinal cords. Such K^+ release can only come from the intracellular compartment, where normal concentrations are over 90 mmol. Traumatic injury, either by disruption of cells or by increasing membrane permeability to K^+, rapidly elevates extracellular K^+ concentration within seconds. Extracellular K^+ levels above 10 mmol effectively block axonal conduction (Cordingley and Somjen, 1978) and release neurotransmitters (Yaksh and Tyce, 1980). Ion-sensitive microelectrodes have been used to directly measure changes in extracellular K^+ concentrations. Young *et al.* (1982) found that, in the lateral white matter columns, it rose from pre-injury levels of <4 mmol to a mean of 54 mmol shortly after impact injury, and then was cleared with a half time of 35–40 min. Evoked potentials disappeared with the rise in extracellular K^+ and then returned as K^+ was cleared.

The clearance rate of K^+, but not the initial rise, appears to depend on white matter blood flow. Prevention of post-traumatic hypoperfusion by paravertebral sympathectomy increased the clearance rate but had no effect on the initial rise. Measurement of total tissue K^+ showed a marked loss from the impact site. There was no secondary rise of extracellular K^+ at 2–3 h after injury when blood flow and the evoked potentials (for the second time) diminished (Lewin, Hansebout and Pappius, 1974; Young, 1985; Young and Koreh, 1986). Extracellular Na^+ ionic activity, in contrast to K^+, falls, while total tissue Na^+ ions increase at the injury site, doubling during the first 1–3 h (Young, 1985). This finding is consistent with Na^+ ions entering cells at the injury site and Na ions coming from blood and surrounding tissues into the lesion site.

Studies of calcium ion fluxes have provided additional insights into the pathophysiology of SCI. Normally a >1000-fold gradient exists between intracellular (<0.1 micromolar) and extracellular (> 1 millimolar) compartments in the CNS, which is strictly maintained by ion transport mechanisms (Baker, 1976; Kretsinger, 1979), to insure proper neuronal function. Trauma-induced changes in membrane calcium permeability permit Ca^{2+} to rush into the injured cells. This would be manifested as a decrease in extracellular Ca^{2+} (Nicholson, 1980).

Role of calcium in spinal cord injury

Unregulated entry of Ca^{2+} into cells has been implicated in cell death in a variety of tissues (Schanne *et al.*, 1979), and has been proposed as a major contributor to neuronal death in the injured spinal cord (Balentine and Hilton, 1980a, 1980b; Happel *et al.*, 1981; Stokes, Fox and Hollinden, 1983). Several observations support this hypothesis: the finding of intra-axonal calcification in injured spinal tissues (Happel *et al.*, 1981), marked elevations of total tissue calcium levels, two-fold by 2 h and five-fold by 8 h (Happel *et al.*, 1981), the finding that superfusion of the spinal cord with hypercalcemic solutions produces pathological changes similar to those seen after trauma (Balentine and Hilton, 1980a), and finally the precipitous and long-lasting fall in extracellular Ca^{2+} concentration following trauma, from 1.0–1.3 mmol to 0.01–0.1 mmol (Young, Yen and Blight, 1982; Stokes, Fox and Hollinden, 1983), implying the rapid entry of Ca^{2+} into cells at the site of injury. This decrease persists in the gray matter, but recovers partially in the white matter (to 0.4 mmol), only to decrease again within 2–3 h.

A direct cause-and-effect relationship between this influx of Ca^{2+} and neuronal cell death has not been definitely established. Many of the above-described Ca^{2+} changes could be a manifestation and not necessarily the cause of cell death. Extracellular Ca^{2+} falls (albeit temporarily) as far as 1 cm from the impact site, but without significant tissue damage at those sites (Young, Yen and Blight, 1982). Also, other CNS phenomena, such as spreading depression, can cause similar Ca^{2+}

influxes without producing cell death (Kraig and Nicholson, 1978; Nicholson, 1980). Therefore, survival may be possible following an initial influx of Ca^{2+}, but, in the injured spinal cord, subsequent events, some of which may be influenced by the high intracellular Ca^{2+}, could prevent this recovery.

What is the fate of the calcium that enters into spinal cord cells, and how does it cause cell death? As mentioned above, despite prolonged extracellular decreases, there is an overall increase in tissue calcium levels and calcium deposits have been noted in ultrastructural studies. This may be due to the binding of Ca^{2+} by anions, such as inorganic phosphate, and its precipitation as hydroxyapatite salt (Stumm and Morgan, 1981). Inorganic phosphate pools would become depleted, decreasing its availability for the regeneration of ATP (Kretsinger, 1979). If mitochondrial calcium-extrusion mechanisms are overwhelmed (Chance, 1965; Carofoli and Lehninger, 1971; Carofoli and Crompton, 1978), calcium also binds to mitochondrial enzymes, and electron transport chains become uncoupled, decreasing the generation of ATP through oxidative phosphorylation. Further ATP depletion could be produced through the stimulation of Na/K-dependent ATPase by the high extracellular K^+ concentration (Astrup, 1982).

Calcium ions entering cells are known to act as intracellular messengers, regulating a wide variety of biological functions (Llinas, 1978; Urry, 1978). These include increases of membrane permeability to ions, protein synthesis, and metabolism through inhibition of phosphorylation mechanisms, all neurotransmitter release, cellular transport, and pH regulation inside cells. Excessive calcium entry may disrupt these cellular functions and cause cell death. In addition, Ca^{2+} entry can initiate pathological mechanisms of cellular destruction. For example, Ca^{2+} activates calcium-dependent phospholipase A, which breaks down membrane lipids to produce arachidonic acid. Metabolites of arachidonic acid include prostaglandins, leukotrienes, thromboxanes and free radical species. These in turn can set in motion a number of harmful, cascading phenomena (Janssen, 1989), such as platelet aggregation, vasospasm, inhibition of neurotransmitter release, stimulation of lysosomal enzyme release, and the destruction of normal cellular membranes. Considering the multitude of deleterious effects ascribed to excessive calcium entry into cells, it is not surprising that agents have been investigated which specifically block this entry (see below).

High doses of corticosteroids have been shown to prevent the secondary decline in extracellular Ca^{2+} in white matter at the site of injury (Young and Flamm, 1982). A hypothesis has been proposed (Young, 1986, 1987) that this may not be desirable, because it maintains a high gradient favoring Ca^{2+} entry into partially damaged but potentially salvageable cells. According to this hypothesis, the fall in extracellular Ca^{2+} actually plays a protective role for the population of cells that have survived the initial trauma. Therefore, a rapid restoration of extracellular Ca^{2+} levels, when spinal cells have accommodated to low levels, may exacerbate the damage to neurons and glia. This hypothesis is similar to the 'calcium paradox' reported in myocardial cells (Boink et al., 1976; Ruigrok, 1982).

Lipid peroxidation and eicosanoids

Membrane lipid peroxidation, with its deleterious effects on membrane integrity and on the production of arachidonic acid metabolites, is potentially one of the principal harmful side effects of excessive calcium entry into cells. A second pathway to lipid peroxidation is through free radical production secondary to spinal cord ischemia. This theory of secondary injury mechanisms has been developed by Demopoulos *et al.* (1979, 1982). Free radicals are molecules with a single, unpaired electron in their outer electron orbit. These molecules are chemically very active, reacting with other molecules to form more free radicals. Free radicals play a role in normal cellular oxidative and lipid metabolism (Fridovich, 1978; Del Maestro, 1980). Endogenous enzyme systems and antioxidants control the production and effects of free radicals.

The most extensively studied free radical system is oxygen. Active oxygen free radical species include the superoxide anion (O_2^-), hydrogen peroxide (H_2O_2) and the hydroxyl radical ($OH\cdot$), produced by the sequential, univalent reduction of oxygen to water. During oxidative metabolism, cytochrome oxidase prevents the formation of the intermediates O_2^- and H_2O_2, except for a small 'univalent leak'. Aerobic organisms have evolved enzymes such as catalases, superoxide dismutase and peroxidases, and substances intercalated within membranes (vitamin E, beta-carotene and cholesterol) and in the cytosol (ascorbic acid, cysteine, and reduced glutathione), to 'scavenge' the excess free radicals. When these systems are overwhelmed, secondary injury may occur.

The production of many free radicals requires the presence of oxygen. Total anoxia, for example, would discourage the production of oxygen free radicals. However, as pointed out above, ischemia is only partial and develops slowly in SCI. Free radical production is also catalysed by the Cu^{2+} and Fe^{2+} present in extra-vasated blood (Demopoulos *et al.*, 1982). Thus, the environment of the injured spinal cord, in addition to the entry of Ca^{2+} into injured cells, is conducive to the formation of damaging free radicals.

There is a considerable body of biochemical evidence for the participation of free radicals and lipid peroxidation in SCI (see Hall and Braughler, 1986, for review). Ascorbic acid and vitamin E levels are decreased in injured spinal cords, as is cholesterol. Free radical reaction products increase, e.g. oxidized cholesterol, cyclic GMP (due to free radical-activation of guanylate cyclase), and malonyldialdehyde, a product of unsaturated fatty acid peroxidation. Certain membrane-bound, phospholipid-dependent enzymes, such as sodium/potassium-dependent ATPase, are also inhibited.

The production of arachidonic acid and its eiconsanoid metabolites (prostaglandins, thromboxanes, and leukotrienes – Wolfe, 1982) by lipid peroxidation may further impair spinal cord blood flow (Raichle, 1983; Banik, Hogan and Hsu, 1985; Hsu *et al.*, 1985, 1986, 1988). The effects of the eicosanoids are complex. Thromboxanes A_2 and B_2 (TxA_2 and TxB_2), mediate vasoconstriction and platelet aggregation, and accumulate post-injury (Jacobs *et al.*, 1987). The formation of prostacyclin (PGI_2), which counteracts the action of TxA_2, is not as affected in injured tissues, and PGI_2 synthesis may even be inhibited by free radicals. Activation of arachidonate metabolism may also affect microvessel wall integrity and then contribute to vasogenic edema, in head injury and cerebral ischemia, as well as in SCI. The relative levels of the different eicosanoid compounds vary with time, so that the thromboxane–prostacyclin balance reverts to favor prostacylin by 18 h post-injury. These changes should be considered in the administration of therapy aimed at reducing eicosanoid activity in SCI. Another eicosanoid family, the leukotrienes, are potent smooth muscle contractors, leading to vasoconstriction. They also alter cell membrane permeability (Wolfe, 1982). A direct effect of arachidonic acid metabolites on edema formation, inflammation, necrosis of oligo-dendroglia and demyelination has also been reported (Horrocks *et al.*, 1985). The effect of corticosteroids in inhibiting arachidonic acid metabolism has been a major impetus in its use in CNS injury (Hall and Braughler, 1986; Saunders *et al.*, 1987).

Receptor-mediated secondary injury

Among the putative neurotransmitters released at the time of injury, the endogenous opioids have received considerable attention as playing a major role in secondary injury. The spinal cord contains high levels of endorphins, enkephalins, and dynorphins (Yaksh, 1987). Interest in these neurotransmitters initially arose because of reports that naloxone, an opiate receptor antagonist, effectively reduced hypotension resulting from endotoxic, hemorrhagic and spinal shock (Holaday and Faden, 1980). Soon after, two independent groups reported that naloxone, given in very high doses, improved neurological outcome and blood flow in animal models of SCI (Faden, Jacobs and Holaday, 1981a; Young *et al.*, 1981). Faden, Jacobs and Holaday (1981) postulated that the large doses of naloxone are necessary because the secondary injury is mediated by non-mu-receptors such as kappa- or delta-receptors.

Particular attention has been focused on the kappa-receptor since its endogenous ligand, dynorphin A (dynA) (Long *et al.*, 1986), is elevated in injured spinal cords. Faden *et al.* (1985) have found progressive increases in dynA with graded SCI, whereas enkephalin levels were unchanged. Furthermore, intrathecal administration of kappa-receptor agonists, and particularly dynorphin, was found to produce paraplegia in rats and kappa-receptor antagonists prevent this paralysis (see below). The mechanisms by which opioids mediate tissue damage and affect spinal cord function remain controversial, since subsequent studies suggest that dextro-forms of dynorphin, which are not stereospecific for opiate receptors, will also induce paralysis. It is not known whether opiates act through secondary effects on spinal cord blood flow or by direct effects on neuronal function, or both. The doses of naloxone required to have a beneficial effect on injured spinal cord are of the order of 1000 times or more than the doses necessary to block mu-receptors in the central nervous system. At these unprecedented high doses, these drugs may have numerous yet poorly understood side effects on membranes.

Faden *et al.* (1988) recently reported that MK801, a selective competitive blocker of the *N*-methyl-D-aspartate (NMDA) receptor in the CNS, significantly reduces the histological and neurological manifestations of tissue damage in the rat SCI model. NMDA receptors are activated by glutamate, kainic acid and other excitatory amino acids. Tissue culture studies have shown that excitatory amino acids kill neurons (Olney, Ho and Rhee, 1971) and that their lethal effects can be blocked by drugs such as MK801 (Meldrum, 1985). Activation of NMDA receptors by these 'excitotoxins' enhances Ca^{2+} ion entry into cultured neurons (MacDermott *et al.*, 1986; Choi, 1987). A link between NMDA receptor activation and deleterious changes in tissue magnesium levels has also been postulated (Gibson and Reif-Lehrer, 1985; Faden *et al.*, 1988). The impetus for trying MK801 in a SCI model stems from reports in the ischemia literature that this drug has significant protective effects in rat and gerbil cerebral ischemia models (Simon *et al.*, 1984; Foster *et al.*, 1987).

All the receptor-mediated secondary injury hypotheses suffer from a common problem. There are no opiate, NMDA or catecholamine receptors on axons. Unless these agents operated through indirect mechanisms, their effects on axons should be minimal. Moreover, it is uncertain what effects they may have on neurons in the gray matter, since the outcome of SCI is usually assessed from behavioral or neurophysiological tests which only reflect long spinal tract function.

One common mechanism through which all these receptor blockers may be acting is the augmentation of SCBF. Additionally, they may act through unsuspected side effects such as lipid peroxidation inhibition. Most of these drugs have to be given in relatively high doses to achieve a beneficial effect. At these doses, the drugs may have effects other than the ones by which they are commonly supposed to act.

Other non-receptor-mediated injury mechanisms

Some studies have suggested a role for the release of lysosomal enzymes such as acid glycosidases, in progressive membrane destruction (Kakari *et al.*, 1976; Abraham *et al.*, 1985). Accumulation of these enzymes occurs late and may, therefore, be a secondary phenomenon (Kao and Chang, 1977). Non-lysosomal proteolytic enzymes, such as neutral proteinase and cathepsin B-like and cathepsin D activities, increase in traumatized spinal cords and were felt by Banik *et al.* (1986) to explain some of the pathological alterations seen in axons and myelin. The contributions of axons, glia, myelin and, later, from invading inflammatory cells, to those enzymatic activities at the injury site are unclear. Neurofilament and myelin protein degradation has been hypothesized to result from release of these enzymes. Neutral proteinases are probably calcium-activated (Malik *et al.*, 1983; Banik *et al.*, 1986), linking this theory to the calcium-entry hypothesis, but the relative importance of the proteinase to the overall scheme of secondary injury is unknown.

Recently, attention has been given to the potential role of the 'heat shock response' in protecting the injured cord. This response occurs ubiquitously, throughout the animal kingdom, in many forms of sublethal cellular trauma (Lindquist, 1986). Initially described as an adaptive response to thermal insult, synthesis of heat shock, or 'stress' proteins, also occurs after other kinds of metabolic stress. This response apparently protects tissue from further ischemic or traumatic injury. The trigger for the synthesis and the mechanism by which the heat shock proteins protect or otherwise benefit the tissue or organism are not well understood. Gower *et al.* (1989) recently demonstrated the synthesis, accumulation and redistribution of a 70 kD stress protein in the spinal cords of rats following SCI, raising the possibility that enhancement of this response could improve post-traumatic spinal cord recovery.

Current theory of spinal cord injury

Figure 12.1 synthesizes the above information into an all-encompassing theory of SCI. In this scheme, loss of energy stores, neurotransmitter release, and electrolyte shifts lead to loss of spinal cord conduction and failure of synaptic transmission. Structural integrity, which is essential for functional integrity, is damaged through direct traumatic forces and, secondarily, through membrane damage and cytoskeletal disruption due to lipid peroxidation, proteinase activation and loss of energy stores needed to repair damage. The linchpin around which these events revolve are mediated by excessive Ca^{2+} influx into cells, free radical production and ischemic hypoxia, all of which are interdependent, secondary effects of the initial traumatic event. The relative importance of each of the pathways is unknown, but therapeutic strategies aimed at each pathway have been developed and are being tested in laboratory and clinical situations. Rational combination and sequencing of physical and pharmacological therapies await a more detailed understanding of the events and their specific time-course (Hall and Wolf, 1986).

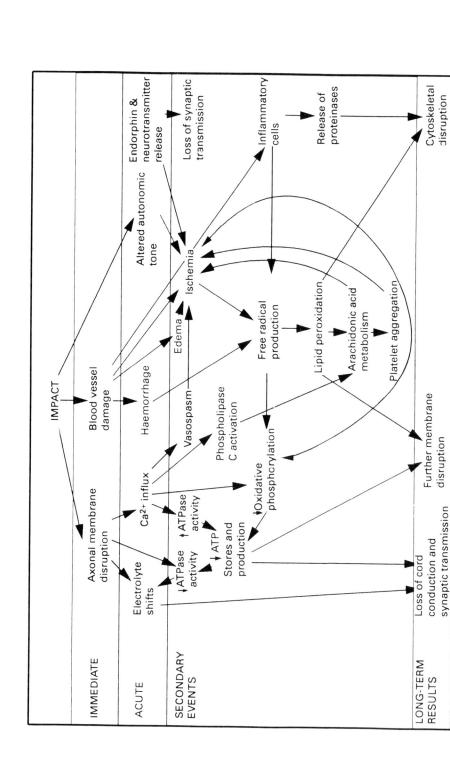

Figure 12.1 Theory of spinal cord injury

Therapeutic strategies

Pharmacological therapies

The different treatments which have been tested in experimental SCI may be divided into three distinct categories: pharmacological, non-pharmacological, and regenerative. The first category is by far the largest. Many of the therapies, having shown promise in the laboratory, are being tested in the clinical setting. None has been proven to be effective in clinical SCI. An impediment to progress in this endeavor has been the diversity of experimental models, the failure to test treatments across a range of doses, and timing of treatments and poorly standardized measurements of therapeutic outcome (e.g. blood flow, morphologic changes, metabolite and ionic concentrations, electrical activity, neurological function, etc.) (Faden, 1985). Additional problems, such as the diverse nature of human SCI and the difficulties of developing rigorous clinical trials, have complicated the situation (Collins, 1983; Bracken and Collins, 1985).

Corticosteroids   Corticosteroids are currently the most widely accepted pharmacological treatment of SCI. A large number of experimental studies have reported the beneficial effects of steroids in animal models of SCI. These include improvements of neurological function and of physiological and pathological parameters (Hansebout, Kuchner and Romero-Sierra, 1975; Green, Kahn and Close, 1980; Means *et al.*, 1981; Young and Flamm, 1982; Anderson *et al.*, 1985; Braughler *et al.*, 1987). However, some studies failed to show such improvements (Parker and Smith, 1976; Faden and Jacobs, 1983). More important, some clinical studies failed to demonstrate a clearcut benefit of the 1 g doses of methylprednisolone, a synthetic corticosteroid, used in experimental studies (Bracken *et al.*, 1985). Detailed studies of the dose response curve of methylprednisolone suggest that such higher doses are required, on the order of 30 mg/kg (Braughler and Hall, 1982; Young and Flamm, 1982; Broakman *et al.*, 1983). These animal results have been incorporated into current trials.

A number of physiological and biochemical effects have been attributed to steroids, which forms the theoretical basis for their use (Hall and Braughler, 1982b; Janssen and Hansebout, 1989). These mechanisms include: the suppression of edema (Hansebout, Kuchner and Romero-Sierra, 1975; Kuchner *et al.*, 1976), improvement of spinal cord blood flow (Means *et al.*, 1981; Anderson *et al.*, 1982; Young and Flamm, 1982; Hall, Wolf and Braughler, 1984), inhibition of the inflammatory response (de la Torre *et al.*, 1975; Janssen and Hansebout, 1989), decreased lipid peroxidation (Braughler, 1982; Hall and Braughler, 1982a, 1982b; Anderson *et al.*, 1985), enhanced Na^+/K^+-ATPase activity (Braughler and Hall, 1982) and recovery of extracellular Ca^{2+} (Means *et al.*, 1981; Young and Flamm, 1982). Recently, reports have been published which demonstrate the effectiveness of U-74006F, a 21-aminosteroid which lacks glucocorticoid or mineralocorticoid activity, in promoting functional recovery from SCI (Anderson *et al.*, 1988; Hall, Braughler and McCall, 1988). The compound was felt to work specifically through its potent inhibition of lipid peroxidation.

Free-radical scavengers and antioxidants   The formation of free radicals after SCI has been both a direct and indirect target of pharmacological control. Indirectly, the use of agents to improve mean arterial blood pressure and spinal cord blood flow is hoped to decrease ischemia-related production of free radicals. More directly, since the presence of extravasated blood in the hemorrhagic, post-traumatic spinal cord may catalyse free-radical generation even in the absence of ischemia, agents have been used to 'scavenge' the free radicals, thereby preventing lipid peroxidation and membrane destabilization. In addition to megadose steroids (Braughler and Hall, 1982; Anderson and Means, 1985; Braughler *et al.*, 1987), such agents have included vitamins C and E (alpha tocopherol) (Anderson *et al.*, 1985; Hall and Wolf, 1986; Anderson *et al.*, 1988), selenium (Anderson *et al.*, 1985), coenzyme Q (Sugigama, Kitazawa and Ozawa, 1980) and high doses of opiate antagonists (Sugigama, Kitazawa and Ozawa, 1980). Alpha tocopherol and selenium were found by Hall and Wolf (1986) to prevent post-traumatic falls in SCBF, and they hypothesized that, in addition to their direct effect on neuronal membrane stability, they also prevented microvascular lipid peroxidation with its attendant effect on microvessel integrity.

Opiate antagonists   As discussed above, the opiate antagonist naloxone was originally used with the rationale that it would prevent the drop in MABP and therefore improve regional SCBF in injured spinal cords. Work by Faden and co-workers (Faden, Jacobs and Holaday, 1980; Faden *et al.*, 1981a, 1981b; Koreh *et al.*, 1981) and others (Matsumiya and Dohi, 1983) suggests that this effect is due to a central action of opioids and their antagonists on autonomic tone. Analysis of electrophysiological and neurological data by several groups (Young *et al.*, 1981; Flamm *et al.*, 1982; Arias, 1985) have suggested beneficial effects of naloxone. A phase I study in humans has been reported (Flamm *et al.*, 1985). However, other investigators have not found similar beneficial effects of naloxone on blood flow (Wallace and Tator, 1986), electrophysiological (Haghighi and Chehrazi, 1987), or neurological (Black *et al.*, 1986b) outcome.

Due to the high doses of naloxone reported to be necessary for beneficial effects in SCI, Faden and co-workers have proposed that the kappa-receptor and its ligand (dynA) are specifically involved in SCI secondary injury mechanisms (Faden *et al.*, 1985, 1988). Very high doses of naloxone are required to block kappa-receptors. They recently studied the effect of a selective kappa-receptor antagonist, nor-binaltorphimine, in SCI and reported significant neurological improvement (Faden, Takemori and Portoghese, 1987). However, the potency of this drug was about the same as the relatively non-selective naloxone, and less than other non-selective opiate antagonists, WIN44, U41-3 and nalmefene. More important, even if the opiate receptor blockers were acting by blocking kappa-receptors, the relationship of these receptors to secondary injury is still unclear.

The mechanisms by which opiate antagonists reduce secondary injury are not known. High doses of naloxone will block the post-traumatic hypotension that occurs after SCI, but these effects are not sufficient to explain improvements in spinal cord blood flow. Thus, a direct effect of naloxone on spinal microcirculation has been postulated (Faden *et al.*, 1983a). In addition, naloxone has been reported to have antioxidant properties at high doses (Koreh *et al.*, 1981; Hall and Braughler, 1982b). Stokes, Fox and Hollinden (1985) have reported that naloxone restores extracellular calcium ionic activity in injured spinal cords. A direct effect of naloxone on membrane characteristics and metabolism has not been ruled out.

The tripeptide thyrotropin-releasing hormone (TRH) has a large variety of physiological effects, among which is the ability to antagonize some effects of endogenous opioids without decreasing their antinociceptive activity (Holaday *et al.*, 1978; Holaday, D'Amato and Faden, 1981). This has been the rationale for testing its efficacy in experimental SCI. Most of the reports have been published by Faden and his colleagues (Faden, Jacobs and Holaday, 1981b; Faden et al., 1983b; Faden, Jacobs and Smith, 1984; Salzman et al., 1987b), who find it to be at least as effective as naloxone, even when administered after 24 h (Faden, Jacobs and Smith, 1984). Because of its ability to reverse leukotriene-induced shock (Lux, Feuerstein and Faden, 1983), which is normally naloxone resistant, at least part of TRH's beneficial effects may reflect an ability to antagonize the activity of leukotrienes, which, as we have seen, have also been implicated, through the lipid peroxidation–arachidonic acid metabolism pathway, in secondary mechanisms of SCI. Based on work with analogs of TRH, it appears that the integrity of the C-terminal end is necessary for its effect in SCI (Faden and Jacobs, 1985; Faden, 1987; Faden, Sacksen and Noble, 1988). The recent report by Salman et al. (1987) postulates that TRH treatment acts centrally to restore pre-injury balances between endogenous TRH and serotonin (which becomes elevated due to the high serotonin content of extravasated platelets), and to decrease vasogenic edema.

Arachidonic acid metabolism inhibitors   Because of the multiplicity of effects that the metabolites of arachidonic acid are felt to have in secondary SCI, there has been some interest in agents which inhibit their formation. These agents may act at a number of different steps along the metabolic pathway. Vitamin E and selenium have already been mentioned as scavengers of free radicals and, therefore, lipid peroxidation inhibitors. Other drugs which have been tested were intended to shift the eicosanoid balance away from the vasoconstrictive and thrombogenic metabolites, such as TxA_2, and in favor of the vasodilator prostacyclin, or PGI_2. These drugs include the cyclo-oxgenase inhibitors ibuprofen and meclofenamate, the thromboxane A_2 synthatase inhibitor furegrelate sodium, and the PGI_2 analog ciprostene calcium (Hall and Wolf, 1986). The clinical applicability of these drugs for SCI is uncertain because most of the studies pretreated the animals prior to SCI. However, the observation that these drugs affect post-traumatic spinal cord blood flow suggests that the balance of eicosanoids may play a role in the pathophysiology of secondary injury and post-traumatic ischemia.

Calcium channel blockers   Inhibition of Ca^{2+} ionic influx has been a rational target for pharmacological intervention. Calcium channel blockers have received considerable attention for the treatment of cerebral ischemia (Allen and Bahr, 1979; Harris et al., 1982; Steen et al., 1983). Agents used in SCI models include nicardipine (Black et al., 1988b; Hitchon et al., 1989), nimodipine (Ford and Malm, 1985; Guha, Tator and Piper, 1987; Haghighi et al., 1988), verapamil, diltiazem and nifedipine (Hall and Wolf, 1986). Most of the studies showed no significant effects of these agents on SCBF, electrophysiological changes, or histopathologic and behavioral outcomes. Calcium channel blockers, however, cause systemic arterial pressure to fall, prompting Guha, Tator and Piper (1987) to recommend giving nimodipine with a hypertensive agent, such as epinephrine (adrenaline). They report that nimodipine will improve post-traumatic blood flow, and histological and neurophysiological outcome of the clip compression SCI model in rats when the fall in blood pressure is prevented.

   Although the original rationale and interest in calcium channel blockers stemmed from the possibility that such drugs may reduce Ca^{2+} influx into injured neurons, little evidence supports this mode of action. The dihydropyridine Ca^{2+} channel blockers, such as nimodipine, block the L-channels which are voltage sensitive and situated mostly on neuronal cell bodies. Although the function of the L-channels is

Table 12.1 Effects of pharmacological agents on spinal cord injury

Pharmacological agent	Potential effects
1. Steroids	Decrease edema
	Enhance SCBF
	Scavenge free radicals
	Inhibit inflammation
2. Mannitol	Decrease edema
	Enhance SCBF
	Scavenge free radicals
3. Vitamin C, vitamin E, selenium	Scavenge free radicals
4. Naloxone, Nor-binaltorphimine	Opioid antagonism
	Anti-hypotension
5. Thyrotropin-releasing hormone (TRH)	Opioid antagonism
6. Ibuprofen, meclofenamate	Arachidonic acid metabolism inhibition
7. Nimodipine, nicardipine, nifedipine, verapamil, diltiazem	Block calcium influx
8. Vasodilators [e.g. aminophylline, isoproterenol (isoprenaline)]	Enhance SCBF
9. Alpha-methyltyrosine	Enhance SCBF
10. Lidocaine (lignocaine), thiopental (thiopentone)	Decrease SC metabolism
11. Dimethyl sulfoxide (DMSO)	Decrease inflammation
	Decrease edema
	Decrease free radical formation and scavenge free radicals
	Decrease membrane lipid peroxidation
	Enhance SCBF
12. Protease inhibition	Decrease cytoskeleton breakdown
13. Enzyme therapy	Decrease scar formation
	Enhance regeneration
14. Hypothermia	Decrease SC metabolism
	Decrease inflammation
	Decrease arachidonic acid metabolism
15. Hyperbaric oxygen	Decrease hypoxia

not well understood, it is clear that these channels are not the presynaptic Ca^{2+} channels nor the leakage channels believed to allow Ca^{2+} into ischemic neurons. Moreover, because calcium is an essential intracellular messenger, truly effective blockade of all Ca^{2+} channels should be inimical to life. Several highly lethal effective Ca^{2+} channel blockers are known, including alpha-conotoxin, a toxin isolated from snails. These blockers are profoundly toxic to organisms.

Table 12.1 shows the effects on SCI of various pharmacological agents.

Other pharmacological therapies   Other pharmacological agents have been used in experimental (and human) SCI (Dohrmann, 1972; Yashon, 1978; de la Torre, 1981; Hansebout, 1982; Janssen and Hansebout, 1989). Most have had little or no success in animal models. Several that have had reported benefits in animal models have had no proven beneficial influence in clinical situations.

Low molecular weight dextran, mannitol, glycerol and urea have been used unsuccessfully to decrease edema formation in injured spinal cords (Joyner and Freeman, 1963; de la Torre *et al.*, 1975; Hedeman and Ranajit, 1979). Lack of success with these hypertonic agents has been attributed to edema being only a component of the cascade of secondary injury mechanisms, and combination therapy is usually advocated. Note, however, that these drugs have not even been conclusively shown to reduce edema formation.

Dimethyl sulfoxide has been advocated for use in SCI because of its actions as a diuretic agent, anti-inflammatory agent, vasodilator, and free radical scavenger (Kajihara *et al.*, 1973; de la Torre *et al.*, 1975). The finding of improved histopathological appearance of canine spinal cords, reported by Kajihara *et al.* (1973), has not been duplicated in other animal models (Eidelberg *et al.*, 1976; Hoerlein *et al.*, 1983).

Aminophylline and isoproterenol (isoprenaline) have been used in combination to try to improve spinal cord blood flow, based on evidence for its effectiveness in reversing neurological deficits caused by cerebral vasospasm following sub-arachnoid hemorrhage (Dow-Edwards *et al.*, 1980). For similar reasons, when the catecholamine hypothesis of post-traumatic spinal cord ischemia was current, anti-adrenergic agents such as alpha-methyltyrosine were tested with contradictory results (Osterholm and Mathews, 1972; Hedeman and Ranajit, 1979). Serotonin antagonists (Howitt and Turnbull, 1972), phenytoin (Gerber, Olson and Harris, 1980) and thyroid hormones (Tator and van der Jogt, 1980; Tator *et al.*, 1983) have also been tried by individual laboratories. None of these drugs has been consistently reported to be effective in animal SCI models.

Other drugs which have recently been tested for their ability to protect against spinal cord ischemia include lidocaine (lignocaine) (Kobrine *et al.*, 1984; Robertson *et al.*, 1986; Haghighi *et al.*, 1987), magnesium (Robertson *et al.*, 1986) and thiopental (thiopentone) (Robertson *et al.*, 1986). These agents have been used in the hopes of reducing tissue metabolism by blocking neuronal activity. Although Kobrine *et al.* (1984) found that systemic lidocaine (lignocaine) prevented loss of evoked potentials and improved histopathological appearance in treated animals compared to the untreated controls, Haghighi *et al.* (1987), using a weight-drop model rather than the epidural balloon model, found no significant differences after intravenous or subarachnoid administration of lidocaine.

Excitatory amino acids are known to be toxic to neurons (Olney, Ho and Rhee, 1971). Recently, much attention has been focused on the NMDA receptor as the basis of selective neuronal vulnerability in cerebral ischemia models (Simon *et al.*, 1984; Meldrum, 1985; Foster *et al.*, 1987). Faden *et al.* (1988) recently reported that MK801, a selective antagonist of the NMDA receptor, improves histological and behavioral outcome after impact trauma to rat spinal cords. Long-term neurological recovery and histopathological appearance were significantly improved by a dose of 1 mg/kg given intravenously 15 min after trauma. A protective effect of MK801 and U-50488H, a kappa-opioid receptor agonist (Hansebout, 1982) in pretreated rats has independently been reported by Gomez-Pinilla *et al.* (1989).

A somewhat different approach has been taken by Iwasaki *et al.* (1987), who attempted to suppress the post-traumatic, calcium-activated degradation of neuro-filament proteins. They administered the neutral protease inhibitors, leupeptin and E-64c, intraperitoneally for 3 days after crush injury in rats. These drugs improved recovery of motor function and decreased axonal degeneration, as measured by automated image analysis. Again, these studies have not yet been reproduced in other laboratories.

Non-pharmacological studies
Non-pharmacological strategies for the treatment of experimental SCI have included surgical maneuvers to ameliorate cord swelling and decrease tissue pressures,

cooling the spinal cord to decrease cellular metabolic rates, and attempts to increase oxygen delivery to the spinal cord.

Many of the surgical therapies have also been used in the clinical setting, but none has proven satisfactory in humans. One of the earliest methods was the mid-line myelotomy to remove the central hemorrhage (Allen, 1914; Benes, 1968; Parker and Smith, 1974). Not only would this alleviate the increased tissue pressure caused by expansion of the cord within its relatively inelastic pial lining, but it would remove much of the Fe^{2+} and Ca^{2+} ions which act to catalyse free radical production. Results in clinical situations have been equivocal, some studies showing improved function but a higher case mortality rate (de la Torre, 1981; Hansebout, 1982, 1986). Incision of the dura in the mid-line, just to relieve pressure, has also been tried unsuccessfully. Simple laminectomy for decompression has been commonly practised in humans, without demonstrated benefit (Bohlmann, 1979; Hansebout, 1982, 1986). These questions, however, have not been adequately tested in double-blind randomized clinical trials. Also, most of the animal studies report that the mid-line myelotomy must be extended to the anterior spinal cord to have a beneficial effect and this has not been assessed clinically in patients yet.

Perfusion of the injured or ischemic spinal cord with a cool, isotonic solution has been used in animal models (Albin *et al.*, 1968; Hansebout, Kuchner and Romero-Sierra, 1975; Robertson *et al.*, 1986), and in humans has shown some promise (Acosta-Rua, 1970; Hansebout, 1982, 1986; Hansebout, Tanner and Romero-Sierra, 1984). The potential beneficial effects are decreased spinal cord metabolism, removal of accumulating toxins, and increased CSF circulation with greater delivery of nutrients to the damaged area. Non-perfusive cooling of the cord with an epidural, self-contained, silastic cooling unit has also been reported (Romero-Sierra *et al.*, 1974). A mathematical description of the effects of this device on spinal fluid circulation indicates that the convection it creates, even around segments of swollen spinal cord, causes significant CSF circulation (Goetz *et al.*, 1988). Further studies in animals and in controlled human trials will be needed before this technique can gain widespread acceptance, as the optimal timing, duration and degree of cooling are unknown, and the use of steroids in the human series has complicated the interpretation of outcome data.

There is some evidence that perfusion of the injured spinal cord with saline at ambient temperatures may decrease edema formation and cord necrosis at the site of injury (Osterholm *et al.*, 1984). This report, more importantly, suggested that the use of an oxygenated fluorocarbon nutrient solution as the perfusate heightened this beneficial effect, and increased post-traumatic levels of ATP and the number of surviving anterior horn cells. In addition to carrying high concentrations of oxygen, this solution contained glucose and essential amino acids, and was slightly hyper-osmolar.

Another potential means of increasing oxygen delivery to ischemic, post-traumatic spinal cord is the use of hyperbaric oxygen. One animal study (Balentine, 1975) has shown that hyperbaric oxygen leads to increased central necrosis. The results of preliminary human studies have been promising but not dramatically so (Jones, Unsworth and Marosszeky, 1978; Gameche *et al.*, 1981; Yeo, 1984). A rigorous randomized trial involving large populations of SCI patients will be necessary to assess this treatment modality.

Ford and Malm (1984) have tested the effects of arterial hypercarbia and hypocarbia on neurological and histological outcome after experimental SCI and found none. Their rationale was that, since normal spinal cord arteries, like the cerebral vasculature, respond to hypercarbia with reflex vasodilatation, then this may be a means of delivering more blood to ischemic spinal cord segments. They did not measure SCBF in this set of experiments. Another physiological manipulation has been to expand blood volume with whole blood, albumin, packed red blood cells, low molecular weight dextran or hetastarch (Wallace and Tator, 1987a; Dyste *et al.*, 1989). Although most of these manipulations elevate cardiac output, their effect on SCBF was variable. In these studies, the animals were sacrificed acutely, so no long-term outcome data was included.

Tator's group has attempted to promote recovery from acute SCI using long-term stimulation of the cord with either direct (Fehlings, Tator and Linden, 1988) or alternating (Wallace and Tator, 1987b) current. The results were felt to be beneficial using direct current in more severe injuries, and no benefit was noted with alternating current. Similar beneficial results with a direct current electrical field were reported by Borgens *et al.* (1986) and by Politis and Zenakis (1988).

Studies of spinal cord regeneration
In contrast to most of the above therapeutic trials, which have sought to reduce secondary injury to the spinal cord, studies of spinal cord regeneration have attempted to improve the chances of regrowth of already damaged spinal cells, or to enhance the plasticity of remaining elements, to bring back lost function through the formation of new connections and networks. The CNS has long been thought to have very limited regenerative capabilities, but the hope remains that, by local manipulation of the environment, axons may be induced to grow back across damaged spinal segments and reform their genetically determined connections (Guth *et al.*, 1983).

As mentioned at the beginning of this chapter, experimental studies of spinal cord regeneration differ from studies of secondary injury in that the models need, in order to permit the unequivocal demonstration of regeneration, to start with the complete physical disruption of the spinal cord, whereas in most clinical cases, and in experimental models of secondary injury, there is at least some physical continuity. A further caveat in regeneration experiments is that dorsal root fiber regeneration can be erroneously interpreted as central axonal regeneration (Tator and Rivlin, 1983).

Most of the work has concentrated on devising means for the regenerating axons to cross the segment of damaged spinal cord. Since glial and connective tissue scarring is present, attempts have been made to remove the scarred segment with sharp dissection and reappose the two severed ends (Windle and Chambers, 1950; Windle *et al.*, 1956), to inject enzymes locally to decrease scar tissue (Matinian and Andreasian, 1976; Guth *et al.*, 1980), to transplant embryonic (Nygren, Olson and Seiger, 1977; Commissiong, 1983; Bernstein, Underberger and Hoovler, 1984; Reier, 1985; Pallini *et al.*, 1989), or peripheral (Wrathall, Kapoor and Kao, 1984) support cells into the segment, or to 'bridge' the gap using peripheral nerve grafts to redirect regenerating axons external to the CNS and then back into the cord (Benfy and Aguayo, 1982; Fernandez *et al.*, 1985; Reier, 1985). An attempt has also been made to promote regeneration by altering the immune response to CNS tissue (Feringa, Vahlsing and Gilbert, 1985). The degree of regrowth of axons is normally measured using the axonal transport of horseradish peroxidase as a histochemical marker.

Although axons are often found to grow through these 'favorable environments', they usually do not grow much further, and studies of neurological function and electrophysiological recovery have not been encouraging (Windle and Chambers, 1950; Windle *et al.*, 1956). This is probably because quantitative axonal regeneration is not the main determinant of functional recovery. Neurological function can be maintained in many circumstances, with very few surviving axons (Windle, Smart and Beers, 1958; Guth *et al.*, 1980). However, even the survival of large numbers of axons does not, in itself, assure function if demyelination (Blight, 1982, 1983) or other factors interfere with their ability to conduct impulses of an appropriate latency and frequency. Functional recovery should therefore be measured not only by morphological but also by electrophysiological and behavioral parameters.

Conclusions

Advances in acute and chronic care for SCI patients have reduced complication rates and mortality, while technological advances in rehabilitation have helped many patients with otherwise devastating neurological deficits to regain a significant degree of social activity. However, reliable means of preventing loss of function, or of increasing return of function, have not been developed. The more we learn about the phenomenology of SCI and CNS regeneration, the more unanswered questions arise. The main questions remaining, each with their myriad of sub-questions, are: (a) to what extent does 'secondary injury' play a role in determining loss of function following SCI; (b) what are the factors which hinder regeneration and recovery of function, and to what extent can either secondary injury or regeneration be influenced by external manipulation in a positive fashion? In order to answer these questions, it is of paramount importance to know how applicable data obtained from animal models are to human SCI. Improved methods for non-invasively monitoring electrophysiological and biochemical phenomena in humans may provide data with which improved animal models can be developed.

References

Abraham, J., Balasubramanian, A.S., Theodore, D.R., Nagarajan, S., Apte, C.A. and Chadi, S. (1985) Spinal cord edema, 5-hydroxytryptamine, lipid peroxidation, and lysosomal enzyme release after acute contusion and compression injury in primates. *CNS Trauma*, **2**, 45–58

Acosta-Rua, G.J. (1970) Treatment of traumatic paraplegic patients by localized cooling of the spinal cord. *Journal of the Iowa Medical Society*, **60**, 326–328

Albin, M.S., White, R.J., Acosta-Rua, G. and Yashon, D. (1968) Study of functional recovery produced by delayed localized cooling after spinal cord injury in primates. *Journal of Neurosurgery*, **29**, 113–120

Alderman, J.L., Osterholm, J.L., D'Amore, B.R. and Williams, H.D. (1980) Catecholamine alterations attending spinal cord injury: a reanalysis. *Neurosurgery*, **6**, 412–417

Allen, A.R. (1914) Remarks on the histopathological changes in the spinal cord due to impact. An experimental study. *Journal of Nervous and Mental Diseases*, **41**, 141–147

Allen, G.S. and Bahr, A.L. (1979) Cerebral artery spasm: Part 10. Reversal of acute and chronic spasm in dogs with orally administered nifedipine. *Neurosurgery*, **4**, 43–47

Anden, N.E., Haggendal, J., Magnusson, T and Rosengren, E. (1964) The time course of the disappearance of noradrenalin and serotonin in the spinal cord after transection. *Acta physiologica scandinavica*, **62**, 115–118

Anderson, D.K., Braughler, J.M., Hall, E.D., Waters, T.R., McCall, J.M. and Means, E.D. (1988) Effects of treatment with U-74006F on neurological outcome following experimental spinal cord injury. *Journal of Neurosurgery*, **69**, 562–567

Anderson, D.K. and Means, E.D. (1985) Iron-induced lipid peroxidation in spinal cord: protection with mannitol and methylprednisolone. *Journal of Free Radical Biological Medicine*, **1**, 59–64

Anderson, D.K., Means, E.D., Waters, T.R. and Green, E.S. (1982) Microvascular perfusion and metabolism in injured spinal cord after methylprednisolone treatment. *Journal of Neurosurgery*, **56**, 106–113

Anderson, D.K., Means, E.D., Waters, T.R. and Spears, C.J. (1980) Spinal cord energy metabolism following compression trauma to the feline spinal cord. *Journal of Neurosurgery*, **53**, 375–380

Anderson, D.K., Saunders, R.D., Demediuk, P., Dugan, L.L., Braughler, J.M., Hall, E.D., Means, E.D. and Horrocks, L.A. (1985) Lipid hydrolysis and peroxidation in injured spinal cord: partial protection with methylprednisolone or vitamin E and selenium. *CNS Trauma*, **2**, 257–267

Arias, M.J. (1985) Effect of naloxone on functional recovery after experimental spinal cord injury in the rat. *Surgical Neurology*, **23**, 440–442

Astrup, J. (1982) Energy requiring cell functions in the ischemic brain. *Journal of Neurosurgery*, **56**, 482–497

Ayer, J.B. (1919) Cerebrospinal fluid in experimental compression of the spinal cord. *Archives of Neurology and Psychiatry*, **2**, 158–164

Baker, P.F. (1976) The regulation of intracellular calcium. *Symposia of the Society for Experimental Biology*, **30**, 67–88

Balentine, J.D. (1975) Central necrosis of the spinal cord induced by hyperbaric oxygen exposure. *Journal of Neurosurgery*, **43**, 150–155

Balentine, J.D. (1978a) Pathology of experimental spinal cord trauma. The necrotic lesion as a function of vascular injury. *Laboratory Investigation*, **39**, 236–253

Balentine, J.D. (1978b) Pathology of experimental spinal cord trauma. II. Ultrastructure of axons and myelin. *Laboratory Investigations*, **39**, 254–266

Balentine, J.D. and Hilton, C.W. (1980a) Ultrastructural pathology of axons and myelin in calcium-induced myelopathy. *Journal of Neuropathology and Experimental Neurology*, **39**, 339

Balentine, J.D. and Hilton, C.W. (1980b) Calcifications of axons in experimental spinal cord trauma. *Annals of Neurology*, **2**, 520–523

Banik, N.L., Hogan, E.L. and Hsu, C.Y. (1985) Molecular and anatomical correlates of spinal cord injury. *CNS Trauma*, **2**, 99–107

Banik, N.L., Hogan, E.L., Powers, J.M. and Smith, K.P. (1986) Proteolytic enzymes in experimental spinal cord injury. *Journal of Neurological Science*, **73**, 245–256

Banik, N.L., Hogan, E.L., Powers, J.M. and Whetstine, L.J. (1982) Degradation of cytoskeletal proteins in experimental spinal cord injury. *Neurochemical Research*, **7**, 1465–1475

Beggs, J.L. and Waggener, J.D. (1976) Transendothelial vesicular transport of protein following compression injury to the spinal cord. *Laboratory Investigations*, **34**, 428–439

Benes, V. (1968) *Spinal Cord Injury*, Ballière, Tindall and Cassell, London, pp. 94–96

Benes, V. Jr and Rokyta, R. (1988) Experimental spinal cord injury: lumbar vertebra resection to shorten the gap between spinal cord stumps. *Acta neurochirurgica*, **90**, 152–156

Benfy, M.L. and Aguayo, A.J. (1982) Extensive elongation of axons from rat brain into peripheral nerve grafts. *Science*, **296**, 150–152

Benoist, G., Kausz, M., Rethelyi, M. and Pasztor, E. (1979) Sensitivity of the short-range spinal interneurons of the cat to experimental spinal cord trauma. *Journal of Neurosurgery*, **51**, 834–840

Bernstein, J.J., Underberger, D. and Hoovler, D.D. (1984) Fetal CNS transplants into adult spinal cord: techniques, initial effects, and caveats. *CNS Trauma*, **1**, 39–46

Black, P., Markowitz, R.S., Cooper, V., Mechanic, A., Kushner, H., Damjanov, I., Finkelstein, S.D. and Wachs, K.C. (1986a) Models of spinal cord injury: Part 1. Static load technique. *Neurosurgery*, **19**, 752–762

Black, P., Markowitz, R.S., Damjanov, I., Finkelstein, S.D., Kushner, H., Gillespie, J. and Feldman, M. (1988a) Models of spinal cord injury: Part 3. Dynamic load technique. *Neurosurgery*, **22**, 57–60

Black, P., Markowitz., R.S., Finkelstein, S.D., McMonagle-Strucko, K. and Gillespie, J.A. (1988b) Experimental spinal cord injury: effect of a calcium channel antagonist (nicardipine). *Neurosurgery*, **22**, 61–66

Black, P., Markowitz., R.S., Keller, S., Wachs, K., Gillespie, J. and Finkelstein, S.D. (1986b) Naloxone and experimental spinal cord injury: Part 2. Megadose treatment in a dynamic load injury model. *Neurosurgery*, **19**, 909–913

Blight, A.R. (1982) To what extent is traumatic paraplegia a demyelinating disease? *Society of Neuroscience* (Abstract), **8**, 31

Blight, A.R. (1983) Axonal physiology of chronic spinal cord injury in the cat: intracellular recording *in vitro*. *Neuroscience*, **10**, 1471–1486

Blight, A.R. (1985) Delayed demyelination and macrophage invasion: a candidate for secondary cell damage in spinal cord injury. *CNS Trauma*, **2**, 299–315

Blight, A.R. and Young, W. (1989a) Central axons in injured cat spinal cord recover electrophysiological function following remyelination by Schwann cells. *Journal of Neurological Science.*, **91**, 15–34

Blight, A.R. and Young, W. (1989b) Axonal morphometric correlates with evoked potentials in experimental spinal cord injury. In *Preventing Intraoperative Neural Injury* (ed. S. Solzman), Humana Press, Philadelphia (in press)

Bohlmann, H.H. (1979) Acute fractures and dislocations of the cervical spine. An analysis of three hundred hospitalized patients and review of the literature. *Journal of Bone and Joint Surgery*, **61-A**, 119–142

Boink, A.B.T.J., Ruigrok, T.J.C., Maas, A.H.J., Zimmerman, A.N.E. (1976) Changes in high energy phosphate compounds of isolated rat hearts during Ca^{++} free perfusion and reperfusion with Ca^{++}. *Journal of Molecular Cell Cardiology*, **8**, 973–979

Borgens, R.B., Blight, A.R., Murphy, D.J. and Stewart, L. (1986) Transected dorsal column axons within the guinea pig spinal cord regenerate in the presence of an applied electric field. *Journal of Comparative Neurology*, **250**, 168–180

Bracken, M.B. and Collins, W.F. (1985) Randomized clinical trials of spinal cord injury treatment. In *Central Nervous System Trauma Status Report* (eds D.P. Becker and J.T. Povlishok), National Institutes of Health, Bethesda, Md, pp. 303–312

Bracken, M.B., Shepard, M.J., Hellenbrand, K.G. *et al.* (1985) Methylprednisolone and neurologic function one year after spinal cord injury. Results of the National Acute Spinal Cord Injury Study. *Journal of Neurosurgery*, **63**, 704–713

Braughler, T.M. and Hall, E.D. (1982) Correlations of methylprednisolone levels in cat spinal cord with its effect on $(Na^+–K^+)$-ATPase, lipid peroxidation and alpha motor neuron function. *Journal of Neurosurgery*, **56**, 838–844

Braughler, J.M. and Hall, E.D. (1983) Lactate and pyruvate metabolism in the injured cat spinal cord before and after a single large intravenous dose of methylprednisolone. *Journal of Neurosurgery*, **59**, 256–261

Braughler, J.M., Hall, E.D., Means, E.D., Waters, T.R. and Anderson, D.K. (1987) Evaluation of an intensive methylprednisolone sodium succinate dosing regimen in experimental spinal cord injury. *Journal of Neurosurgery*, **67**, 102–105

Bresnahan, J.C., Beattie, M.S., Todd, F.D., III and Noyes, D.H. (1987) A behavioral and anatomical analysis of spinal cord injury produced by a feedback-controlled impaction device. *Experimental Neurology*, **95**, 548–570

Brightman, M.W., Klatzo, I., Olsson, Y. and Reese, T.S. (1970) The blood brain barrier to proteins under normal and pathologic conditions. *Journal of Neurological Science*, **10**, 215–240

Broakman, R., Schouten, H.J.A., Blaauw-van Dishoek, M. and Minderhoud, J.M. (1983) Megadose steroids in severe head injury. Results of a prospective double-blind clinical trial. *Journal of Neurosurgery*, **58**, 326–330

Brodner, R.A. and Dohrmann, G.J. (1977) Norepinephrine, dopamine and serotonin in experimental spinal cord trauma: current status. *Paraplegia*, **15**, 166–171

Carofoli, E. and Crompton, M. (1978) The regulation of intracellular calcium by mitochondria. *Annals of the New York Academy of Sciences*, **307**, 269–284

Carofoli, E. and Lehninger, A.L. (1971) A survey of the interactions of calcium ions with mitochondria from different tissues and species. *Biochemical Journal*, **122**, 681–690

Cawthon, D.F., Senter, H.J. and Stewart, W.B. (1980) Comparison of hydrogen clearance and 14-C-antipyrine autoradiography in the measurement of spinal cord blood flow after severe impact injury. *Journal of Neurosurgery*, **37**, 591–593

Chance, B. (1965) The energy-linked reaction of calcium with mitochondria. *Journal of Biological Chemistry*, **240**, 2729–2748

Choi, D.W. (1987) Ionic dependence of glutamate neurotoxicity. *Journal of Neuroscience*, **7**, 369–379

Clendenon, N.R., Allen, N., Gordon, W.A. and Bingham, W.G. Jr (1978) Inhibition of Na-K-activated ATPase following experimental spinal cord trauma. *Journal of Neurosurgery*, **49**, 563–568

Collins, W.F. (1983) A review and update of experimental and clinical studies of spinal cord injury. *Paraplegia*, **21**, 204–219

Commissiong, J.W. (1983) Fetal locus coeruleus transplanted into the transected spinal cord of the adult rat. *Brain Research*, **271**, 174–179

Cordingley, G.E. and Somjen, G.G. (1978) The clearing of excess potassium from extracellular space in spinal cord and cerebral cortex. *Brain Research*, **151**, 291–306

Cusick, J.F., Mycklebust, J.B., Larson, S.J. and Sances, A. Jr (1979) Spinal cord evaluation with cortical evoked responses. *Archives of Neurology*, **36**, 140–143

Deecke, L. and Tator, C.H. (1973) Neurophysiological assessment of afferent and efferent conduction in the injured spinal cord of monkeys. *Journal of Neurosurgery*, **39**, 65–74

Del Maestro, R.F. (1980) An approach to free radicals in medicine and biology. *Acta physiologica scandinavica* (Suppl.), **492**, 153–168

Demopoulos, H.B., Flamm, E.S., Seligman, M.L., Mitamura, J.A. and Ransohoff, J. (1979) Membrane perturbations in central nervous system injury: theoretical basis for free radical damage and a review of the experimental data. In *Neural Trauma* (eds A.J. Popp, R.S. Bourke, L.R. Nelson and H.K. Kimelberg), Raven Press, New York, pp. 63–78

Demopoulos, H.B., Flamm, E., Seligman, M. and Pietronigro, D.D. (1982) Oxygen free radicals in central nervous system ischemia and trauma. In *Pathology of Oxygen* (ed. A.P. Autor), Academic Press, New York, pp. 127–155

Dohrmann, G.J. (1972) Experimental spinal cord trauma: a historical review. *Archives of Neurology*, **27**, 468–474

Dohrman, G.J., Wagner, F.C. and Bucy, P.C. (1971) The microvasculature in transitory traumatic paraplegia. *Journal of Neurosurgery*, **35**, 263–271

Dolan, E.J. and Tator, C.H. (1979) A new method for testing the force of clips for aneurysms or experimental spinal cord compression. *Journal of Neurosurgery*, **51**, 229–233

Dow-Edwards, D., De Crescito, V., Tomasula, J.J. and Flamm, E.S. (1980) Effect of aminophylline and isoproterenol on spinal cord blood flow after impact injury. *Journal of Neurosurgery*, **53**, 385–390

Dyste, G.N., Hitchon, P.W., Girton, R.A. and Chapman, M. (1989) Effect of hetastarch, mannitol and phenylephrine on spinal cord blood flow following experimental spinal injury. *Neurosurgery*, **24**, 228–234

Eidelberg, E., Staten, E., Watkin, C.J. and Smith, J.S. (1976) Treatment of experimental spinal cord injury in ferrets. *Surgical Neurology*, **6**, 243–246

Eidelberg, E., Sullivan, J. and Brigham, A. (1975) Immediate consequences of spinal cord injury. Possible role of potassium in axonal conduction block. *Surgical Neurology*, **3**, 317–321

Evans, D.E., Alter, W.A. III, Shatsky, S.A. and Gunby, E.N. (1976) Cardiac arrhythmias resulting from experimental head injury. *Journal of Neurosurgery*, **45**, 609–616

Evans, D.E., Kobrine, A.L. and Rizzoli, H.V. (1980) Cardiac arrhythmias accompanying acute compression of the spinal cord. *Journal of Neurosurgery*, **52**, 52–59

Faden, A.L. (1985) Pharmacological therapy in acute spinal cord injury: experimental strategies and future directions. In *Central Nervous System Trauma Status Report* (eds D.P. Becker and I.T. Povlishok), National Institutes of Health, Bethesda, Md, pp. 481–485

Faden, A. (1987) Opiate receptor antagonists, thyrotropin-releasing hormone (TRH), and TRH analogs in the treatment of spinal cord injury. *CNS Trauma*, **4**, 217–226

Faden, A.L. and Jacobs, T.P. (1983) High dose corticosteroid therapy in experimental spinal injury: increased mortality and failure to improve neurological recovery. *Neurology*, **33** (Suppl. 2), 192

Faden, A.L. and Jacobs, T.P. (1985) Effect of TRH analogs on neurological recovery after experimental spinal trauma. *Neurology*, **35**, 1331–1334

Faden, A.L., Jacobs, T.P., Feuerstein, G. and Holaday, J.W. (1981b) Dopamine partially mediates the cardiovascular effects of naloxone after spinal injury. *Brain Research*, **213**, 415–421

Faden, A.L., Jacobs, T.P. and Holaday, J.W. (1980) Endorphin-parasympathetic interactions in spinal shock. *Journal of the Autonomic Nervous System*, **2**, 295–304

Faden, A.L., Jacobs, T.P. and Holaday, J.W. (1981a) Opiate antagonist improves neurologic recovery after spinal injury. *Science*, **211**, 493–494

Faden, A.L., Jacobs, T.P. and Holaday, J.W. (1981b) Thyrotropin-releasing hormone improves neurologic recovery after spinal cord injury in cats. *New England Journal of Medicine*, **305**, 1063–1067

Faden, A.L., Jacobs, T.P., Mougey, E. and Holaday, J.W. (1981a) Endorphins in experimental spinal injury. Therapeutic effect of naloxone. *Annals of Neurology*, **10**, 326–332

Faden, A.L., Jacobs, T.P., Smith, M.T. and Holaday, J.W. (1983b) Comparison of thyrotropin-releasing hormone (TRH), naloxone and dexamethasone treatments in experimental spinal injury. *Neurology*, **33**, 673–678

Faden, A.L., Jacobs, T.P. and Smith, M.T. (1984) Thyrotropin-releasing hormone in experimental spinal injury: dose response and late treatment. *Neurology*, **34**, 1280–1284

Faden, A.L., Jacobs, T.P., Smith, G.P., Green, B.A. and Zivin, J.A. (1983a) Neuropeptides in spinal cord injury: comparative experimental models. *Peptides*, **4**, 631–634

Faden, A.L., Lemke, M., Simon, R.P. and Noble, L.J. (1988) N-methyl-D-aspartate antagonist MK801 improves outcome following traumatic spinal cord injury in rats: behavioral, anatomic and neurochemical studies. *Journal of Neurotrauma*, **5**, 33–45

Faden, A.L., Molineaux, C.J., Rosenberger, J.G., Jacobs, T.P. and Cox, B.M. (1985) Endogenous opioid immunoreactivity in rat spinal cord following traumatic injury. *Annals of Neurology*, **17**, 386–390

Faden, A.I., Sacksen, I. and Noble, L.J. (1988) Structure activity relationships of TRH analogs in rat spinal cord injury. *Brain Research*, **448**, 287–293

Faden, A.I., Takemori, A.E. and Portoghese, P.S. (1987) Kappa-selective opiate antagonist nor-binaltorphimine improves outcome after traumatic spinal cord injury in rats. *CNS Trauma*, **4**, 227–234

Fehlings, M.G., Tator, C.H. and Linden, R.D. (1988) The effect of direct current field on recovery from experimental spinal cord injury. *Journal of Neurosurgery*, **68**, 781–792

Fehlings, M.G., Tator, C.H., Linden, R.D. and Piper, I.R. (1987) Motor evoked potentials recorded from normal and spinal cord-injured rats. *Neurosurgery*, **20**, 125–130

Feringa, E.R., Vahlsing, H.L. and Gilbert, W.J. (1985) Failure to promote spinal cord regeneration in rats with immunosuppressive therapy. *Journal of Neurology, Neurosurgery and Psychiatry*, **48**, 723–725

Fernandez, E., Pallini, R., Maira, G. and Rossi, G.F. (1985) Peripheral nerve autografts to the injured spinal cord of the rat: an experimental model for the study of spinal cord regeneration. *Acta neurochirurgica*, **78**, 57–64

Flamm, E.S., Young, W., Collins, W.F., Piepmeier, J., Clifton, G.L. and Fischer, B. (1985) A phase I trial of naloxone treatment in acute spinal cord injury. *Journal of Neurosurgery*, **63**, 390–397

Flamm, E.S., Young, W., Demopoulos, H.B., De Crescito, V. and Tomasulo, J.J. (1982) Experimental spinal cord injury: treatment with naloxone. *Neurosurgery*, **10**, 227–231

Fontaine, R., Mandel, P. and Dany, A. (1954) Etude du deséquilibre biochimique provoque par les traumatismes médullaires, chez l'homme et chez le chien. *Lyon chirurgical*, **49**, 395–408

Ford, R.W.J. and Malm, D.N. (1984) Therapeutic trial of hypercarbia and hypocarbia in acute experimental spinal cord injury. *Journal of Neurosurgery*, **61**, 925–930

Ford, R.W.J. and Malm, D.N. (1985) Failure of nimodipine to reverse acute experimental spinal cord injury. *CNS Trauma*, **2**, 9–17

Foster, A.C., Gill, R., Iversen, L. and Woodruff, G.N. (1987) Systemic administration of MK801 protects against ischemia-induced hippocampal neurodegeneration in the gerbil. *British Journal of Pharmacology*, **90**, 9P

Fridovich, I. (1978) The biology of oxygen radicals. *Science*, **201**, 875–880

Gale, K., Kerasidis, H. and Wrathall, J.R. (1985) Spinal cord contusion in the rat: behavioral analysis of functional neurological impairment. *Experimental Neurology*, **88**, 123–134

Gamache, F.W. Jr, Meyers, R.A.M., Ducker, T.B. and Cowley, R.A. (1981) The clinical application of hyperbaric oxygen therapy in spinal cord injury: a preliminary report. *Surgical Neurology*, **15**, 85–87

Gerber, A.M., Olson, W.L. and Harris, J.H. (1980) Effect of phenytoin on functional recovery after experimental spinal cord injury in dogs. *Neurosurgery*, **7**, 472–476

Gibson, B.L. and Reif-Lehrer, L. (1985) Mg^{2+} reduces N-methyl-D-aspartate neurotoxicity in embryonic chick neural retina *in vitro. Neuroscience Letters*, **57**, 13–18

Goetz, T., Romero-Sierra, C., Ethier, R. and Henriksen, R.N. (1988) Modeling of therapeutic dialysis of cerebrospinal fluid by epidural cooling in spinal cord injuries. *Journal of Neurotrauma*, **5**, 139–150

Goldman, S.S., Elowitz, E. and Flamm, E.S. (1983) Effect of traumatic injury on membrane phosphatase activity in the cat spinal cord. *Experimental Neurology*, **82**, 650–662

Gomez-Pinilla, F., Ren, H., Cotman, C.W. and Nieto-Sampedro, M. (1989) Neuroprotective effect of MK801 and U-50488H after contusive spinal cord injury. *Experimental Neurology*, **104**, 118–124

Goodman, J.H., Bingham, W.G. and Hunt, W.E. (1978) Platelet aggregation in experimental spinal cord injury. *Archives of Neurology*, **36**, 197–201

Gower, D.J., Hollman, C., Lee, S. and Tytell, M. (1989) Spinal cord injury and the stress protein response. *Journal of Neurosurgery*, **70**, 605–611

Green, B.A., Kahn, T. and Klose, K.J. (1980) A comparative study of steroid therapy in acute experimental spinal cord injury. *Surgical Neurology*, **13**, 91–97

Griffiths, I.R. (1975) Vasogenic edema following acute and chronic spinal cord compression in the dog. *Journal of Neurosurgery*, **42**, 155–165

Griffiths, I.R. and Miller, R. (1974) Vascular permeability to protein and vasogenic oedema in experimental concussive injuries to the canine spinal cord. *Journal of Neurological Science*, **22**, 291–304

Griffiths, I.R., Trench, J.G. and Crawford, R.A. (1979) Spinal cord blood flow and conduction during experimental cord compression in normotensive and hypotensive dogs. *Journal of Neurosurgery*, **50**, 353–360

Guha, A. and Tator, C.H. (1988) Acute cardiovascular effects of experimental spinal cord injury. *Journal of Trauma*, **28**, 481–490

Guha, A., Tator, C.H. and Piper, I. (1987) Effect of a calcium channel blocker on posttraumatic spinal cord blood flow. *Journal of Neurosurgery*, **66**, 423–430

Guth, L., Albuquerque, E.X., Deshpande, S.S., Barrett, C.P., Donati, E.J. and Warnick, J.E. (1980a) Ineffectiveness of enzyme therapy on regeneration in the spinal cord of the rat. *Journal of Neurosurgery*, **52**, 73–86

Guth, L., Brewer, C.R., Collins, W.F., Goldberger, M.E. and Perl, E.R. (1980b) Criteria for evaluating spinal cord regeneration experiments. *Experimental Neurology*, **69**, 1–3

Guth, L., Reier, P., Barrett, C.P. and Donati, E.J. (1983) Repair of the mammalian spinal cord. *TINS*, **6**, 20–24

Haghighi, S.S. and Chehrazi, B. (1987) Effect of naloxone in experimental acute spinal cord injury. *Neurosurgery*, **20**, 385–388

Haghighi, S.S., Chehrazi, B.B., Higgins, R.S., Remington, W.J. and Wagner, F.C. (1987) Effect of lidocaine treatment on acute spinal cord injury. *Neurosurgery*, **20**, 536–541

Haghighi, S.S., Chehrazi, B.B. and Wagner, F.C. Jr (1988) Effect of nimodipine-associated hypotension on recovery from acute spinal cord injury in cats. *Surgical Neurology*, **29**, 293–297

Hall, E.D., Braughler, J.M. (1982a) Effects of methylprednisolone on spinal cord lipid peroxidation and (Na^+/K^+)-ATPase activity. *Journal of Neurosurgery*, **57**, 247–253

Hall, E.D. and Braughler, J.M. (1982b) Glucocorticoid mechanisms in acute spinal cord injury: a review and therapeutic rationale. *Surgical Neurology*, **18**, 320–327

Hall, E.D. and Braughler, J.M. (1986) Role of lipid peroxidation in post-traumatic spinal cord degeneration: a review. *CNS Trauma*, **3**, 281–294

Hall, E.D., Braughler, J.M. and McCall, J.M. (1988) New pharmacological treatment of acute spinal cord trauma. *Journal of Neurotrauma*, **5**, 81–89

Hall, E.D. and Wolf, D.L. (1986) A pharmacological analysis of the pathophysiological mechanisms of posttraumatic spinal cord ischemia. *Journal of Neurosurgery*, **64**, 951–961

Hall, E.D., Wolf, D.L. and Braughler, J.M. (1984) Effects of a single large dose of methylprednisolone sodium succinate on experimental posttraumatic spinal cord ischemia. *Journal of Neurosurgery*, **61**, 124–130

Hansebout, R.R. (1982) A comprehensive review of methods of improving cord recovery after acute spinal cord injury. In *Early Management of Acute Spinal Cord Injury* (ed. C.H. Tator), Raven Press, New York, pp. 181–196

Hansebout, R.R. (1986) The neurosurgical management of cord injuries. In *Management of Spinal Cord Injuries* (eds R. Block and M. Basbaum), Williams and Wilkins, Baltimore, pp. 1–27

Hansebout, R.R., Kuchner, E.F. and Romero-Sierra, C. (1975) Effects of local hypothermia and of steroids upon recovery from experimental spinal cord compression injury. *Surgical Neurology*, **4**, 531–536

Hansebout, R.R., Tanner, J.A. and Romero-Sierra, C. (1984) Current status of spinal cord cooling in the treatment of spinal cord injury. *Spine*, **9**, 508–511

Happel, E.D., Smith,K.P., Banik, M.C., Powers, J.M., Hogan, E.L. and Balentine, J.D. (1981) Ca^{++} accumulation in experimental spinal cord trauma. *Brain Research*, **211**, 476–479

Harris, R.J., Branston, N.M., Symon, L., Bayhan, M. and Watson, A. (1982) The effects of a calcium antagonist, nimodipine, upon physiological responses of the cerebral vasculature and its possible influence upon focal cerebral edema. *Stroke*, **13**, 759–766

Hartwell, J.B. (1917) An analysis of 133 fractures of the spine treated at the Massachusetts General Hospital. *Boston Medical and Surgical Journal*, **177**, 31–41

Hayashi, N., de la Torre, J. and Green, B. (1980) Regional spinal cord blood flow and tissue oxygen content after spinal cord trauma. *Surgical Forum*, **31**, 461–463

Hedeman, L.S. and Ranajit, S. (1979) Studies in experimental spinal cord trauma: Part 2: Comparison of treatment with steroids, low molecular weight dextran and catecholamine blockade. *Journal of Neurosurgery*, **40**, 44–51

Hitchon, P.W., Hansen, T., McKay, T. Girton, R.A., Dyste, G.N., Sokoll, M.D. (1989) Nicardipine after spinal cord compression in the lamb. *Surgical Neurology*, **31**, 101–110

Hoerlein, B.F., Redding, R.W., Hoff, E.J. and McGuire, J.A. (1983) Evaluation of dexamethasone, DMSO, mannitol and sercoseryl in acute spinal cord trauma. *Journal of the American Animal Hospital Association*, **19**, 216–226

Holaday, J.W., D'Amato, R.D. and Faden, A.I. (1981) Thyrotropin-releasing hormone improves cardiovascular function in experimental endotoxic and hemorrhagic shock. *Science*, **213**, 216–218

Holaday, J.W. and Faden, A.I. (1980) Naloxone acts at central opiate receptors to reverse hypotension, hypothermia and hypoventilation in spinal shock. *Brain Research*, **189**, 295–299

Holaday, J.W., Tseng, L.-F., Loh, H.H., Li, C.H. (1978) Thyrotropin-releasing hormone antagonizes β-endorphin hypothermia and catalepsy. *Life Sciences*, **22**, 1537–1543

Holtz, A., Nystrom, B. and Gerdin, B. (1989) Spinal cord blood flow measured by 14-C-iodo-antipyrine autoradiography during and after graded spinal cord compression in rats. *Surgical Neurology*, **31**, 350–360

Horrocks, L.A., Demediuk, P., Saunders, R.D., Dugan, L., Clendenon, N.R., Means, E.D. and Anderson, D.K. (1985) The degradation of phospholipids, formation of metabolites of arachidonic acid, and demyelination following experimental spinal cord injury. *CNS Trauma*, **2**, 115–120

Howitt, W.M. and Turnbull, I.M. (1972) Effects of hypothermia and methysergide on recovery from experimental paraplegia. *Canadian Journal of Surgery*, **15**, 179–186

Hsu, C.Y., Halushka, P.V., Hogan, E.L., Banik, N.L., Lee, W.A. and Perot, P.L., Jr (1985) Alteration of thromboxane and prostacyclin levels in experimental spinal cord injury. *Neurology*, **35**, 1003–1009

Hsu, C.Y., Halushka, P.V., Hogan, E.L. and Cox, R.D. (1986) Increased thromboxane level in experimental spinal cord injury. *Journal of Neurological Science*, **74**, 289–296

Hsu, C.Y., Halushka, P.V., Spicer, K.M., Hogan, E.L. and Martin, H.F. (1988) Temporal profile of thromboxane-prostacyclin imbalance in experimental spinal cord injury. *Journal of Neurological Science*, **83**, 55–62

Iizuka, H., Yamamoto, T., Iwasaki, Y., Konno, H. and Kadoya, S. (1986) Experimental spinal cord injury: quantitation of axonal damage by automated image analysis. *Journal of Neurosurgery*, **64**, 304–308

Iizuka, H., Yamamoto, H., Iwasaki, Y., Yamamoto, T. and Konno, H. (1987) Evolution of tissue damage in compressive spinal cord injury in rats. *Journal of Neurosurgery*, **66**, 595–603

Ito, T., Allen, N. and Yashon, D. (1978) A mitochondrial lesion in experimental spinal cord trauma. *Journal of Neurosurgery*, **49**, 563–568

Iwasaki, Y., Yamamoto, H., Iizuka, H., Yamamoto, T. and Konno, H. (1987) Suppression of neurofilament degradation by protease inhibitors in experimental spinal cord injury. *Brain Research*, **406**, 99–104

Jacobs, T.P., Shohami, E., Baze, W., Burgard, E., Gunderson, C., Hallenbeck, J. and Feuerstein, G. (1987) Thromboxane and S-Hete increase after experimental spinal cord injury in rabbits. *CNS Trauma*, **4**, 95–118

Janssen, L. and Hansebout, R.R. (1989) Pathogenesis of spinal cord injury and newer treatments. A review. *Spine*, **14**, 23–32

Jones, R.F., Unsworth, I.P. and Marosszeky, J.E. (1978) Hyperbaric oxygen and acute spinal cord injuries in humans. *Medical Journal of Australia*, **2**, 573–575

Joyner, J. and Freeman, L.W. (1963) Urea and spinal cord trauma. *Neurology*, **13**, 69–72

Kajihara, K., Kawanaga, H., de la Torre, J.C. and Mullan, S. (1973) Dimethyl sulfoxide in the treatment of experimental acute spinal cord injury. *Surgical Neurology*, **1**, 16–22

Kakari, S., DeCrescito, V., Tomasula, J.J., Flamm, E.S. and Ransohoff, J. (1976) Long term studies of histochemical and cytochemical changes in the contused feline spinal cord. *Journal of Neuropathology and Experimental Neurology*, **35**, 109

Kao, C.C. and Chang, L.W. (1977) The mechanism of spinal cord cavitation following spinal cord transection. Part 1: A correlated histochemical study. *Journal of Neurosurgery*, **46**, 197–209

Kapadia, S.E. (1984) Ultrastructural alterations in blood vessels of the white matter after experimental spinal cord trauma. *Journal of Neurosurgery*, **61**, 539–544

Khan, M. and Griebel, R. (1983) Acute spinal cord injury in the rat: comparison of three experimental techniques. *Canadian Journal of Neurological Science*, **10**, 161–165

Kobrine, A.I. and Doyle, T.F. (1976) Role of histamine in posttraumatic luxury perfusion. *Journal of Neurosurgery*, **44**, 16–20

Kobrine, A.I., Doyle, T.F. and Martins, A.N. (1975) Local spinal cord blood flow in experimental traumatic myelopathy. *Journal of Neurosurgery*, **42**, 144–149

Kobrine, A.I., Evans, D.E., LeGrys, D.C., Yaffe, L.J. and Bradley, M.E. (1984) Effect of intravenous lidocaine on experimental spinal cord injury. *Journal of Neurosurgery*, **60**, 595–601

Koozekanani, S.H., Vise, W.M. and McGhee, R.B. (1976) Possible mechanisms for observed pathophysiological variability in experimental spinal cord injury by the method of Allen. *Journal of Neurosurgery*, **44**, 429–434

Koreh, K., Seligman, M.L., Flamm, E.S. and Demopoulos, H.B. (1981) Lipid antioxidant effects of naloxone *in vitro*. *Biochemical and Biophysical Research Communications*, **102**, 1317–1322

Kraig, R.P. and Nicholson, C. (1978) Extracellular ionic variation during spreading depression. *Neuroscience*, **3**, 1045–1059

Kretsinger, R.H. (1979) Calcium in neurobiology: a general theory of its function and evolution. In *The Neurosciences – Fourth Study Program* (eds F.O. Schmitt and F.G. Worden), MIT Press, Cambridge, Mass., pp. 617–622

Kuchner, E.F., Mercer, I.D., Pappius, H.M. and Hansebout, R.R. (1976) Experimental spinal cord injury: effects of steroids and/or cooling on edema, electrolyte and motor recovery. In *Dynamics of Brain Edema* (eds H.M. Pappins and W. Feindel), Springer-Verlag, Berlin, pp. 315–322

Kurihara, M. (1985) Role of monoamines in experimental spinal cord injury in rats. Relationship between Na-K-ATPase and lipid peroxidation. *Journal of Neurosurgery*, **62**, 743–749

Kuruvilla, A., Theodore, D.R. and Abraham, J. (1985) Changes in norepinephrine and histamine in monkey spinal cords traumatized by weight drop and compression. *CNS Trauma*, **2**, 61–68

Kushner, H., Markowitz, R.S., Mechanic, A. and Black, P. (1986) Models of spinal cord injury: Part 2. A mathematical model. *Neurosurgery*, **19**, 763–766

Kwo, S., Young, W. and De Crescito, V. (1989) Spinal cord sodium, potassium, calcium and water concentration changes in rats after graded contusion injury. *Journal of Neurotrauma*, **6**, 13–24

Lehman, K.G., Lane, J.G., Peipmeier, J.M. and Batsford, W.P. (1987) Cardiovascular abnormalities accompanying acute spinal cord injury in humans: incidence, time course and severity. *Journal of the American College of Cardiologists*, **10**, 46–52

Lewin, M.G., Hansebout, R.R. and Pappius, H.M. (1974) Chemical characteristics of traumatic spinal cord edema in cats. Effects of steroids on potassium depletion. *Journal of Neurosurgery*, **40**, 65–75

Lindquist, S. (1986) The heat shock response. *American Review of Biochemistry*, **55**, 1151–1191

Llinas, R. (1978) The role of calcium in neuronal function. In *The Neurosciences – Fourth Study Program* (eds F.O. Schmitt and F.G. Worden), MIT Press, Cambridge, Mass., pp. 555–572

Lohse, D.C., Senter, H.J., Kauer, J.S. and Wohns, R. (1980) Spinal cord blood flow in experimental transient traumatic paraplegia. *Journal of Neurosurgery*, **52**, 335–345

Long, J.B., Martinez-Arizala, A., Petras, J.M. and Holaday, J.W. (1986) Endogenous opioids in spinal cord injury: a critical evaluation. *CNS Trauma*, **3**, 295–315

Lux, W.E., Feuerstein, G. and Faden, A.I. (1983) Alteration of leukotriene D4 hypotension by thyrotropin-releasing hormone. *Nature*, **302**, 822–824

MacDermott, A.B., Mayer, M.L., Westbrook, G.L., Smith, S.J. and Barker, J.L. (1986) NMDA-receptor activation increases cytoplasmic calcium concentration in culture spinal cord neurons. *Nature*, **321**, 519–522

McVeigh, J.F. (1923) Experimental cord crushes with special reference to the mechanical factors involved and subsequent changes in the areas of the cord affected. *Archives of Surgery*, **7**, 573–600

Malik, M., Fenko, M.D., Iqbal, K. and Wisniewski, H.M. (1983) Purification of two forms of Ca^{++}-activated neutral protease from calf brain. *Journal of Biological Chemistry*, **258**, 8955–8962

Martin, S.H. and Bloedel, J.R. (1973) Evaluation of experimental spinal cord injury using cortical evoked potentials. *Journal of Neurosurgery*, **39**, 75–81

Matinian, L.A. and Andreasian, A.S. (1976) *Enzyme Therapy in Organic Lesions of the Spinal Cord*, Academia Nauk Armenian SSR, 1973, 94 pp. (English translation: Brain Information Service, University of California, Los Angeles, 156 pp.)

Matsumiya, N. and Dohi, S. (1983) Effects of intravenous or subarachnoid morphine on cerebral and spinal cord hemodynamics and antagonism with naloxone in dogs. *Anesthesiology*, **59**, 175–181

Maynard, F.M., Reynolds, G.G., Fountain, S., Wilmot, C. and Hamilton, R. (1979) Neurologic prognosis after traumatic quadriplegia. *Journal of Neurosurgery*, **50**, 611–619

Means, E.D. and Anderson, D.K. (1983) Neuronophagia by leukocytes in experimental spinal cord injury. *Journal of Neuropathology and Experimental Neurology*, **42**, 707–719

Means, E.D., Anderson, D.K. and Gutierrez, C. (1976) Light and electron microscopy of grey matter following experimental spinal cord compression injury. *Journal of Neuropathology and Experimental Neurology*, **35**, 348

Means, E.D., Anderson, D.K., Waters, T.R. and Kalaf, L. (1981) Effect of methylprednisolone in compression trauma to the feline spinal cord. *Journal of Neurosurgery*, **55**, 200–208

Meldrum, B. (1985) Possible therapeutic applications of antagonists of excitatory amino acid neurotransmitters. *Clinical Science*, **68**, 113–122

Misra, S.S., Singh, K.S. and Bhargava, K.P. (1967) Estimation of serotonin (5-HT) level in cerebrospinal fluid of patients with intracranial/spinal lesions. *Journal of Neurology, Neurosurgery and Psychiatry*, **30**, 163–165

Naftchi, N.E., Abrahams, S.J., St. Paul, H.M., Lowman, E.W. and Schlosser, W. (1978) Localization and changes of substance P in spinal cord of paraplegic rats. *Brain Research*, **153**, 507–513

Naftchi, N.E., Demeny, M., DeCrescito, V., Tomasula, J.J., Flamm, E.S. and Campbell, J.B. (1974) Biogenic amine concentrations in traumatized spinal cords of cats. Effect of drug therapy. *Journal of Neurosurgery*, **40**, 52–57

Nemecek, S., Petr, T., Suba, P., Rozsival, V. and Melka, O. (1977) Longitudinal extension of oedema in experimental spinal cord injury – evidence for two types of post-traumatic oedema. *Acta neurochirurgica*, **37**, 7–16

Nicholson, C. (1980) Modulation of extracellular calcium and its functional implications. *Federation Proceedings*, **39**, 1519–1523

Noble, L.J. and Wrathall, J.R. (1985) Spinal cord contusion in the rat: morphometric analysis of alterations in the spinal cord. *Experimental Neurology*, **88**, 134–149

Noyes, D.H. (1987a) Electromechanical impactor for producing experimental spinal cord injury in animals. *Medical and Biological Engineering and Computing*, **25**, 335–340

Noyes, D.H. (1987b) Correlation between parameters of spinal cord impact and resultant injury. *Experimental Neurology*, **95**, 535–547

Nygren, L.G., Olson, L. and Seiger, A. (1977) Monoamine reinnervation of the transected spinal cord by homologous fetal brain tissue. *Brain Research*, **124**, 227–235

Olney, J.W., Ho, O.L. and Rhee, V. (1971) Cytotoxic effects of acidic and sulfur-containing amino acids on the infant mouse central nervous system. *Experimental Brain Research*, **14**, 61–76

Osterholm, J.L. (1974) The pathophysiological response to spinal cord injury. *Journal of Neurosurgery*, **40**, 5–33

Osterholm, J.L., Alderman, J.B., Triolo, A.J., D'Amore, B.R. and Williams, H.D. (1984) Oxygenated fluorocarbon nutrient solution in the treatment of experimental spinal cord injury. *Neurosurgery*, **15**, 373–380

Osterholm, J.L. and Mathews, G.J. (1972) Altered norepinephrine metabolism following experimental spinal cord injury. Part 2: Protection against traumatic spinal cord hemorrhagic necrosis by norepinephrine synthesis blockade with alpha-methyltyrosine. *Journal of Neurosurgery*, **36**, 395–401

Pallini, R., Fernandez, E., Gangitano, C., Del Fa, A., Oliveri-Sangiacomo, C. and Sbriccoli, A. (1989) Studies on embryonic transplants to the transected spinal cord of adult rats. *Journal of Neurosurgery*, **70**, 454–462

Pallini, R., Fernandez, E. and Sbriccoli, A. (1988) Retrograde degeneration of corticospinal axons following transection of the spinal cord in rats. A quantitative study with anterogradely transported horseradish peroxidase. *Journal of Neurosurgery*, **68**, 124–128

Parker, A.J. and Smith, C.W. (1974) Functional recovery from spinal cord trauma following incision of spinal meninges in dogs. *Research in Veterinary Science*, **16**, 276–279

Parker, A.J. and Smith, C.W. (1976) Functional recovery from spinal cord trauma following dexamethasone and chlorpromazine therapy in dogs. *Research in Veterinary Science*, **21**, 246–247

Phillipi, R., Kuhn, W., Zach, G.A., Jacob-Chia, D., Dollfus, P. and Mole, J.P. (1980) Survey of the neurological evaluation of 300 spinal cord injuries seen within 24 hours after injury. *Paraplegia*, **18**, 337–346

Politis, M.J. and Zenakis, M.F. (1988) Short term efficacy of applied electric field in the repair of the damaged rodent spinal cord: behavioral and morphological results. *Neurosurgery*, **23**, 582–588

Raichle, M.E. (1983) The pathophysiology of brain ischemia. *Annals of Neurology*, **13**, 2–10

Raines, A., Dretchen, K.L., Marx, K. and Wrathall, J.R. (1988) Spinal cord contusion in the rat: somatosensory evoked potentials as a function of graded injury. *Journal of Neurotrauma*, **5**, 151–160

Reier, P.J. (1985) Neural tissue graft and repair of the injured spinal cord. *Neuropathology and Applied Neurobiology*, **11**, 81–104

Rivlin, A.S. and Tator, C. (1977) Objective clinical assessment of motor function after experimental spinal cord injury in the rat. *Journal of Neurosurgery*, **49**, 577–581

Rivlin, A.S. and Tator, C.H. (1978) Regional spinal cord blood flow in rats after severe cord trauma. *Journal of Neurosurgery*, **49**, 844–853

Robertson, C.S., Foltz, R., Grossman, R.G. and Goodman, J.C. (1986) Protection against experimental ischemic spinal cord injury. *Journal of Neurosurgery*, **64**, 633–642

Romero-Sierra, C., Sierhuis, A., Hansebout, R.R. and Lewin, M. (1974) A new method for localized cord cooling. In *Medical and Biological Engineering*, National Research Council of Canada, Ottawa, pp. 188–193

Rosenthal, M., LaManna, J., Yamada, S., Younts, W. and Somjen, G. (1979) Oxidative metabolism, extracellular potassium and sustained potential shifts in cat spinal cord *in situ*. *Brain Research*, **162**, 113–127

Rowed, D.W. (1982) Value of somatosensory evoked potentials for prognosis in partial cord injuries. In *Early Management of Acute Spinal Cord Injury* (ed. C.H. Tator), Raven Press, New York, pp. 167–180

Ruigrok, T.J.C. (1982) The calcium paradox: mechanisms and clinical relevance. In *The Role of Calcium in Biological Systems*, Vol. II (eds L.J. Anghilari and A.M. Tuffet-Anghileri), CRC Press, Boca Raton, Florida, pp. 133–141

Salzman, S.K., Hirofugi, E., Knight, P.B., Llados-Eckman, C., Beckman, A.L. and Winokur, A. (1987b) Treatment of experimental spinal trauma with thyrotropin-releasing hormone: central serotonergic and vascular mechanisms of action. *CNS Trauma*, **4**, 181–196

Salzman, S.K., Hirofuji, E., Llados-Eckman, C., MacEwen, G.D. and Beckman, A.L. (1987a) Monoaminergic responses to spinal trauma. Participation of serotonin in posttraumatic progression of neural damage. *Journal of Neurosurgery*, **66**, 431–439

Sandler, A.N. and Tator, C.H. (1976) Review of the effects of spinal cord trauma on vessels and blood flow in the spinal cord. *Journal of Neurosurgery*, **45**, 638–646

Saunders, R.D., Dugan, L.L., Demediuk, P., Means, E.D., Horrocks, L.A. and Anderson, D.K. (1987) Effects of methylprednisolone and the combination of α-tocopherol and selenium on arachidonic acid metabolism and lipid peroxidation in traumatized spinal cord tissue. *Journal of Neurochemistry*, **49**, 24–31

Schanne, F., Kane, A.B., Young, E.E. and Farber, J.L. (1979) Calcium dependence of toxic cell death: a final common pathway. *Science*, **206**, 700–702

Schoultz, T.W., DeLucca, D.C. and Reding, D.L. (1976) Norepinephrine levels in traumatized spinal cord of catecholamine-depleted cats. *Brain Research*, **109**, 367–374

Schramm, J., Krause, T., Shigeno, T. and Brock, M. (1983) Experimental investigation on the spinal cord evoked injury potential. *Journal of Neurosurgery*, **59**, 485–492

Senter, H.J. and Venes, J.L. (1978) Altered blood flow and secondary injury in experimental spinal cord trauma. *Journal of Neurosurgery*, **49**, 569–578

Simon, R.P., Swan, J.H., Griffiths, T. and Meldrum, B.S. (1984) Blockade of N-methyl-D-aspartate receptors may protect against ischemic damage in the brain. *Science*, **226**, 850–852

Smith, A.J.K., McCreery, D.B., Bloedel, J.R. and Chou, S.N. (1978) Hyperemia, CO_2 responsivity, and autoregulation in the white matter following experimental spinal cord injury. *Journal of Neurosurgery*, **48**, 239–251

Steen, P.A., Newberg, L.A., Milde, J.H. and Michenfelder, J.D. (1983) Cerebral blood flow and neurologic outcome when nimodipine is given after complete cerebral ischemia in the dog. *Journal of Cerebral Blood Flow Metabolism*, **3**, 38–43

Stewart, W.B. (1985) Edema in spinal cord injury. In *Central Nervous System Trauma Status Report* (eds D.P. Becker and J.T. Povlishok), National Institutes of Health, Bethesda, Md, pp. 475–479

Stokes, B.T., Fox, P. and Hollinden, G. (1983) Extracellular calcium activity in the injured spinal cord. *Experimental Neurology*, **80**, 561–572

Stokes, B.T., Fox, P. and Hollinden, G. (1985) Extracellular metabolites: their measurement and role in the acute phase of spinal cord injury. In *Proceedings of the Fifth Neurotrauma Conference* (ed. J. Jane), Raven Press, New York, pp. 309–324

Stumm, W. and Morgan, J.J. (1981) *Aquatic Chemistry – An Introduction Emphasizing Chemical Equilibria in Natural Waters*, John Wiley, New York, pp. 230–322

Sugigama, S., Kitazawa, M. and Ozawa, T. (1980) Anti-oxidative effect of coenzyme Q. *Experientia*, **36**, 1002–1003

Tarlov, I.M. (1957) *Spinal Cord Compression: Mechanism of Paralysis and Treatment*, Charles C. Thomas, Springfield, Ill.

Tarlov, I.M., Klinger, H. and Vitale, S. (1953) Spinal cord compression studies: 1. Experimental techniques to produce acute and gradual compression. *Archives of Neurology and Psychiatry*, **70**, 813–819

Tator, C.H. (1973) Acute spinal cord injury in primates produced by an inflatable extradural cuff. *Canadian Journal of Surgery*, **16**, 222–231

Tator, C.H. and van der Jagt, R.H.C. (1980) The effect of exogenous thyroid hormones on functional recovery of the rat after acute spinal cord compression injury. *Journal of Neurosurgery*, **53**, 381–384

Tator, C.H. and Rivlin, A.S. (1983) Elimination of root regeneration in studies of spinal cord regeneration. *Surgical Neurology*, **19**, 255–259

Tator, C.H., Rivlin, A.S., Lewis, A.J. and Schmoll, B. (1983) Effect of triiodo-L-thyronine in axonal regeneration in the rat spinal cord after acute compression injury. *Journal of Neurosurgery*, **58**, 406–410

Thompson, J.E. (1923) Pathological changes occurring in the spinal cord following fracture dislocation of the vertebrae. *Annals of Surgery*, **78**, 260–293

de la Torre, J.C. (1981) Spinal cord injury: review of basic and applied research. *Spine*, **6**, 315–334

de la Torre, J.C. (1984) Spinal cord injury models. *Progress in Neurobiology*, **22**, 289–344

de la Torre, J.C. and Boggan, J.E. (1980) Neurophysiological recording in rat spinal cord trauma. *Experimental Neurology*, **70**, 356–370

de la Torre, J.C., Johnson, C.M., Goode, D.J. and Mullan, S. (1975) Pharmacologic treatment and evaluation of permanent experimental spinal cord trauma. *Neurology*, **25**, 508–514

Urry, D.W. (1978) Basic aspects of calcium chemistry and membrane interaction: on the messenger role of calcium. *Annals of the New York Academy of Sciences*, **307**, 3–27

Wagner, F.C. and Stewart, W.B. (1981) Effect of trauma dose on spinal cord edema. *Journal of Neurosurgery*, **54**, 802–806

Walker, J.G., Yates, R.R. and Yashon, D. (1979) Regional canine spinal cord energy state after experimental trauma. *Journal of Neurochemistry*, **33**, 397–401

Wallace, M.C. and Tator, C.H. (1986) Failure of naloxone to improve spinal cord blood flow and cardiac output after spinal cord injury. *Neurosurgery*, **18**, 428–432

Wallace, M.C. and Tator, C.H. (1987a) Successful improvement of blood pressure, cardiac output, and spinal cord blood flow after experimental spinal cord injury. *Neurosurgery*, **20**, 710–715

Wallace, M.C. and Tator, C.H. (1987b) Effect of alternating current stimulation of the spinal cord on recovery from acute spinal cord injury in rats. *Surgical Neurology*, **28**, 269–276

Wallace, M.C., Tator, C.H. and Frazee, P. (1986) Relationship between posttraumatic ischemia and hemorrhage in the injured rat spinal cord as shown by colloidal carbon angiography. *Neurosurgery*, **18**, 433–439

Windle, W.F. (1980) Concussion, contusion and severance of the spinal cord. In *The Spinal Cord and Its Reaction to Traumatic Injury* (ed. W.F. Windle), Marcel Dekker, New York, pp. 205–217

Windle, W.F. and Chambers, W.W. (1950) Regeneration in the spinal cord of the cat and dog. *Journal of Comparative Neurology*, **67**, 493–509

Windle, W.F., Littrell, J.L., Smart, J.O. and Joralemon, J. (1956) Regeneration in the cord of spinal monkeys. *Neurology*, **6**, 420–428

Windle, W.F., Smart, J.O. and Beers, J.J. (1958) Residual function after subtotal spinal cord transection in adult cats. *Neurology*, **8**, 518–521

Wolfe, L.S. (1982) Eicosanoids: prostaglandin, thromboxanes, leukotrienes and other derivatives of carbon-20 unsaturated fatty acids. *Journal of Neurochemistry*, **38**, 1–14

Wrathall, J.R., Kapoor, V. and Kao, C.C. (1984) Observation of cultured peripheral non-neuronal cells implanted into the transected spinal cord. *Acta neuropathologica (Berlin)*, **64**, 203–212

Yaksh, T.L. (1987) Opioid receptor systems and the endorphins: a review of their spinal organization. *Journal of Neurosurgery*, **67**, 157–176

Yaksh, T.L. and Tyce, G.M. (1980) Resting and K^+ evoked release of serotonin and norepinephrine *in vivo* from the rat and cat spinal cord. *Brain Research*, **192**, 133–146

Yashon, D. (1978) Pathogenesis of spinal cord injury. *Orthopedic Clinics of North America*, **9**, 247–261

Yashon, D., Bingham, W.D. Jr. Faddoul, E.M. and Hunt, W.E. (1973) Edema of the spinal cord following experimental impact trauma. *Journal of Neurosurgery*, **38**, 693–697

Yeo, J.D. (1984) The use of hyperbaric oxygen to modify the effects of recent contusion injury to the spinal cord. *CNS Trauma*, **1**, 161–165

Yeo, J., Payne, W. and Hinwood, B. (1975) The experimental contusion injury of the spinal cord in sheep. *Paraplegia*, **12**, 275–296

Young, W. (1982) Correlation of somatosensory evoked potentials and neurological findings in spinal cord injury. In *Early Management of Acute Spinal Cord Injury* (ed. C.H. Tator), Raven Press, New York, pp. 153–165

Young, W. (1985) Blood flow, metabolic and neurophysiologic mechanisms in spinal cord injury. In *Central Nervous System Trauma Status Report* (eds. D.P. Becker and J.T. Povlishok), National Institutes of Health, Bethesda, Md, pp. 463–473

Young, W. (1986) Ca paradox in neural injury: a hypothesis. *CNS Trauma*, **3**, 235–251

Young, W. (1987) Post-injury responses in trauma and ischemia: secondary injury or protective mechanisms? *CNS Trauma*, **4**, 27–51

Young, W., De Crescito, V., Tomasula, J.J. and Ho, V. (1980) The role of the sympathetic nervous system in pressor responses induced by spinal injury. *Journal of Neurosurgery*, **52**, 473–481

Young, W. and Flamm, E.S. (1982) Effect of high dose corticosteroid therapy on blood flow, evoked potentials and extracellular calcium in experimental spinal injury. *Journal of Neurosurgery*, **57**, 667–673

Young, W., Flamm, E.S., Demopoulos, H.B., Tomasula, J.J. and DeCrescito, V. (1981) Effect of naloxone on post-traumatic ischemia in experimental spinal contusion. *Journal of Neurosurgery*, **55**, 209–219

Young, W. and Koreh, I. (1986) Potassium and calcium changes in injured spinal cords. *Brain Research*, **365**, 42–53

Young, W., Koreh, I., Yen, V. and Lindsay, A. (1982) Effect of sympathectomy on extracellular potassium activity and blood flow in experimental spinal cord contusion. *Brain Research,* **253**, 115–125

Young, W., Tomasula, J.J., DeCrescito, V., Flamm, E.S. and Ransohoff, J. (1980) Vestibulospinal monitoring in experimental spinal trauma. *Journal of Neurosurgery,* **52**, 64–72

Young, W., Yen, V. and Blight, A.R. (1982) Extracellular calcium activity in experimental spinal contusion. *Brain Research,* **253**, 115–125

Chapter 13

Moral and legal issues in the treatment of patients with spinal cord injuries

Kathleen Marie Dixon

Introduction

Traumatic spinal cord injuries (SCIs) are catastrophic and unexpected events. Patients and families are shocked by the abrupt or violent aspect of this tragedy. Few, if any, are prepared for a dramatic intrusion of disability into their lives. Spinal cord injuries present substantial challenges to patients who must address the impact of physical handicap on their concept of self and sense of personal value. Patients must not only confront new physical restrictions, but must surmount tremendous social barriers that limit the opportunities available to the disabled.

Treatment of patients with SCIs forces physicians to develop acceptable responses to perplexing moral and legal questions. Four of these questions will be considered in this chapter. First, how is the doctrine of informed consent best applied to the treatment of spinal cord injured patients? Second, what should be done when a spinal cord injured patient wishes to die? Third, what are the moral and legal foundations of third parties' entitlements to determine care for incompetent spinal cord injured patients? Finally, how may standards for minimally adequate quality of life be determined? Two case histories have been constructed in order to illustrate effective deliberation and analysis of these moral issues.

Profiles of spinal cord injury: when should patient dissent be considered definitive?
   Robert Williams is a 30-year-old master cabinet maker who has worked with a local builder for the past 10 years. Mr Williams has been married for 7 years. His wife, June, is a 28-year-old librarian who works part-time at the neighborhood elementary school. The couple have three children, Jeremy, age 6; Sarah, age 4; and Rachel, age 2½. Robert was driving the company truck to a home in order to supervise the installation of new cabinets and wall units when his vehicle was struck by a drunk driver. The force of the collision sent Mr Williams' truck careering across the highway into oncoming traffic where it was struck several times, from the side and the rear. Mr Williams had been wearing a lap and shoulder harness at the time of the accident. He sustained damage to his arms, legs and torso. Mr Williams retained consciousness. He was surprised to find that he had no pain from the lacerations on his arms, legs and trunk. He attempted to release his harness and climb from the car, but when he found that he was unable to move, he fainted. Emergency medical technicians transported Mr Williams to the emergency ward of City Hospital where he was assessed. Physicians noted swelling and bruising of the spinal cord at C3. They discovered a fracture of the

cervical vertebrae at C4. Mr Williams also sustained a fracture of the distal portion of the left tibia.

Mr Williams recovered consciousness in the emergency room. The anesthesiologist on the ward, Dr Patricia Edwards, informed him that he had been in a car accident and had sustained injury to his spinal cord. She indicated that he needed treatment to stabilize his spinal column. A conservative, non-surgical treatment would be attempted. She gently explained that a special device would be fitted to his skull so that traction could be applied to his neck. A tracheostomy might be performed if his breathing became labored and difficult. Dr Edwards told him that ventilators were available to assist him with his breathing should it become necessary. Finally, she told Mr Williams that he would be placed on a special bed that would help to immobilize his spine and prevent him from getting bed sores. Mr Williams listened and said, 'Doctor, I can't feel anything in my chest or legs? Am I paralyzed? Will I walk again?' Dr Edwards told him that they had visualized damage to the spinal cord and vertebrae at points on his neck. She said they did not yet know if the lesion was partial or complete. Mr Williams asked Dr Edwards to do everything possible to restore him to function.

Mr Williams subsequently found himself in a hospital room, unable to move his head or his body. He could only stare at a point on the ceiling. He felt like a balloon, he thought he was floating, his legs felt as if they were rising off the bed (Trieschmann, 1988). The only thing that held him down was the tube that attached him to the machine. He was comforted by the realization that the machine was his anchor. He wouldn't float away. Mrs Williams noticed that her husband was awake. She told him that a tracheostomy had been performed. He was attached to a ventilator. She asked him if he was in any pain. While Mr Williams was not suffering from his injuries, he did feel disoriented and stunned. He was relieved to find that his wife had been informed. Mrs Williams related the story of the accident to him and described the initial care he had received. He lay in bed for what seemed to be a long time, trying to grapple with what had occurred. He dozed off and was stunned when he awoke and found himself facing the floor.

Dr Trevor Montgomery, attending physician in the intensive care unit, stopped to examine and interview Mr Williams on his afternoon rounds. He found the patient responsive and anxious to learn about his medical condition. Dr Montgomery explained that Mr Williams had suffered a number of injuries in the accident. He had a concussion, two ribs were broken, he had a fracture of the large bone in the lower part of his left leg, and he had a number of lacerations. These were all being treated. Dr Montgomery explained that the lack of feeling and inability to move that so disturbed Mr Williams was the result of an injury to his spinal cord. He indicated that until the damage to the cervical vertebrae was corrected and the bones were healed, they would not be able to be certain about the level of the lesion and extent of neurological damage (Trieschmann, 1988). Mr Williams indicated, 'Doctor, will I ever walk again?' Dr Montgomery paused and said, 'I can't imagine what this must be like for you. I want to be honest, you *are paralyzed* and won't be able to walk, but perhaps *you won't always be on a ventilator* and you *may be able to use your shoulder muscles*.' Dr Montgomery continued for a few moments, but Mr Williams only heard a dull droning. The word 'paralyzed' was echoing in his brain. With a jolt he thought, 'Oh, God! I'm going to be this way for the rest of my life.'

Mr Williams' primary nurse noted that although he cooperated with requests and responded to questions, he seemed withdrawn and anxious the rest of the day. When Dr Montgomery came to see him the following afternoon, Mr Williams indicated that he wanted all treatment to be discontinued. By signs he said, 'If what you told me yesterday is true, the damage to my spinal cord cannot be reversed. I am not going to get any better. Please understand me, I am not ungrateful for what you have done. But, I don't want to live this way – it will be far too great a strain on myself and my family. I don't want to live the rest of my life as a *helpless cripple*. Please let me die!'

Models of decision-making in the clinical setting: the doctrine of informed consent reconsidered

This case raises the question of the foundation and extent of patients' entitlements to determine the course of their medical care. In so doing it forces physicians to chart a reasonable course between twin perils. If physicians adopt a libertarian moral framework, asserting that the fundamental right of competent individuals is to be left alone, they may allow Mr Williams to die. This interpretation of the moral requirements of respect for patient autonomy will result in unnecessary loss of life. It prioritizes the current preferences of the patient and precludes subsequent restoration to a sense of the significance or value of life. If physicians adopt a paternalistic approach, they will override Mr Williams' objections to treatment. He will be forced to endure a rigorous and prolonged course of therapy and rehabilitation. Absence of control over his own fate may deepen feelings of inadequacy and vulnerability. Treatment will become an ordeal coercively imposed by others. For a patient who remains unconvinced of the beneficent motives or ends of treatment, continued care can be seen as torture. Nurses and physicians will become the patient's jailers and wardens.

Mr Williams' case challenges us to reconsider traditional paradigms for consent. Most models presume that the consenting party is an adequate independent decision-maker. This person is thought to require only case specific data in order to make an appropriate choice. Patients are thought to have stable, well-deliberated or authentic life-plans and goals that might be expressed as functions. Diagnoses, prognoses, and treatment options serve as dependent variables in these functions. Thus, it is thought that if a patient is to make a reasonable treatment decision, he or she must have access to information about: the inherent and potential hazards of proposed treatments, the results of a failure to obtain treatment, and the benefits that can be reasonably expected from each treatment option*. These data are then inserted into the functions as values for the dependent variables in the patient's case. This process is thought to result in an autonomous choice.

Analogous justification can be made for professional authority. Physicians have readier access to and greater facility with technical data. Their knowledge of the nuances of diagnosis allows for a more subtle understanding of the patient's medical status. Their training and experience permit them to refine distinctions between various courses of medical care, arriving at an independent evaluation of attendant risks and benefits. Thus, it is thought that physicians' formulae only require patient specific data on socio-moral values in order to be complete. Physicians possessing this information could insert it in pre-existing functions and derive an appropriate treatment decision.

* *Canterbury v. Spence*, 464 F. 2d 772, 785 (D.C. Cir. 1972).

In acute treatment of SCI, neither patient nor physician is a fully adequate independent decision-maker. Individuals admitted to emergency wards or intensive care units for post-trauma care experience medical and psychological complications that limit their ability to dictate the course of their medical care. Stover and Fine (1986) reported that diagnoses of coma or stupor were made in 5.2% of patients admitted for treatment of SCI. An additional 2% had suffered cerebral laceration and contusion.

Trieschmann (1988) suggests that in the majority of cases of SCI, initial awareness of the damage is followed by a period of shock. Thus, patients may not be able to absorb much of the information initially presented to them. They may feel strangely distanced from the flurry of medical activity around them. Like Mr Williams, they may not yet appreciate the significance or implications of the information provided.

During the period initially following injury, the patient's deliberations and choices may be influenced by anger or situational depression (McGowan and Roth, 1987). Dembo, Leviton and Wright (1975) argue that adjustment to disability should be seen as a process of mourning and, eventually, resolution of grief. Thus, it could be argued that spinal cord injured individuals must reach a psychological and emotional accommodation to the loss of certain physical abilities. Only then will they be restored to effective and personally satisfying function in their world.

Another feature of the social landscape of disability further distances the individual with SCI from the philosophical ideal of the completely rational and dispassionate deliberator. Those with handicapping conditions frequently experience a dramatic loss of self-esteem as they acquire a 'stigmatized identity' (Goffman, 1963). The list of capacities and accomplishments that help to form the backbone of personal identity are irrevocably changed. It is more difficult to maintain one's position as a peer in the social and moral community when one can no longer perform the simplest tasks of personal care. Patients' perceptions of themselves as competent and valuable individuals are further eroded as they appreciate the adverse impact that disability has on many of their relationships. Many able-bodied persons are unfamiliar with acceptable patterns of behavior governing interaction with the handicapped. As a result, friends and acquaintances are suddenly uncomfortable in the patient's presence. They are unable to converse or find common ground. This isolation reinforces the patient's perceptions of self as 'damaged goods'. Patients attempting to reject this classification may be unable to engage in a reconstruction of the meaning of disability that preserves personal identity. Like Mr Williams, they may believe that only death will preserve personal integrity and dignity.

Factors that limit adequate or effective deliberation by spinal cord injured patients are widely discussed in the professional literature (Wittkower et al., 1954; Gunther, 1969; Dembo, Leviton and Wright, 1975). Consideration of analogous deficits in providers' perceptions or patterns of reasoning are more difficult to find. The adequacy of independent decision-making by medical authorities is dependent upon providers' abilities to assess patients' situations accurately. They must subsequently identify and employ patients' schedules of social and moral values. Trieschmann (1988) has challenged professionals' characterizations of patients' mental and emotional states. She reviews the literature describing stages of adjustment to SCI concluding:

It is important to note that each of the preceding descriptions of stages of adjustment is based on the *clinical impressions of the particular author, and that no data have been presented in any of these articles to demonstrate reliably and validly the existence, sequence, or duration of these stages.*

Trieschmann (1988) suggests that professionals have an exaggerated sense of the distress and psychological difficulty associated with SCI. They impose inappropriate interpretative frameworks on patient behavior, confusing hope or inattention to pain with denial (Goldiamond, 1973) and lack of facility in verbal expression with depression (Rohe and Athelstan, 1982). While professionals' explanatory models may be clumsy indicators of the nature of individual patients' experiences, they may be more accurate expressions of the providers' own values. This point is illustrated in Wright's notion of the 'requirement of mourning'. Wright argues that individuals need to emphasize a passive response to disability in order to sustain their own system of values. Wright (1960) states:

When a person has a need to safeguard his values, he will either (1) insist that the person he considers unfortunate is suffering (even when he seems not to be suffering) or (2) devaluate the unfortunate person because he ought to suffer and he does not.

Thus, physicians and other health care providers should take great care to avoid interpretative frameworks that project onto patients providers' own assessments of the limited value and competence of the disabled. Not only do such theories reinforce destructive stereotypes, but they allow individuals to engage in a psychological distancing that encourages abuse through the avoidance of responsibility. This theme is represented in the work of spinal cord injured authors. Goldiamond (1973) observes:

Reaction to one's own injury is supposed to cause depression. By considering apathy, depression, or aggression as inevitable developmental stages in injury (or aging or illness), the professional staff can avoid asking how their actions might have been causal.

Physicians' adequacy as independent decision-makers for spinal cord injured patients has been contested on the grounds that their ability to assess two important parts of the patient's world view accurately, i.e. the patient's mental and emotional states, is insufficiently developed. Providers' adequacy as independent decision-makers can be challenged on another front. Physicians are unlikely to have access to any *external* source of complete and reliable information about patient values. In the emergency ward or intensive care unit, physicians and patients are strangers, encountering each other for the first time. Thus, there will be virtually no pre-existing appreciation for the details of the patient's value system. Alternate sources of information about the patient's moral commitments may not be available. While many individuals have discussed with family or friends their preferences for care should they be faced with incurable illness, few have indicated how they would wish to be treated if they were to suffer SCI resulting in quadriplegia or paraplegia. Patients who have said that they do not wish to have ventilators employed in a context of terminal illness may have given no indication of their views about temporary respiratory assistance or permanent dependence on portable ventilators installed in wheelchairs. Finally, physicians providing emergency care to spinal cord injured patients may either not have access to a living will enacted by the patient or may be unable to obtain meaningful direction from a vague or poorly executed document.

Recognition that neither physicians or patients are fully adequate independent decision-makers propels us toward a truly collaborative model of medical care. Both parties must candidly admit limitations on the freedom or effectiveness of their deliberations. They must also express their commitment to acknowledge and respect other points of view. Only then will they avoid the twin perils of atomistic individualism and professional authoritarianism. In so doing, they will be able to give fullest expression to the fundamental moral principle supporting requirements to obtain informed and voluntary consent from competent persons considering medical care, the principle of respect for persons. For this principle prohibits us from treating an entity capable of rational self-direction as a mere means to any given end. Respect for individuals' capacity for self-direction requires us to recognize mutual consent as the foundation of all rules governing the interaction of competent individuals. At the same time, we express the unconditional value of the capacity for rational thought and action by attempting to identify and overcome barriers to effective deliberation. Parties adopting this moral framework will attempt to reach a negotiated settlement in which they extend the horizons of their own concerns and expand their intellectual and behavioral repertoires.

How might these insights be applied to the case of Mr Williams? Let us begin with an examination of the models of disclosure presented in the case. Dr Edwards offers Mr Williams an overview of his injuries and sketch of medical care phrased in simple language, accessible to almost any patient. Only occasionally does she resort to technical terms. She provides information in order to orient the patient to his situation. In so doing, she reduces his confusion and anxiety. She does not offer Mr Williams information on the risks of treatment. Thus, she does not attempt to obtain a legally valid, informed and voluntary consent from the patient at this time.

This decision should not put the doctor and her colleagues in legal jeopardy. For when patients require emergency medical assistance and an attempt to gain consent would delay treatment, placing the patient's life and health at significant risk, consent can be presumed. American law usually requires that the attending physician have no reason to believe that the patient would reject essential medical care (Faden and Beauchamp, 1986). This provision has been readily fulfilled through Mr Williams' request for maximally aggressive treatment.

Although disclosure was not sufficient to support an informed and voluntary consent by the patient, it was adequate to support a less demanding standard of ratification of treatment. His request should be considered a morally meaningful *assent* to medical care. For Mr Williams is arguably capable of appreciating his situation, making reasonably free choices, and communicating these selections clearly and unambiguously (Levine, 1981). It should be noted, however, that when a patient would not be unduly hazarded by the delay, physicians are legally required to seek proxy consent to medical intervention (Faden and Beauchamp, 1986).

Dr Edwards and Dr Montgomery achieve an effective balance between the reliability of available data and the genuine uncertainty of subsequent outcome in their representations of the level and extent of neurological damage. In so doing, they provide accurate data in a compassionate and supportive manner. They do not attempt to purchase amelioration of Mr Williams' present distress at the price of subsequent depression and loss of trust. Thus, they avoid holding out false hopes that he might walk again. Their judicious use of review further assists Mr Williams in his effort to come to terms with his situation. Dr Edwards' and Dr Montgomery's decisions to review the sequence of events and schedule of care with Mr Williams represent conscious and appropriate attempts to combat the disorienting features of sudden, severe injury and hospitalization.

If a truly collaborative model of medical care is to be applied in Mr Williams' case, one that acknowledges the limitations on the deliberations of physicians and patient, then all parties will have to commit to participation in sustained and respectful dialogue regarding available options. Parties must also recognize that negotiation of treatment is no less important than actual provision of care. Collaboration is not to be reduced to the status of a sham to elicit patient consent.

Collaborative model of medical care and the right to die

How should Dr Montgomery respond to Mr Williams' request that all treatment be discontinued and he be permitted to die? He might do well to begin by reassuring Mr Williams that he will not be forced to endure a prolonged and difficult course of treatment or rehabilitation against his will. He might also indicate that he and his colleagues recognize that individuals have different levels of tolerance for pain and frustration. Although education, counseling, and medical intervention can help to improve our level of tolerance, we cannot compel individuals to avail themselves of these opportunities. Neither can we chastise those who pursue decisions for death after obtaining no relief despite consistent and appropriate use of techniques derived from these disciplines. Dr Montgomery might suggest that the most that anyone can ask of individuals facing an ordeal is that they make their best effort to respond to the challenges presented while preserving their personal integrity and capacity to find meaning or value in life.

Once these fundamental commitments have been acknowledged, Dr Montgomery can go on to address factors that limit the adequacy or effectiveness of independent deliberations by participants. He can readily admit that despite his considerable expertise in the treatment of patients with SCI and his familiarity with an interdisciplinary literature on the subject, he does not *know how it feels* to have one's world turned upside down in this manner. Neither can he predict Mr Williams' precise response to common problems and hurdles. Dr Montgomery can indicate that he will rely on Mr Williams to share his thoughts and experiences with members of the health care team. In this way, patient and physician can achieve an optimal balance of challenges and resources. Thus, both parties will be able to make maximal use of their abilities in the realization of a negotiated outcome.

At this point, the stage has been set for a discussion of limitations in the patient's ability to make fully adequate independent determinations of his own fate. Dr Montgomery should step gingerly here. He must first help Mr Williams to recognize the factors that presently shape or influence his response. These may then be identified either as essential components of any rational decision or impediments to completely effective deliberation. Dr Montgomery will have to make good use of active listening and other interview skills. He will have to avoid prejudgment, maintaining an open mind. Provider and patient should work together to reach a joint evaluation of the factors influencing their perceptions and thought. Throughout this process Dr Montgomery must express and reinforce his appreciation of Mr Williams as a fully franchised member of the moral community, accorded equal dignity and respect.

We should take a few moments now to consider some of the factors that might be influencing Mr Williams' decision to reject further treatment. Mr Williams states that he realizes that he will not get any better. While it is true that he will never recover his ability to make conscious and voluntary use of the muscles in his chest, trunk or lower extremities, his medical condition may well 'improve'. If subsequent tests reveal that his level of normal neurological function is C4, he is capable of independent respiration and may be successfully weaned from the ventilator (Trieschmann, 1988). This might significantly improve his assessment of his quality of life.

Mr Williams is worried about the impact of his disability on his family. He may feel that requirements for his care represent an unwarranted financial burden for them, one that will deprive them of needed goods and services. This is not a wild or inappropriate concern. Mr Williams probably does not yet appreciate the full extent of the costs associated with treatment in the USA for SCI. Whiteneck et al. (1985) report a mean total expense for acute and rehabilitative care of $305 801 for respirator-dependent patients and $108 028 for patients capable of independent respiration. Mr Williams has, as of yet, no way of calculating the costs of living with a SCI. There are a number of services he may require after discharge: rehospitalization, perhaps for treatment of urinary tract infections or pressure sores; outpatient treatment; a personal attendant to assist in activities of daily living; a specially equipped car or van, and modifications to the family dwelling. Whiteneck et al. (1985) report that average annual disability related expenses for a respirator-dependent individuals with high quadriplegia are $101 246. The same figure for patients capable of independent respiration is $27 607. Any candid evaluator will acknowledge that this is a grim situation. These costs are far too significant to fail to be appreciated by most families. Even so, Mr Williams is more fortunate than many of the spinal cord injured patients treated in the USA. He may be eligible for Worker's Compensation. He may also recover disability-related expenses by proceeding with litigation against the drunk driver. Compensatory and punitive damages for such an extensive injury would be high. They would help to further defray costs of his care and maintenance.

We would do Mr Williams a disservice if we made no attempt to put these financial costs into a broader perspective. What is the value of a person's life? Without doubt, Mr Williams' world has been altered by SCI. He has suffered a substantial loss that will make his life more difficult. Yet, he and his family need not be seen as victims helplessly playing out some scripted roles in a tragedy. Mr Williams' intellectual powers are undiminished; he retains the capacity to find, make or experience intrinsic value (Attig, 1979). Some avenues of enjoyment or expression have been cut off, but many others remain. Mr Williams can be a co-director and an active participant in the development and life of his family. He can give love, support, and direction to his wife and children.

It may well be that Mr Williams appreciates these factors and intends to sacrifice his own opportunities for meaning and development to protect his family from pain or financial hardship. Dr Montgomery might want to help Mr Williams to free himself from falsely dichotomous thinking. We cannot determine the prospects of this patient or family with any certainty. But we can see that their future is not neatly divided into two alternatives – one a Dickensian story of poverty and social distress caused by physical handicap and the other a happy tale of a young single parent sailing through life with three small children. Dr Montgomery should inform Mr Williams that he is engaging in paternalism in his attempt to determine fully his family's fate even as he struggles to maintain and exercise autonomy in his interactions with health care professionals. Mr Williams is considering a momentous and irreversible course of action that will have a major impact on his family's future. Certainly his wife is entitled to participate in these deliberations and discussions. Although the children are quite young, their concerns and interests should not be ignored. If Mr Williams were to attempt to purchase a brighter future for his family by ending his life, they might well rue the decision and consider it a poor bargain.

Presentation of some hard data might improve the value of this exchange and help participants to reach more reasonable conclusions. Many studies have been conducted on the marriages and family lives of spinal cord injured patients. Abrams looked at the impact on marriage of adult onset paraplegia (Abrams, 1981). No picture of general or unavoidable devastation emerged. Spinal cord injury does not rigidly determine the future of marital partners. Their responses to pre-existing family systems, changes in marital roles and communication patterns, and reactions to stress will determine the nature of their experience. Trieschmann (1988) describes the responses of wives of spinal cord injured men:

The spinal injury provided an opportunity to clarify the couples' values, particularly in regard to the marriage. Usually, a commitment to the marriage was specifically talked about and affirmed publicly. Value changes in regard to future planning also occurred. While these women were quite security conscious, security now derived from *not* planning too far ahead. Furthermore, while few considered the adaptation to the crisis of the husband's disability to be a personal triumph, the opposite, lack of coping, would have been viewed as a personal failure. These women were not necessarily happy with the changes that had occurred in their lives, yet they viewed them as an opportunity to mature and grow.

It is much the same situation with respect to parenting. Buck and Hohmann (1981) compared the emotional adjustment and stability of children raised with a spinal cord injured father to peers in non-disabled families. No adverse effect on the children was detected. Indeed, the children with spinal cord injured fathers received more physical and verbal affection from their fathers than did the control group. These children tended to be more obedient and to play a greater supportive role within the family than peers raised by non-disabled parents (Buck and Hohmann, 1981). Trieschmann (1988) concludes that children of a disabled parent have more developed senses of personal responsibility and more profound interpersonal involvement with their parents.

Few families with spinal cord injured members believe that the costs of care are not adequately compensated by the psychosocial benefits of having their loved one continue as an active participant in family life. Gardner *et al.* (1985) conducted a study in which they interviewed relatives of patients treated over a 26-year period at a regional SCI center in Great Britain. Sixteen of the 21 relatives of patients still alive at the time the interviews were conducted indicated that they were glad that the lives of their family member had been sustained with a ventilator. They were glad that the individual was not allowed to die. Thirteen of 21 relatives reported that their lives would not have been better if their family member had been permitted to die. An important note of caution relevant to Mr Williams' case must be sounded, however. Gardner *et al.* (1985) provided the following information about relatives who were dissatisfied with or unhappy about maintenance of their family member on a ventilator:

The nine relatives who were not glad that ventilation had been carried out fell into three groups. Firstly, those whose relative had died while on the ventilator considered that everyone had suffered in vain. Secondly, those whose paralyzed relative was aged stated that the patient would never recover from the loss of independence. Thirdly, young wives with young children who said that their own loss of dignity, independence, and lifestyle, coupled with the inevitable deprivation of the children, outweighed any benefits accrued by the patient, especially when the support of family and friends drifted away.

Dr Montgomery should encourage Mr Williams to contact some of the hospital's other spinal cord injured patients, especially those who have been rehabilitated and discharged into the community. He could also help Mr Williams to get in touch with self-help groups for spinal cord injured persons. Mr Williams should have discussions with other spinal cord injured individuals and their family members and hear their views of the relative trials and benefits of family life. Dr Montgomery can also identify support agencies that will assist families by providing respite care, technical assistance or financial support. This information will give Mr Williams a fuller, richer sense of the possibilities and challenges that spinal cord injured persons face in our society. In the end, Mr Williams must realize that while the impressions he is compiling are helpful and informative, each individual's experience is unique. The life histories of other spinal cord injured patients cannot be used to predict or determine his own path with certainty.

One final issue should be discussed before the participants attempt to negotiate a solution to the question Mr Williams' case has proposed. Just as Mr Williams is experiencing some distortions in his body image, his perceptions of his capacities and status as a spinal cord injured person may also be skewed. He stated that he does not wish to live his life as a 'helpless cripple'. Dr Montgomery should give Mr Williams information revealing the range of physical function available to him with the use of various support devices. Mr Williams would certainly be able to use a mouthstick or sip-and-puff mechanism to operate an electronic wheelchair. He could also use a mouthstick to operate a computer or an environmental control unit. Voice-activated computers are also available that greatly expand the employment, educational and leisure opportunities of disabled persons (Trieschmann, 1988).

Dr Montgomery should discuss the effectiveness of rehabilitation with Mr Williams. While his capacities to care for himself will be very limited, rehabilitative treatments should enable him to at least assist in a broad range of activities in daily living. Dr Montgomery might want to discuss with Mr Williams the implications of a recent study of rehabilitative outcomes of patients with complete C5 quadriplegia. Yarkony et al. (1988) report that at discharge only 4.8% of patients were dependent on others to drink from a cup, 90.5% of patients required some assistance but were able to perform half the effort of the task themselves, and 4.8% of patients were independent in the performance of this task. These authors also indicate that at discharge only 6.3% of their subjects were dependent on others to eat from a dish, 88.9% could feed themselves when the tray was provided, the meat cut, and beverages poured, and 4.8% of their subjects were independent in this area. Finally, after rehabilitation 98.4% of the patients could manage urinary drainage devices on their own without spills, and 76.2% could similarly maintain bowel continence (Yarkony et al., 1988).

These statistics are significant not because Mr Williams can presently expect to duplicate the achievements of the patients who attained functional independence in these areas, for these patients had good or normal deltoid and bicep strength bilaterally. They are interesting because they represent an evolution in professional perceptions of the rehabilitative potential of quadriplegic patients. Professional wisdom once was that only the exceptional C5 patient was capable of performing limited feeding functions with special hand devices (Yarkony et al., 1988). Perhaps with additional developments in rehabilitative medicine, proportional gains can be made by patients with high quadriplegia.

Even if Mr Williams were to fail in his attempts to master components of Barthel-type tasks, he would not be 'helpless', for he will not fit the image that this word conveys. He will not be incompetent or ineffective. Neither will he be weak. Mr Williams is capable of productive employment and effective contribution to his family and society. His status as an autonomous adult and fully franchised member of the moral community remains unaltered.

Mr Williams is the one who bears ultimate responsibility for the course and direction of his life. Others can, and some invariably will, make his road more difficult by discriminating against him and limiting his opportunities. Only he can choose how he will respond to this stigmatization.

Some advocates for the handicapped would argue that a choice for death represents a capitulation to the proponents of discrimination. They would think that Mr Williams has conceded that because of his physical impairment, his life has less significance or value. It is doubtful, however, that the matter can be so simply resolved. Decisions for death can serve as ultimate expressions of the individual's control over his or her own fate. They can reflect the primacy of subjective standards of quality of life.

The most that anyone can ask of individuals facing an ordeal is that they make their best effort to respond to challenges while preserving their personal integrity and capacity to find meaning or value in life. An assessment of the concerns of the participants in this case suggests the following as a reasonable compromise between competing interests and desires. Mr Williams should agree to attempt a trial of treatment and rehabilitation. In return, Dr Montgomery would pledge to review present care policies and alter any practices that limit effective contribution by patients to the course of their care. Similarly, he and other health care providers should agree to reconsider the models of communication and interaction they adopt with handicapped patients. Practices that reinforce dependence and regressive behavior should be abandoned. We must insure that the enlightened goals of rehabilitative medicine are implemented in daily practice on the ward.

One final provision would complete the covenant. Should Mr Williams find his resources so exhausted by the struggle to maintain the minimal conditions of human existence that he is no longer capable of deriving meaning or satisfaction from his life, then he may forgo further treatment or take steps to end his own life. Health care providers may temporarily intervene in order to determine that these conditions have been fulfilled. After this assessment has been made, physicians and other health care professionals should either stand aside or do what they can to assist Mr Williams in his efforts to achieve a dignified and appropriate death.

Profiles of spinal cord injury: proxy consent and social utility

Margie Wilkins is a bright, outgoing 17-year-old high school senior, member of the honor society and star of the school's 'all-state' volleyball team. Margie was on a weekend outing with some of her friends and classmates, spending a hot summer's afternoon in the countryside when she had her accident. The group had stumbled across an abandoned quarry whose waters looked cool and inviting. Margie couldn't resist. She picked her way down the rocks until she was about 15 ft (4.5 m) above the surface of the water. She called to her friends and dove in. The water was much shallower than Margie had expected. She tried unsuccessfully to pull her dive up short. She struck submerged rocks and everything went black.

For a few moments, no one moved. The youths simply stared at the surface of the water in shock. The first to recover yelled to the others, 'Pull Margie out!' He then ran to summon the rescue squad. Her friends began to climb down the rock face to the water. They pulled her head above the surface, got her out of the water. Only then did they discover that she wasn't breathing. They carried her to a large boulder, put her down and performed mouth-to-mouth resuscitation. The rescue squad removed Margie from the quarry and took her to Metro General Hospital.

Margie's mother, Alice Wilkins, a 49-year-old clerk-typist, arrived at the hospital as Margie was being admitted. Mr Ted Wilkins, a 50-year-old accountant, arrived shortly afterwards. Physicians informed Mrs Wilkins that Margie had sustained substantial injury to her cervical vertebiae and spinal cord. Even more tragic, her brain had been damaged as a result of hypoxia. Tests would have to be performed to determine the extent of the dysfunction. Mrs Wilkins authorized physicians to pursue aggressive treatment. Accordingly, Margie was admitted to the intensive care unit and placed on a respirator. Test results subsequently confirmed that Margie had a complete lesion of the spinal cord at C5. When the diagnosis of severe hypoxic encephalopathy was made, physicians began to question the appropriateness of aggressive management. They felt that the cost–benefit ratio of continued intervention was too high. Margie's physicians wondered whether it would be acceptable for them to approach Mr and Mrs Wilkins with a request to remove life support systems from their daughter.

Proxy consent and advance directives

This case raises the question of the foundation and extent of third parties' entitlements to determine the course of others' medical care. There is a generally acknowledged exception to the requirement to gain the patient's informed and voluntary acceptance of medical treatment. This exception governs the delivery of care to incompetent patients. Incompetence can be a statutory matter, as when legislatures stipulate that minors not meeting criteria of independence or maturity may not consent to medical care. By contrast, declarations of incompetence reflect medical and judicial assessments of patients' levels of cognitive function. In the USA physicians treating incompetent patients are required to obtain the consent of a proxy to any non-emergency medical care (Faden and Beauchamp, 1986).

At one time, proxies were court-appointed guardians who had no familial or social relationship to the patient. Recently, courts and legislatures in the USA have recognized families' rights to make treatment decisions for incompetent loved ones (Appelbaum, Lidz and Meisel, 1987)*. In many states in the USA families are no longer required to seek specific approval for proxy status by the court. It should be noted, however, that in most jurisdictions incompetent patients must have a terminal illness or be in a persistent vegetative state before family members can present themselves as proxies without prior approval by the courts (Areen, 1987).

Two approved standards of deliberation are available for proxies' use. The preferred standard, 'substituted judgment', requires the proxy to adopt the patient's pattern of reasoning and value scheme (Wichman and Dixon, 1990). Thus, the proxy first attempts to identify and subsequently pursues the same treatment option the patient would have selected were she or he capable of making the decision. The

* Judith Areen notes that many legislatures have responded to the absence of common-law justification for the practice of obtaining consent from family members by passing statutes that authorize specific family members to consent to necessary medical treatment for non-communicative adult family members. Areen cites: Ark Stat Ann 82-363; Ga Code Ann 31-9-1; Idaho Code 39-4303; La Rev Stat 40: 1299.53; Md Code Ann 20-107; Miss Code Ann 41-41-3, and Utah Code Ann 78-14-5 (Areen, 1987).

'reasonable person standard' should be adopted when available information does not permit the proxy to duplicate patient choice. Under this standard the proxy selects the treatment that a reasonable person would choose after a thorough and careful analysis of the likely results of available alternatives. In this way, it is hoped that the best interests of the patient will be served.

Two legal vehicles have recently emerged in the USA that expand options for end-of-life decision-making. Areen (1987) notes that 38 states and the District of Columbia have passed natural death acts that permit competent adults to prepare directions that will govern their care should they become terminally ill and unable to speak for themselves. These statutes place various limitations on the preparation or implementation of advance directives. Areen (1987) writes:

Under most statutes, the directive becomes operative only if and when the patient is determined to be terminally ill by more than one physician. In some states, a directive is legally binding only if, after the onset of terminal illness but before the onset of incompetence, the patient reaffirms the directive.

While these documents reveal patients' general wishes, they frequently employ terminology that is so vague that they offer physicians little useful guidance about specific treatment options (Wichman and Dixon, 1990). Popular versions of living wills express patients' desires to forgo 'heroic treatments' or 'extraordinary care', leaving physicians and family members to struggle with the classification of proposed interventions.

Patients can attempt to avoid such difficulties by designating an individual who will serve as their legal proxy when they become unconscious or incompetent to determine their medical care (Areen, 1987). Areen (1987) notes that 12 states have enacted statutes that explicitly authorize this delegation of decision-making authority*. She indicates that the remaining states have statutes governing the execution of durable powers of attorney. These appear to be broad enough to permit the designation of an individual to act as the patient's proxy for the purpose of making treatment decisions (Areen, 1987).

Unfortunately, we have no advance directive to guide us in our resolution of the case at hand. While many older persons have decided to draft living wills, far fewer healthy adolescents or young adults undertake such a task. Although as a dependent minor Margie may have lacked statutory entitlement to draft a living will, such a document would have provided morally relevant instruction to her parents. Jurisdictions in the USA generally recognize the authority of a parent or legal guardian to consent to medical care for dependent minors (Faden and Beauchamp, 1986). Thus, Mr and Mrs Wilkins are legally responsible for Margie's care.

They may try to identify appropriate interventions by a process of extrapolation, drawing on their knowledge of Margie's personality, values, and life experiences. In such a manner they attempt, as far as possible, to replicate her pattern of deliberation and determine a patient authentic choice. This mode of reasoning has much to recommend it. It would demonstrate their respect for the burgeoning autonomy their teenage daughter had demonstrated in happier times. It would express their recognition of her prior efforts to formulate independent standards of value. Finally, it would serve as a powerful expression of their appreciation of the integrity of her thought.

* Areen cites Cal Civil Code 2430-2444; Col Rev Stat 15-14-1501; 20 Pa Cons Stat Ann 5603(h) and provides a secondary reference that gives textual support to the existence of statutes in Delaware, Florida, Indiana, Iowa, Louisiana, Texas, Utah, Virginia and Wyoming (Areen, 1987).

Should such efforts fail, the Wilkins may resort to the hypothetical construct of the reasonable person to determine an appropriate course of action. They would try to identify a rank ordering of goods or schedule of values that any reasonable individual would be willing to adopt. Thus, they might assign ultimate priority to the support or protection of life that meets certain minimal qualitative criteria. Once they have identified a primary good, or established a hierarchy of values, they must evaluate treatment options on the basis of their ability to promote the relevant value(s). This construct presumes that a rational individual would select the treatment option that maximizes net production of the primary value. In so doing, it places ultimate emphasis on rational warrant for choice. This construct does not require us to mimic Margie's selection. Perhaps her decision would have been rash or capricious. Neither are we bound to use her characteristic processes of thought. To do so might preserve irrational or defective patterns of reasoning. We instead identify and pursue the instrumentally rational choice.

Quality of life arguments and the limitation of technological invervention

The fundamental moral obligation of physicians has traditionally been expressed in terms of a commandment to employ the science and art of medicine in a helpful, or at least benign, fashion*. This noble professional norm was eclipsed by the technological imperative of our post-war decades. Seduced by our new found power, we embarked on a professional reconstruction of the meaning of technology. The tool became an end in itself and patients found themselves ensnared by machines. They were doomed to a twilight existence, too ill and debilitated to live, apparently incapable of dying. We have been brought, with some trepidation, to a reconsideration of the role of technology in medicine. However, we measure our progress carefully, fearful that we might jump from one unacceptable extreme to another.

Both of the cases discussed in this chapter turn on the question of the appropriateness and necessity of technological intervention. In the case of Mr Robert Williams, physicians had to determine whether they would contest a competent patient's refusal of further treatment. Adequate resolution of the case was thought to require use of a truly collaborative model of medical care. Treatment and rehabilitation were to be viewed as means to support Mr Williams' capacities to find meaning and value in life. When the struggle to sustain the minimal conditions of human existence exhausted the patient's capacities for meaning, treatment could be appropriately refused. Mr Williams' capacities for meaningful life were challenged by the injuries he sustained to his spinal cord. Margie Wilkins' accident may have left her without any potential for meaningful life.

Mrs Wilkins authorized aggressive medical management at a time when doctors were unsure of the extent of the damage done to Margie's brain. In the absence of reliable data predicting the patient's level of cognitive functioning, physicians believed maximal intervention was warranted. When they subsequently made a diagnosis of severe hypoxic encephalopathy, they began to question the wisdom of an aggressive approach.

* In 'Epidemics', Hippocrates instructs physicians to: 'Declare the past, diagnose the present, foretell the future; practice these acts. As to diseases, make a habit of two things – to help, or at least to do no harm' (Jones, 1962).

Margie's physicians should engage her parents in candid discussions of the assets and liabilities various care plans. They should explain the significance of the diagnosis in functional terms that the parents can readily understand. The physicians may want to begin by describing Margie's present cognitive capacities. They should accurately represent the possibility of recovery of specific cognitive functions. Margie's physicians will also want to insure that her parents have an adequate understanding of the implications of complete C5 quadriplegia. They will have to describe the extent of physical impairment associated with this level of lesion. They should review the various treatments of fractures of the cervical vertebrae and discuss associated risks and benefits. Finally, they should realistically examine Margie's capacity for successful rehabilitation. Discussion should focus on the rehabilitative implications of Margie's cognitive impairment.

Three very different arguments could support the physicians' conclusion that the cost–benefit ratio of treatment was too high. The first argument is built on the premise that Margie is not *capable* of deriving any benefit from the application of medical technology. If neurological examination of the patient indicates that she is irreversibly unconscious, the argument would be sound and respiratory support should be discontinued. The end of any medical intervention is either the benefit of a particular patient or the preservation of public health. If Margie is irreversibly unconscious she is, in a fundamental way, beyond the reach of medical care. While we can apply countless treatments to her cognitively inert body, she as an individual can derive no benefit from them. Without the capacity to experience herself as a subject interacting with a broader physical and social world, Margie's existence would have meaning only for others.

The second argument begins with a slightly more optimistic prognosis for cognitive functioning. It premises that Margie would not actually derive any net benefit from the application of medical technology. Here physicians would argue that while they can treat the injury sustained to her spinal cord, they will not be successful in their attempts to rehabilitate her. For although she may be restored to consciousness, her level of intellectual functioning has been dramatically reduced. She no longer has the cognitive capacity to understand and appropriately respond to complex commands or directions. She would be unable to learn or remember the sequence of choreographed movements required to accomplish transfers, feeding, or other aspects of personal care. Margie would also lack the ability to comprehend the nature or cause of her physical restriction. She obviously would not be able to evaluate her experience in an attempt to sustain or expand existing sources of meaning. Consequently, her world would consist of a very narrowly circumscribed range of pleasures and pains. Indeed, frustration might become her predominant experience.

Many would find this line of reasoning persuasive. Yet the argument is only completed with an application of Margie's beliefs, preferences, and goals. When physicians confer with Mr and Mrs Wilkins, all parties might agree that Margie held that three things made life meaningful and valuable: intellectual challenge and exertion, the physical activity and competition of sports, and relationships with others. The extent of her injuries precludes realization of meaning or derivation of value by either of the first two modes. Will the quality of her relationships be sufficient to compensate the losses in the other areas? Will it even offset the discomfort and difficulties associated with the medical intervention required to sustain her life? Given the speculative nature of *a priori* answers to these questions, Margie's physicians and parents might want to consider a trial of treatment with subsequent review.

The third argument is based on social utility. Its proponents claim that the costs of medical treatment for those with substantial physical and cognitive impairments are not compensated by any subsequent social contributions these individuals may make. The plausibility of this claim rests on an assertion that an individual's worth depends exclusively on the economic value of the material products of his or her labor. For those with physical and mental handicaps are obviously capable of making profound emotional, psychological, and moral contributions to the welfare and development of their families and communities.

One might also argue that those who make this assertion have incorrectly applied the notion of constraint. Those with physical and mental handicaps are not incapable of making a significant economic contribution to society. There are many economically productive modes of labor that they can perform. There are many jobs in our workforce that they could adequately fill. The constraints that prohibit them from making full application of their capacities are social ones. Many employers are unwilling to hire members of stigmatized groups, fearful of possible adverse reaction by customers. Many employers and workers do not want to include handicapped persons in their working environments because their presence might make them feel uncomfortable or awkward. These individuals apparently believe that the disabled are not deserving of equal respect and consideration. They seem to presume that their interests are not as significant as those of the able-bodied and that their rights need not be aggressively protected. The central premise of this argument is fatally flawed. It contradicts a fundamental moral principle, the principle of respect for persons. This moral norm prohibits us from reducing persons to the status of mere means to ends. This is exactly what stigmatization and discrimination against the handicapped entail.

Mr and Mrs Wilkins are living every parent's worst nightmare. They must contemplate withdrawing technological support from a child they dearly love and are utterly unable to help. If they are to make effective decisions they will need the understanding and support of physicians and other health care professionals. We should recognize that two features of this case add considerably to the parents' difficulties. The injury resulted from an accident that the parents could neither have predicted nor prevented. They were caught unaware, horribly shocked. Thus, they may need some additional time for the reality of the situation to settle in. This tragic accident was also the result of a rash choice by their daughter. Margie's responsibility or complicity in her injury may create feelings of anger and subsequently guilt in her parents. These tangled emotions complicate the process of deliberation and may make it more difficult for the parents to authorize withdrawal of life support. Health care providers should help Mr and Mrs Wilkins to express and acknowledge their feelings. Physicians may want to encourage the couple to consult the hospital chaplain, or unit psychologist. These individuals could legitimate their experiences and ultimately help Mr and Mrs Wilkins to release or redirect their anger.

References

Abrams, K.S. (1981) Impact on marriages of adult-onset paraplegia. *Paraplegia*, **19**, 253–259

Appelbaum, P.S., Lidz, C.W. and Meisel, A. (1987) *Informed Consent: Legal Theory and Clinical Practice*, Oxford University Press, New York

Areen, J. (1987) The legal status of consent obtained from families of adult patients to withhold or withdraw treatment. *Journal of the American Medical Association*, **258**, 229–235

Attig, T. (1979) Death, respect and vulnerability. In *The Dying Human* (eds A. de Vries and A. Carmi), Turtledove Publishing, Ramat Gan, Israel, pp. 3–15

Buck, F.M. and Hohmann, G.W. (1981) Child adjustment as related to financial security and employment status of fathers with spinal cord injury. *Archives of Physiological Medicine and Rehabilitation (Chicago)*, **62**, 432–438

Dembo, T., Leviton, G. and Wright, B. (1975) Adjustment to misfortune – a problem of social-psychological rehabilitation. *Rehabilitation Psychology*, **22**, 1–100

Faden, R. and Beauchamp, T.L. (1986) *A History and Theory of Informed Consent*, Oxford University Press, New York

Gardner, B., Theocleous, F., Watt, J.W.H. and Krishnan, K.R. (1985) Ventilation or dignified death for patients with high tetraplegia. *British Medical Journal*, **291**, 1620–1622

Goffman, I. (1963) *Stigma: Notes on the Management of Spoiled Identity*, Prentice Hall, Englewood Cliffs, New Jersey

Goldiamond, I. (1973) A diary of self-modification. *Psychology Today*, **7**, 95–102

Gunther, M. (1969) Emotional aspects. In *Spinal Cord Injuries* (ed. R. Ruge), Charles C. Thomas, Springfield, Illinois, pp. 93–108

Jones, W.H.S. (1962) *Hippocrates*, Epidemics, I, XII, Harvard University Press, Cambridge, Mass., pp. 10–15

Levine, R.J. (1981) *Ethics and Regulation and Clinical Research*, Urban and Schwarzenberg, Baltimore

McGowan, M.B. and Roth, S. (1987) Family functioning and functional independence in spinal cord injury adjustment. *Paraplegia*, **25**, 357–365

Rohe, D. and Athelstan, G. (1982) Vocational interests of persons with spinal cord injury. *Journal of Counselling Psychology*, **29**, 283–291

Stover, S. and Fine, R. (eds) (1986) *Spinal Cord Injury: the Facts and Figures*, University of Alabama, Birmingham, Alabama

Trieschmann, R.B. (1988) *Spinal Cord Injuries: Psychological, Social, and Vocational Rehabilitation*, 2nd edn, Demos Publications, New York

Whiteneck, G., Carter, R., Charlifue, S., Hall, K., Menter, R., Wilkerson, M. *et al.* (1985) *A Collaborative Study of High Quadriplegia*, National Institute of Handicapped Research, as cited in Trieschmann (1988)

Wichman, A. and Dixon, K.M. (1990) Ethical issues in critical care. In *Current Therapy in Critical Care Medicine* (ed. J.E. Parillo), B.C. Decker, Toronto (forthcoming)

Wittkower, E., Gingras, G., Mergler, L., Wigdor, B. and Lepine, A. (1954) A combined psychological study of spinal cord lesions. *Canadian Medical Association Journal*, **71**, 109–115

Wright, B. (1960) *Physical Disability – A Psychological Approach*, Harper and Row, New York

Yarkony, G.M., Roth, E., Lovell, L., Heinemann, A., Katz, R.T. and Yeongchi, W. (1988) Rehabilitation outcomes in complete C5 quadriplegia. *American Journal of Physical Medicine and Rehabilitation*, **67**, 73–76

Index